Orthopedic Management of Cerebral Palsy

Guest Editor

HENRY CHAMBERS, MD

ORTHOPEDIC CLINICS OF NORTH AMERICA

www.orthopedic.theclinics.com

October 2010 • Volume 41 • Number 4

SAUNDERS an imprint of ELSEVIER, Inc.

W.B. SAUNDERS COMPANY
A Division of Elsevier Inc.

1600 John F. Kennedy Blvd. ● Suite 1800 ● Philadelphia, PA 19103-2899.

http://www.orthopedic.theclinics.com

ORTHOPEDIC CLINICS OF NORTH AMERICA Volume 41, Number 4
October 2010 ISSN 0030-5898, ISBN-13: 978-1-4377-2475-2

Editor: Debora Dellapena

Orthopedic Clinics of North America (ISSN 0030-5898) is published quarterly by Elsevier Inc., 360 Park Avenue South, New York, NY 10010-1710. Months of issue are January, April, July, and October. Business and Editorial Offices: 1600 John F. Kennedy Blvd., Suite 1800, Philadelphia, PA 19103-2899. Customer Service Office: 3251 Riverport Lane, Maryland Heights, MO 63043. Periodicals postage paid at New York, NY and additional mailing offices. Subscription prices are $269.00 per year for (US individuals), $513.00 per year for (US institutions), $318.00 per year (Canadian individuals), $615.00 per year (Canadian institutions), $392.00 per year (international individuals), $615.00 per year (international institutions), $132.00 per year (US students), $191.00 per year (Canadian and international students). Foreign air speed delivery is included in all *Clinics* subscription prices. All prices are subject to change without notice. **POSTMASTER: Send change of address to** *Orthopedic Clinics of North America*, **Elsevier Health Sciences Division, Subscription Customer Service, 3251 Riverport Lane, Maryland Heights, MO 63043. Customer Service (orders, claims, online, change of address): Elsevier Health Sciences Division, Subscription Customer Service, 3251 Riverport Lane, Maryland Heights, MO 63043. Tel: 1-800-654-2452 (U.S. and Canada); 314-447-8871 (outside U.S. and Canada). Fax: 314-447-8029. E-mail: journalscustomerservice-usa@elsevier. com (for print support); journalsonlinesupport-usa@elsevier.com (for online support).**

Reprints. For copies of 100 or more, of articles in this publication, please contact the Commercial Reprints Department, Elsevier Inc., 360 Park Avenue South, New York, NY 10010-1710. Tel.: 212-633-3812; Fax: 212-462-1935; E-mail: reprints@elsevier. com.

Orthopedic Clinics of North America is covered in *MEDLINE/PubMed* (*Index Medicus*), *Cinahl, Excerpta Medica,* and *Cumulative Index to Nursing and Allied Health Literature.*

Printed and bound by CPI Group (UK) Ltd, Croydon, CR0 4YY
Transferred to Digital Print 2011

Contributors

GUEST EDITOR

HENRY CHAMBERS, MD
Professor of Clinical Orthopedic Surgery,
University of California at San Diego; David H.
Sutherland MD, Director of Cerebral Palsy
Studies Medical Director, Motion Analysis
Laboratory Rady Children's Hospital,
San Diego, California

AUTHORS

EVE BLAIR, PhD
Adjunct Associate Professor, Centre
for Child Health Research, University
of Western Australia, Telethon Institute
for Child Health Research,
Western Australia, Australia

JAMES J. CAROLLO, PhD, PE
Director, Center for Gait and Movement
Analysis, The Children's Hospital, Aurora;
Director, Musculoskeletal Research Center,
The Children's Hospital, Denver; Associate
Professor, Departments of Physical Medicine
and Rehabilitation and Orthopaedics;
Bioengineering, University of Colorado
School of Medicine, Aurora,
Colorado

FRANK M. CHANG, MD
Professor of Orthopaedic Surgery,
Rehabilitation Medicine and Pediatrics,
University of Colorado School of Medicine;
Director, Orthopedic Surgery, Co-Medical
Director, Center for Gait and Movement
Analysis, The Children's Hospital, Aurora,
Colorado

JON R. DAVIDS, MD
Chief of Staff, Medical Director, Motion
Analysis Laboratory, Shriners Hospital for
Children, Greenville, South Carolina

LAURA L. DEON, MD
Pediatric Rehabilitation Fellow, Pediatric
Physical Medicine and Rehabilitation,
Rehabilitation Institute of Chicago at
Northwestern University, Chicago, Illinois

KATHERINE M. FLYNN, BA
Center for Gait and Movement Analysis,
The Children's Hospital, Aurora, Colorado

DEBORAH GAEBLER-SPIRA, MD
Director, Cerebral Palsy Program; Professor,
Pediatrics and Physical Medicine and
Rehabilitation, Rehabilitation Institute of
Chicago at Northwestern University,
Chicago, Illinois

H. KERR GRAHAM, MD, FRCS (Ed), FRACS
Professor of Orthopaedic Surgery,
Orthopaedic Department, University
of Melbourne and Murdoch Childrens
Research Institute, Victoria; Director of the
Hugh Williamson Gait Laboratory, The Royal
Children's Hospital, Melbourne; Chief
Investigator, National Health and Medical
Research Council Centre of Research
Excellence in Gait Rehabilitation,
Victoria, Australia

MEGHAN N. IMRIE, MD
Department of Orthopaedic Surgery, Stanford
University and Lucile Packard Children's
Hospital, Palo Alto, California

ROBERT M. KAY, MD
Childrens Orthopedic Center, Childrens
Hospital Los Angeles; Associate Professor of
Orthopedic Surgery, Keck School of Medicine,
University of Southern California, Los Angeles,
California

L. ANDREW KOMAN, MD
Professor and Chair, Department of
Orthopedic Surgery, Wake Forest University
School of Medicine, Winston-Salem,
North Carolina

KEVIN P. MURPHY, MD
Medical Director, Gillette Specialty
Healthcare Northern Clinics; Associate
Professor, Department Physical Medicine and
Rehabilitation, University of Minnesota Medical
School; Colonel, Minnesota Army National
Guard Medical Corps, Deputy Medical
Commander, State of Minnesota, Duluth,
Minnesota

TOM F. NOVACHECK, MD
Director, James R. Gage Center for Gait and
Motion Analysis, Gillette Children's Specialty
Healthcare, St Paul; Clinical Associate
Professor of Orthopaedics, University of
Minnesota, Minneapolis, Minnesota

SUSAN A. RETHLEFSEN, PT
Childrens Orthopaedic Center, Childrens
Hospital Los Angeles, Los Angeles,
California

JASON T. RHODES, MD, MS
Orthopedic Surgery, The Children's Hospital;
Assistant Professor of Orthopaedic Surgery,
University of Colorado School
of Medicine, Aurora, Colorado

JILL RODDA, PhD
Senior Clinical Physiotherapist, Hugh
Williamson Gait Laboratory, The Royal
Children's Hospital, Melbourne, Australia

ERICH RUTZ, MD
Orthopaedic Fellow, Orthopaedic
Department, The Royal Children's Hospital,
Melbourne, Australia

DEIRDRE D. RYAN, MD
Childrens Orthopaedic Center, Childrens
Hospital Los Angeles; Keck School of
Medicine, University of Southern California,
Los Angeles, California

THOMAS SARLIKIOTIS, MD
Postdoctoral Fellow, Department of
Orthopedic Surgery, Wake Forest University
School of Medicine, Winston-Salem,
North Carolina

PAULO SELBER, MD, FRACS
Consultant Orthopaedic Surgeon,
Orthopaedic Department, The Royal Children's
Hospital, Parkville, Melbourne; Consultant
Orthopaedic Surgeon, Orthopaedic
Department, The Children's Hospital at
Westmead, Sydney, Australia

BETH P. SMITH, PhD
Associate Professor, Department of
Orthopedic Surgery, Wake Forest University
School of Medicine, Winston-Salem,
North Carolina

SUE SOHRWEIDE, PT
James R. Gage Center for Gait and Motion
Analysis, Gillette Children's Specialty
Healthcare, St Paul, Minnesota

JOYCE P. TROST, PT
Research Administration, James R. Gage
Center for Gait and Motion Analysis, Gillette
Children's Specialty Healthcare, St Paul,
Minnesota

FRANCISCO G. VALENCIA, MD
Pediatric Orthopedic Surgeon, Clinical
Assistant Professor of Orthopedic Surgery,
University of Arizona, Tucson, Arizona

BURT YASZAY, MD
Department of Orthopaedic Surgery, Rady
Children's Hospital and Health Center;
Assistant Clinical Professor, University
of California, San Diego, California

JEFFREY L. YOUNG, MD
Orthopaedic Fellow, Orthopaedic
Department, The Royal Children's Hospital,
Parkville, Melbourne, Australia

Contents

Preface: Orthopedic Management of Cerebral Palsy   ix

Henry Chambers

Epidemiology of the Cerebral Palsies   441

Eve Blair

Half of the most severe cases of cerebral palsy (CP) survive to adulthood, but because this longevity is relatively recent, there is no empirical experience of their life expectancy past middle age. The last 2 decades have seen significant developments in the management of persons with CP, involving specialist services from an increasing number of disciplines that require coordination to maximize their effectiveness. This article provides an overview of CP. The author discusses definitions of CP, its epidemiology, pathologies, and range of possible clinical descriptions, and briefly touches on management and prevention.

Classification Systems in Cerebral Palsy   457

Susan A. Rethlefsen, Deirdre D. Ryan, and Robert M. Kay

Because of increasing interest in conducting large-scale, multicenter investigations into the epidemiology of cerebral palsy and its prevention and treatment, efforts have been made to establish a standard definition and classification systems for cerebral palsy. In recent years there has also been increased focus on measurement of functional status of patients and new classifications for gross and fine motor function have been developed. The purpose of this article is to update the orthopaedic community on the current classification systems for patients with cerebral palsy. This information will be of value to surgeons in determining patients' suitability for certain treatments and will also assist them in reviewing current literature in cerebral palsy.

Examination of the Child with Cerebral Palsy   469

Tom F. Novacheck, Joyce P. Trost, and Sue Sohrweide

This article describes the balanced combination of medical history, detailed physical examination, functional assessment, imaging, observational gait analysis, computerized gait analysis, and assessment of patient and family goals that are necessary to prepare treatment plans and accurately assess outcomes of treatment of children with cerebral palsy.

The Role of Gait Analysis in Treating Gait Abnormalities in Cerebral Palsy   489

Frank M. Chang, Jason T. Rhodes, Katherine M. Flynn, and James J. Carollo

Individuals with cerebral palsy (CP) cannot take a normal activity like walking for granted. CP is the most common pediatric neurologic disorder, with an incidence of 3.6 per 1000 live births. The current trend in the treatment of individuals with CP is to perform a thorough evaluation including a complete patient history from birth to present, a comprehensive physical examination, appropriate radiographs, consultation with other medical specialists, and analysis of gait.

Assessment and Treatment of Movement Disorders in Children with Cerebral Palsy   507

Laura L. Deon and Deborah Gaebler-Spira

> Cerebral palsy is the most common motor disability in childhood. Orthopedic care depends on the appreciation and the identification of muscle tone abnormalities and how they affect growth and development of the child. Abnormal muscle tone is a common diagnostic feature of cerebral palsy and can include hypotonia or hypertonia. Hypertonia is the most frequent tone abnormality in children with cerebral palsy. This article reviews hypertonia and provides information on discriminating between spasticity, dystonia, and rigidity. Medication and neurosurgical options for the management of hypertonia are presented and compared.

Surgery of the Upper Extremity in Cerebral Palsy   519

L. Andrew Koman, Thomas Sarlikiotis, and Beth P. Smith

> Functional activities of the upper extremity are limited in most individuals with a diagnosis of cerebral palsy (CP). However, surgical interventions are applied in less than 20% of pediatric patients with an upper extremity affected by CP. This article covers the surgical interventions used for the reconstruction of the upper limb in patients with CP. The optimal surgical approach for each deformity type is described. In addition, the various evaluation techniques of the upper extremity, the general principles of an operative treatment plan, and the appropriate postoperative care of these patients is presented.

Management of Spinal Deformity in Cerebral Palsy   531

Meghan N. Imrie and Burt Yaszay

> An understanding of the three-dimensional components of spinal deformity in children with cerebral palsy is necessary to recommend treatments that will positively affect these patients' quality of life. Management of these deformities can be challenging and orthopedic surgeons should be familiar with the different treatments available for this patient population. This article discusses the incidence, causes, natural history, and treatment of patients with scoliosis.

Management of Hip Deformities in Cerebral Palsy   549

Francisco G. Valencia

> Hip abnormalities affect most children with cerebral palsy. Dedicated surveillance programs have been shown to be effective means of identifying hips at risk and preventing pathologic dislocation. Patients who are ambulatory and correlate with Gross Motor Function Classification Score I and II experience deformities that affect mobility and gait, but rarely dislocations. Marginal and nonambulatory patients have an increasing risk of dislocation. Once subluxation has been identified, early surgical intervention is indicated. Long-term postoperative follow-up is needed to monitor for recurrence. Individuals who recur or who do not respond to initial soft tissue releases benefit from bony surgery. Comprehensive reconstruction of the hip has become the predominant treatment approach when acetabular and proximal femoral dysplasia is present. The painful arthritic dislocated hip has numerous treatment options. Hip arthroplasty procedures show promising results and may supplant other salvage options in the future.

Management of the Knee in Spastic Diplegia: What is the Dose?   561

Jeffrey L. Young, Jill Rodda, Paulo Selber, Erich Rutz, and H. Kerr Graham

This article discusses the sagittal gait patterns in children with spastic diplegia, with an emphasis on the knee, as well as the concept of the "dose" of surgery that is required to correct different gait pathologies. The authors list the various interventions in the order of their increasing dose. The concept of dose is useful in the consideration of the management of knee dysfunction.

The Foot and Ankle in Cerebral Palsy   579

Jon R. Davids

Clinical decision making for the management of foot deformities in children with cerebral palsy is based on the collection and integration of data from 5 sources: the clinical history, physical examination, plain radiographs, observational gait analysis, and quantitative gait analysis (which includes kinematic/kinetic analyses, dynamic electromyography, and dynamic pedobarography). The 3 most common foot segmental malalignments in children with CP are equinus, equinoplanovalgus, and equinocavovarus. The 2 most common associated deformities are ankle valgus and hallux valgus. Foot and ankle deformities caused by dynamic overactivity and imbalance of muscles are best treated with pharmacologic or neurosurgical interventions designed to manage muscle tone and spasticity, or muscle tendon unit transfers. Deformities caused by fixed or myostatic soft tissue imbalance without fixed skeletal malalignment are best treated with muscle tendon unit lengthening surgery. Deformities characterized by structural skeletal malalignment associated with fixed or myostatic soft tissue imbalance are best treated with a combination of soft tissue and skeletal surgeries.

The Adult with Cerebral Palsy   595

Kevin P. Murphy

Advances in medical and surgical care over the past 20 years have resulted in children who formerly would have died at birth or infancy now surviving well into adulthood, many with permanent physical disabilities, including those caused by cerebral palsy. Inadequate medical and surgical diagnoses and intervention are prevalent in the adult cerebral palsy population. Decreased physical activity and participation in physical therapy and fitness programs, along with loss of strength, contractures, and pain are common factors in the loss of functional weight bearing, self-care, and daily performance over time. Increased awareness of these problems is needed by adult health care providers who provide care to these individuals and also by pediatric providers who may be able to intervene and prevent some of the long-term problems. Early identification and intervention in the child and younger adult remain the ideal in the pursuit of optimal musculoskeletal function and lifestyle throughout the adult years.

Index   607

Orthopedic Clinics of North America

FORTHCOMING ISSUES

January 2011

Obesity in Orthopaedics
George V. Russell, MD, *Guest Editor*

April 2011

Current Status of Metal on Metal Hip Resurfacing
Harlan C. Amstutz, MD, Joshua Jacobs, MD,
and Edward Ebramzadeh, PhD,
Guest Editors

July 2011

Lumbar Intervertebral Disc Degeneration
Dino Samartzis, MD, and
Kenneth M.C. Cheung, MD,
Guest Editors

RECENT ISSUES

July 2010

Shoulder Instability
William N. Levine, MD, *Guest Editor*

April 2010

Evidence Based Medicine in Orthopedic Surgery
Safdar N. Khan, MD, Mark A. Lee, MD, and
Munish C. Gupta, MD, *Guest Editors*

January 2010

**Autologous Techniques to Fill Bone Defects
for Acute Fractures and Nonunions**
Hans C. Pape, MD, FACS,
and Timothy G. Weber, MD,
Guest Editors

THE CLINICS ARE NOW AVAILABLE ONLINE!

Access your subscription at:
www.theclinics.com

Preface
Orthopedic Management of Cerebral Palsy

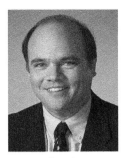

Henry Chambers, MD
Guest Editor

Cerebral palsy is the most common childhood motor disorder. Orthopedic surgeons have historically been the physicians who provide the most care for these patients and their families, although more of our medical colleagues in neurology, physiatry, developmental pediatrics, and therapies have taken a larger and perhaps central role in their care.

In this edition of *Orthopedic Clinics of North America* we are fortunate to have the world's experts provide state-of-the-art articles on this vast field. Eve Blair from Australia is one of the world's leading epidemiologists and tells you her position on why cerebral palsy should really be called the "cerebral palsies," as this definition encompasses many different etiologies and variable brain involvement. Susan Rethlefsen and her team from Los Angeles Children's Hospital update you on the new classification schema that has been developed in the last 10 years. The use of these classifications has revolutionized the field of cerebral palsy and I encourage you to learn them to communicate with your colleagues and appreciate the new literature in the field. It will also help you reinterpret old literature. Tom Novacheck and the team of experts from Gillette Children's Hospital and their world-renowned gait analysis laboratory share their complete physical examination techniques to allow the reader to approach these complex patients with a standardized evaluation. Frank Chang and the motion lab staff from Denver Children's Hospital make a case for the use of computerized gait analysis

for complex ambulatory patients but also provide a systematic way to evaluate the gait of your patient should you not have access to a three-dimensional motion analysis laboratory.

The treatment of cerebral palsy has evolved significantly in the past 20 years with increasingly sophisticated ways to treat the movement disorders of spasticity and dystonia. Deborah Gaebler-Spira and her group from the Rehabilitation Institute of Chicago have been leaders on the forefront of this field and share their clinical insights into the management of these complex movement disorders. Andrew Koman from Wake Forest, one of the original researchers into the use of botulinum toxin in children with cerebral palsy, is also one of the world's experts in upper extremity surgery in children with cerebral palsy. He presents a very understandable approach to this very complex problem. The spinal deformities of the more involved patients are very challenging to treat and Burt Yaszay and Meghan Imrie share their experience from Rady Children's Hospital in San Diego. Treatment of the hip, particularly in the nonambulatory patient, is very controversial. Francisco Valencia from Tucson shares his experience with treatment of ambulatory and nonambulatory patients with long-term follow-up. The Cerebral Palsy Group from the Royal Children's Hospital in Melbourne, Australia is one of the leading research and clinical consortia in the world. Under the leadership of Kerr Graham, they have changed the way that we evaluate and treat children with cerebral palsy. They share their

Orthop Clin N Am 41 (2010) ix–x
doi:10.1016/j.ocl.2010.08.001

orthopedic.theclinics.com

approach to the knee in cerebral palsy. Jon Davids from the Shriner's Hospital in Greenville, South Carolina is known as one of the most intellectual and didactic surgeons in the world. He shares his research and experience in managing foot problems in children with cerebral palsy. An increasingly difficult area to deal with is the adult with cerebral palsy. Most adults with cerebral palsy are not seen by pediatric orthopedic surgeons who have most of the expertise in this area. Adult providers are often overwhelmed by the complexity of these patients. Kevin Murphy has devoted his academic life to understanding the unique problems of young and older adults with cerebral palsy. This area, which needs much more research, continues to be a challenge for all of us who care for people with cerebral palsy.

It has been an honor to compile these articles for this edition of *Orthopedic Clinics of North America*. I have been honored to have mentors such as David Sutherland, Jacquelin Perry, Jim Gage, and Peter Rosenbaum. A large part of all of our education has come from our colleagues in the American Academy for Cerebral Palsy and Developmental Medicine. My best education has come from my patients and I dedicate this edition to my son, Sean, who is 28 and has total body involvement cerebral palsy (GMFCS IV). He has inspired me to do all that I can to teach others about how to care for children and adults with cerebral palsy.

Henry Chambers, MD
University of California at San Diego
San Diego, CA, USA

Motion Analysis Laboratory
Rady Children's Hospital
3030 Children's Way, Suite 410
San Diego, CA 92123, USA

E-mail address:
hchambers@rchsd.org

Epidemiology of the Cerebral Palsies

Eve Blair, PhD

KEYWORDS

- Cerebral palsy • Definition • Classification • Epidemiology
- Etiology • Management • Review

This article provides an overview of cerebral palsy (CP). The author discusses definitions of CP, its epidemiology, pathologies, and range of possible clinical descriptions, and briefly touches on management and prevention.

CP can no longer be considered a disease of children. For the last 50 years the routine use of antibiotics has protected even the most severely impaired from the previously inevitable early death from pneumonia. Now half of the most severely impaired survive to adulthood, but because this longevity is relatively recent, there is no empirical experience of their life expectancy past middle age. The last 2 decades have seen significant developments in the management of persons with CP, involving specialist services from an increasing number of disciplines that require coordination to maximize their effectiveness. Because the role of coordinator seems increasingly to be falling to the general practitioner, a sound understanding of the concept of CP is becoming mandatory.

WHAT IS CEREBRAL PALSY?

Many publications attempt to define CP (see for example Refs.[1–3]). *Definition* is defined as *a precise statement of the essential nature of a thing*[4] and *the clear determination of the limits of anything*.[5] A definition should therefore describe what a thing is and what it is not, precisely and clearly. No publication has yet achieved this, but there is agreement that CP is an "umbrella term" covering a wide variety of clinical conditions that meet 4 criteria:

- Presence of a disorder of movement or posture
- Secondary to a cerebral abnormality
- Arising early in development
- By the time movement impairment exists, the cerebral abnormality is static.

There is no test, genetic, metabolic, immunologic, or otherwise, that demonstrates the existence or absence of CP because there is no specified cause, cerebral pathology, or even type of motor impairment—only that motor impairment exists resulting from nonprogressive cerebral pathology acquired early in life. It is not a single disease. Even as a clinical description these criteria fail in several aspects to achieve the precision required of a definition,[6,7] such as specifying the age at which development is no longer considered "early." There is no agreement on this age, but most surveillance systems distinguish cases in which motor impairment is obviously acquired postneonatally, typically following cerebral infection or head trauma.[8,9] Because it is difficult to definitively differentiate between pre- and neonatally acquired brain damage, all those not postneonatally acquired are usually considered together.

The 4 criteria cannot be addressed until (a) motor development can be clearly recognized as being normal or disordered, and (b) the possibility of progressive cerebral disease can be excluded. Signs suggesting disordered motor control may be recognized very early in life, but accurate

Eve Blair is supported by National Health and Medical Research Council of Australia Program grant #003209.
Division of Population Sciences, Centre for Child Health Research, University of Western Australia at The Telethon Institute for Child Health Research, PO Box 855, West Perth, WA 6872, Australia
E-mail address: eve@ichr.uwa.edu.au

Orthop Clin N Am 41 (2010) 441–455
doi:10.1016/j.ocl.2010.06.004
0030-5898/10/$ – see front matter © 2010 Elsevier Inc. All rights reserved.

prediction has only been confirmed by trained observers in the small proportion of persons with CP born very preterm.[10] Acquisition of the cerebral abnormality may precede recognition of the motor disorder by many months or even years. However, brain-impaired infants, particularly the most severely impaired, are at increased risk of dying before reaching an age at which the criteria for CP can be confirmed. Early death is a competing outcome. On the other hand, it is difficult to definitively exclude the possibility of progression or resolution at any age. Even if cerebral pathology is static, motor abilities change in all children over time, even if that development is grossly abnormal, making functional change an unreliable marker for progressive cerebral pathology. Conversely, a proportion of children described as CP at an early age catch up with their normally developing peers at a later age[11] and the CP label is withdrawn. Therefore, the choice of an age that must be attained before being counted as CP, as well as the age beyond which development is no longer *early*, is arbitrary and depends on the interest in using the CP label. Treating clinicians are more flexible in applying the CP label, because their primary concern is to balance the psychological effects of labeling a child as having CP with the therapeutic opportunities that the label can afford. This balance can change with time. For example, the increasing frequency of children labeled as having CP of minimal severity in Western Australia[12] is attributed to approval of botulinum toxin therapy for the release of hypertonia in lower limbs, but only for those labeled as CP. Before the availability of this therapy, there was little advantage for a minimally impaired toe walker to be labeled as CP.

By contrast, those responsible for population-based CP registers or surveillance systems[13] need to know exactly whom to count. The compilers adhere strictly to self-imposed limits chosen to facilitate reliability over time and between observers contributing to their database. However, different registers face different problems. Registers with a long life span require primarily a constant definition over time, and this was the guiding principle of the recommendation by Badawi and colleagues[14] that conditions historically excluded from CP (not "diagnosed" as CP on account of having another diagnosis) continue to be excluded, even if meeting the criteria for CP. By contrast, reliability between current observers is the guiding principle of the more recent multicenter surveillance system in Europe, which adopted a flow chart driven by dichotomous responses.[15] The reality of barriers to achieving interobserver agreement of classification is demonstrated by the relatively poor agreement achieved with this flow chart, even when initial observations were standardized by presenting classifiers with written descriptions.[16]

EPIDEMIOLOGY

The reported population-based prevalences of CP depend on the definition, ascertainment proportion, rates of early mortality, and choice of denominator as well as the frequency of underlying brain abnormality. Comparisons of rates cannot be assumed to reflect relative rates of brain abnormality without careful scrutiny of the methods of estimation. However, trends are not similarly dependent. A valid trend constitutes a series of frequencies (each estimated with the same methods) that vary systematically with another variable (typically calendar time). Thus 2 valid trends may be meaningfully compared, even if generated by different methods. By contrast, comparing one CP frequency with another generated by different methods may inform primarily of the consequences of the variation in methods. A serious challenge to valid comparisons is the increasing demand for registers to obtain consent of the potential registrant/carers before registration is permitted, leading to unquantifiable and undoubtedly biased[17] underascertainment that may change with time, undermining the value of such registers.[18] Passive consent (opt-out systems)[19] would significantly reduce, and statutory notification status for CP eliminate, such underascertainment, but are rarely used.

Population-based prevalences of CP have been reported from several areas in the developed world with adequate population-based reporting systems of birth, death, and impairment. Recently published rates from geographically defined populations (**Table 1**) show significant differences, due primarily to variations in methods.[13] Variations within a reporting system over time tend to be small (see **Table 1**) without any consistent change over the last 50 years being reported by the longest standing registers (**Fig. 1**).

With CP prevalences much less than 1%, trends are susceptible to the statistical uncertainty associated with small numbers, but several trends are reported consistently. Males are at higher risk of CP, perhaps because of gender-specific neuronal vulnerabilities recently identified.[20] The proportion of children described as CP increases with decreasing gestational age at birth. The advent of mechanical ventilation to neonatal intensive care has allowed survival of increasingly preterm births, creating a new source of high-risk neonates, and perhaps a new cause of brain damage.[21] In most locations, gestation-specific prevalences of CP

Table 1
Recently published rates of CP[a] from population-based samples

Geographic Area	Birth Cohorts	No. of Cases	Rate per 1000
Norway[114]	1996–1998	374	2.1
Western Sweden[115]	1995–1998	170	1.9
BC, Canada[116]	1991–1995		2.7
UK, 4 counties[117]	1984–2002	1301	2.0
	1984–1988		2.5
	1999–2001		1.2
South Australia[118]	1993–2000	344	2.3[b]
		251	1.6[c]
Victoria, Australia[119]	1970–1998	2950	1.61
	1970–1972		1.4
	1996–1998		1.4
Western Australia[12]	1960–1999	2278	2.6
	1960–1964	222	2.6
	1995–1999	352	2.8
USA, 3 areas[120]	2002	416	3.6

[a] Includes postneonatally acquired.
[b] All ascertained cases (maximum).
[c] All cases confirmed at 5 years of age (minimum).

increase as each new gestational survival boundary is crossed, and then decline as gestationally appropriate neonatal management techniques are refined, but remain severalfold higher than rates observed in term and near-term births (**Fig. 2**). Rates around 10% of survivors, the iatrogenic nature of very preterm survival, and the investment in neonatal intensive care that such survival requires has encouraged much attention to be devoted to CP in infants born before 32 weeks' gestation. However, because births before 32 weeks contribute less than 2% of neonatal survivors, they contribute a minority, approximately 20% to 25%, of all CP in developed countries (see for example Refs.[12,22]). Most CP cases are born at term.

The risks of CP increase fourfold in twins and 18-fold in triplets,[23–25] Increasing maternal age and use of assisted reproduction technologies (ART) has increased the proportion of all births that are multiple. Concomitantly, their contribution to CP has risen from 4% in the 1960s to 10% in the 1990s.[12] The increasing proportion of the population of triplets and higher multiples were attributable exclusively to ART. This increase has been halted in many developed countries, where the number of

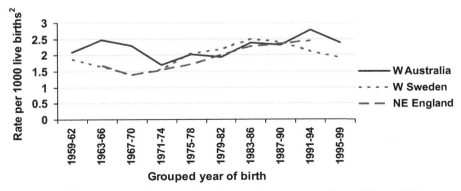

1 NE England data 1964-93, grouped years approximate fit: 1964-68, 1969-73, 1974-78, 1979-83, 1984-88, 1989-93. Final period for Swedish data 1995-98.

2 NE England rates per 1000 neonatal survivors

Fig. 1. Cerebral palsy rates in 3 populations, 1959 to 1999. (*Courtesy of* Linda Watson.)

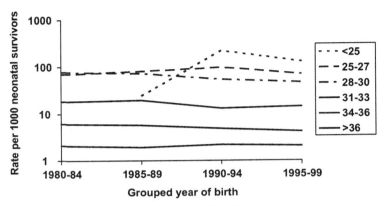

* Excludes cerebral palsy due to post-neonatal causes

Fig. 2. Gestation-specific cerebral palsy rates in Western Australia, 1980 to 1999. (*Courtesy of* Linda Watson.)

transferred embryos in any one cycle has been statutorily limited. The exception is the United States, where the transfer of multiple embryos is encouraged by market forces, despite awareness of the attendant risks[26]; risks that selective fetal reduction may not reverse once pregnancy is achieved.[27] The lower birth weights and shorter gestations associated with multiple birth contribute significantly to their higher risk of CP, but cannot be the only relevant factors because gestation-specific rates are higher for multiples than for singletons born at term or extremely preterm.[24] A biologically plausible mechanism of cerebral damage, specific to monochorionic multiples with placental anastomoses, has been proposed to account for the increased risk of CP in a multiple conception in which one fetus dies antenatally.[28] This mechanism requires monochorionic multiples, which must necessarily be of like gender, as is frequently[23] but not always[24] observed. It may be that CP following cofetal death in multichorionic multiple pregnancies is the result of a single insult that causes both the death of one twin and independently causes brain damage in the other.

A great number of additional potentially etiologic risk factors have been associated with CP in some populations including, but not limited to: parental consanguinity[29,30]; social disadvantage[31,32]; maternal thrombophilia[33]; prior reproductive loss[34,35]; maternal thyroid problems[34,36]; pregnancy conditions including severe antepartum hemorrhage,[34] preeclampsia,[37] cytomegalovirus infection[38]; and other infections,[39] particularly genital tract infections[40] and infections of the fetal membranes in both very preterm infants[41] and infants born later.[42] When reviewing this literature, it must be remembered that any factor causing a very preterm birth lies on a potential causal path to CP. Many etiologic studies control or stratify for

gestation of delivery or limit their samples to very preterm births, thus comparing only neonates of the same gestational age and masking the causal potential of any factor that reduces gestational duration.[37] In the fetus, CP has been associated with intrauterine growth restriction,[43,44] inherited thrombophilias,[33,45] transient neonatal hypothyroxinemia,[36] and congenital anomalies not only of the brain and head, eyes, and face, but also with noncerebral anomalies (in the apparent absence of cerebral anomalies), particularly of the heart and limbs and skeleton.[46,47] The risk of CP also increases with the number of suboptimal factors affecting a pregnancy.[48,49]

The heterogeneity of diseases grouped under the CP label is central to the following discussion.

DIAGNOSIS/CLINICAL DESCRIPTION

Diagnosis is defined as "the art of distinguishing one disease from another, or determining the nature of a case of disease."[5] The CP label groups several diseases, rather than distinguishing them, and reveals little about the nature of either the cause or prognosis of the conditions to which it is attached. It is immaterial to the acquisition of the label how the cerebral abnormality arose and, if the cerebral abnormality should progress or resolve, it is the label of CP that is withdrawn—it is static by definition, not by empirical observation. To call the CP label a diagnosis stretches the definition of diagnosis and can be misleading. As might be anticipated from its definition, diagnoses are frequently considered mutually exclusive, but the CP label is compatible with many etiologic diagnoses. Despite the uncertainty about the causal pathways to many cases of CP, several uncontroversial causes have been identified including kernicterus following maternal Rhesus isoimmunization (now rare in developed countries but still a significant cause in less developed countries),[29] maternal methyl mercury exposure (Minamata disease),[50] maternal iodine deficiency (cretinism),[51,52] acute hypoxia following a sentinel intrapartum event,[53] and Moyamoya disease.[14] These and many other diagnoses will persist whether or not the individual meets criteria for the CP label. Such diagnoses are informative about etiology, pathology, and frequently about final clinical presentation. These diagnoses tend to be mutually exclusive, whereas for each person categorized as CP an additional etiologic diagnosis must exist, whether or not it has been made. The author therefore considers that the CP label refers to clinical description rather than a diagnosis.

The range of clinical descriptions covered by the CP label is very wide in terms of the type, severity, and bodily distribution of primary motor impairment, of associated nonmotor neurologic and behavioral impairments, functional deficits, and cerebral pathology. It is seldom productive to consider the group as a whole. Subcategorization is sometimes referred to as differential diagnosis, though the term differential description is more accurate. However, agreement in categorizing people with CP has proved extremely difficult.

Whatever the responsible insult, the extent and severity of brain impairment can be variable and although specific insults can target specific areas of the brain, the area targeted frequently varies with the gestational age at which the insult occurs. Although some specific syndromes exist,[14] the impairments associated with CP may more generally be described as a series of continua of impairment in many dimensions, rather than a discrete set of syndromes.

To be useful, categorization systems must be reliable (people agree which category each person belongs to). Reliability requires that a person fit into one and only one category; this is only possible if categories are defined by a limited number of criteria and all empirically possible combinations of criteria are represented within the categorization system. In conditions that comprise discrete syndromes, clinical features may be sharply defined and the number of possible combinations of clinical features limited. Such is not the case with CP, so attempting to reliably categorize individuals with CP on the basis of the sum of their clinical features is doomed to failure. However, there are several possible reasons for categorization and each tends to focus on a different clinical feature, or limited set of features. It is therefore likely to be both more attainable and more useful to aim for reliable categorization systems for each of the clinical features associated with CP than for a reliable categorization system for individuals with CP.

A little progress has been made toward this goal. The shining example is the Gross Motor Function Classification System (GMFCS) devised for children with CP.[54] The GMFCS classifies *only* gross motor function, primarily ambulatory ability and its precursors, into 5 possible categories. It is well documented with age-specific criteria, recently augmented by illustrations (**Fig. 3**). The GMFCS has enormous success firstly because the degree of assistance required with ambulation is very important and useful for service provision, and secondly, because the limited aim allows reliable, tessellated categories defined by a single factor. It has been followed by a similar system for upper limb function, the Manual Abilities Classification System (MACS),[55] and similar systems for communication ability are currently being developed[56] or tested for reliability.[57]

However, the very success of such classification systems risks their misuse. The GMFCS is sometimes used to classify people with CP rather than their gross motor function. Although the severity of different impairments tends to correlate within the CP population, such correlations cannot be assumed at the individual level.[58] Furthermore, these simple categorization systems are descriptive: they enable communication between the members of the multidisciplinary teams that manage individuals with CP[59] and may suggest the types of treatment likely to be required, but they are inadequate to determine the details of management[60] or to evaluate change in response to interventions, because the anticipated degree of change is usually too small to cross these broad categories.

Functional ability has a significant impact on quality of life and is a universally understood concept, so it is unsurprising that it has been the first to be successfully classified. Primary impairments do not share these advantages. Spasticity is the primary impairment in most persons with C,P but the tools currently used to assess its severity cannot measure spasticity as it is usually defined, and therefore lack validity as well as reliability.[61] These shortcomings have been addressed by the Australian Spasticity Assessment Scale, which has promising reliability performance.[62] Moreover, the relative contributions of primary impairments to functional performance, participation, or overall quality of life are under debate, with the suggestion that more emphasis be placed on improving strength and physical fitness.[63]

GMFCS E & R between 6th and 12th birthday: Descriptors and illustrations

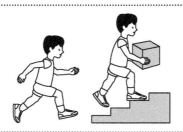

GMFCS Level I

Children walk at home, school, outdoors and in the community. They can climb stairs without the use of a railing. Children perform gross motor skills such as running and jumping, but speed, balance and coordination are limited

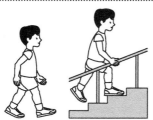

GMFCS Level II

Children walk in most settings and climb stairs holding onto a railing. They may experience difficulty walking long distances and balancing on uneven terrain, inclines, in crowded areas or confined spaces. Children may walk with physical assistance, a hand-held mobility device or used wheeled mobility over long distances. Children have only minimal ability to perform gross motor skills such as running and jumping.

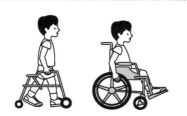

GMFCS Level III

Children walk using a hand-held mobility device in most indoor settings. They may climb stairs holding onto a railing with supervision or assistance. Children use wheeled mobility when traveling long distances and may self-propel for shorter distances.

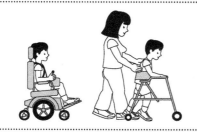

GMFCS Level IV

Children use methods of mobility that require physical assistance or powered mobility in most settings. They may walk for short distances at home with physical assistance or use powered mobility or a body support walker when positioned. At school, outdoors and in the community children are transported in a manual wheelchair or use powered mobility.

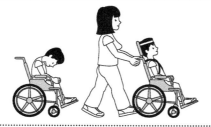

GMFCS Level V

Children are transported in a manual wheelchair in all settings. Children are limited in their ability to maintain antigravity head and trunk postures and control leg and arm movements.

GMFCS descriptors: Palisano et al. (1997) Dev Med Child Neurol 39:214-23
CanChild: www.canchild.ca

Illustrations copyright © Kerr Graham, Bill Reid and Adrienne Harvey,
The Royal Children's Hospital, Melbourne

Fig. 3. Age-specific example of criteria for the Gross Motor Function Classification System (GMFCS). (*Courtesy of Kerr Graham, MD, The Royal Children's Hospital, Melbourne, Australia.*)

PATHOPHYSIOLOGY
Cerebral

By definition, the primary pathology responsible for CP is in the brain. Advances in cerebral imaging, using ultrasound, computed tomography, and now magnetic resonance imaging (MRI) technology have allowed a greater understanding of the variety of cerebral pathologies associated with CP. Because by definition every person with CP has some cerebral pathology, it may be surprising that the pathology remains unidentified in 10% to 20% of cases investigated, more often those with ataxia or with less severe bilateral impairments.[64–66]

Early prediction is highly desirable in high-risk neonatal survivors, and because cerebral ultrasonography could be brought into the nursery, ultrasonography was the first imaging modality brought to focus on early brain impairment. Ultrasonography has been used extensively in very preterm born infants, in whom periventricular white matter injury is common.[67] Patterns of white matter injury associated with increased risks of CP have been identified (see for example Ref.[68]) but although useful, early ultrasonography has not proved very specific in predicting CP nor is it as sensitive as is sometimes assumed.[69] Because the acoustic window is limited to the fontanelles, ultrasonography is well suited to imaging the central regions of the neonatal brain but is less useful for cortical and cerebellar structures and impossible once the fontanelles have closed, precluding imaging final pathology. MRI provides clearer images, can image all parts of the brain at all ages, has become more accessible and user friendly in recent years, and can retrospectively suggest both the very approximate timing of the insult(s) and possible causes.[70] There are strong correlations between cerebral pathology and clinical description of motor impairment: unilateral pathology is associated with unilateral impairment, periventricular white matter damage with lower limb spastic impairment increasingly affecting the upper limbs with increasing extent of the damage, and basal ganglia damage with dyskinetic impairment. However, accurate prediction of CP has not proved possible with any imaging modality, even in high-risk very preterm infants. Moreover, MRI remains expensive, usually requires sedation, if not general anesthesia, to attain the required duration of immobility and, although of great interest to etiologic research, may provide little clinical benefit to the impaired individual. The possibility of identifying genetic causes may be of considerable importance for genetic counseling concerning subsequent pregnancies to the parents, but applies to only a small fraction of cases in areas with little parental consanguinity. Cerebral imaging studies therefore tend to recruit convenience samples of persons with CP who have a suitable cerebral MRI study as part of their clinical workup.[64,65] In studies of total population samples, the proportion of CP cases with such studies has not exceeded 60% to 70%.[66,71] Despite the heterogeneity of published samples, studies agree that the cerebral pathology is varied, no damage is apparent in 10% to 20%, cerebral malformations originating in early pregnancy are seen in approximately 10%, and that damage acquired after organogenesis can occur in periventricular white matter, cortex, basal ganglia, thalamus, or in several locations. Further comparisons are hampered by inconsistent methods of imaging and of describing and classifying the findings.[64,65] Categories of cerebral anomalies are variously defined by location, by nature or extent of the abnormality, by (presumed) proximal cause, and/or by (approximate) timing of

Table 2
Frequency of impairments in total population samples[a] of persons with CP

Impairment		% of All CP Affected
Motor		100
Spasticity		77–93
Dyskinesias		2–15
Ataxia		2–8
Isolated hypotonia[b]		0.7–2.6
GMFCS	I	32–51
	II	17–21
	III	9–12
	IV	10–15
	V	12–19
IQ <70[c]		17–60
Ongoing epilepsy		31–40
Visual impairment		21–63
Blind		1–7
Hearing impairment		11–13
Deaf		1.7–3

[a] Populations cited in **Table 1** were perused for this table. Data were not available for all impairments from all sources.
[b] Some surveillance systems specifically exclude isolated hypotonia.
[c] May be estimated if formal assessment is not possible.

the cause, according to the aims of the classifier.

The cerebral damage found in persons with CP need not be limited to motor centers. More extensive brain damage results in additional neurologic impairments, with frequencies in total population-based samples shown in **Table 2**. CP has also been associated with increased rates of impaired proprioception[72–74] and tactile appreciation,[75] but these sensory abilities are not routinely assessed in population surveillance systems and their prevalence in CP populations is unknown. The wide variation in proportions of disability (see **Table 2**) reflect primarily the different severity of impairment criteria required for registration because, in persons with spasticity, the number of associated impairments tends to increase with the severity of motor impairment. The variation in proportion with dyskinesias reflects that spasticity frequently coexists with dyskinesia and that mixed signs are sometimes included with spasticity and sometimes with dyskinesia.

Musculoskeletal

The cerebral pathology responsible for CP is, by definition, static after the period of acquisition, but the pathologic effects on the developing child are not. The effects on the musculoskeletal system vary with the specific types and distributions of motor impairments. Sometimes categorized as bilateral or unilateral or by the number of limbs affected, in fact topographic continua are observed. It is rare to find spastic hemiplegia with no signs of impairment on the less affected side, bilateral spasticity that is perfectly symmetric, or diplegia with no signs of impairment in the arms; from a functional perspective the degrees of involvement of the trunk, neck, and head are extremely important. Whatever body parts are affected, increased muscle tone inhibits muscle growth, resulting in a progressive failure for muscle length to keep pace with bone length. Untreated, this can result in fixed muscle contractures in which the mismatch between bone and muscle length precludes movement at the joint, leading to joint contracture. Imbalances of muscle tone can lead to deformities such as scoliosis or progressive hip displacement (failure to maintain the head of the femur in the acetabulum) and ultimately, hip dislocation. Paradoxically, hypertonicity is frequently accompanied by muscular weakness, which is exacerbated by the difficulties of engaging in gross motor exercise, particularly in the nonambulant.

Musculoskeletal pathology develops over time and can have devastating consequences on quality of life, not only in terms of motor limitations but also for a person never destined to achieve any functional motor abilities. Hip dislocation can be painful and preclude sitting, and hence normal toileting, or the possibility of observation from an upright position, thus limiting the possibilities for social interaction. Severe contracture can preclude normal hygiene skin care, rendering the person vulnerable to skin breakdown and infection.

Dyskinetic motor impairment arises from involuntary changes in muscle tone producing athetoid or dystonic movements. Dyskinetic movements can be frequent and forceful, and may generate considerable strength. Violent activity, seen particularly in athetoid CP, has been associated with premature aging of the joints, particularly in the cervical spine, necessitating surgical interventions by middle age.[76,77]

Maintaining musculoskeletal health has assumed increasing importance with the survival to adulthood of those with even the most severe impairment.[78] However, musculoskeletal pathologies are secondary, and considerable attention is being devoted to devising strategies whereby they may be minimized or prevented: for example, guidelines for hip surveillance in children with CP have recently become electronically available.[79]

VULNERABILITY TO PNEUMONIA AND MALNUTRITION

Lack of coordination is another source of secondary pathology, quite apart from injury due to falls. Persons with severe CP are frequently unable to expectorate effectively and are hence vulnerable to pneumonia, the most common cause of death in persons with CP. For those with oropharyngeal involvement, the possibility of aspiration adds to the risk of pneumonia.

Difficulties with swallowing can make feeding both time consuming and unpleasant for subject and caregiver, and is responsible for the poor nutritional status of many persons with CP. Nutritional status declines with increasing GMFCS category,[80] even among the ambulatory.[81] Intervention trials have indicated that extreme underweight and poor growth predisposes to infection,[82] and may be associated with gastrointestinal disorders such as reflux and chronic constipation and with decreased motor function.[83] In recent years malnutrition has been addressed with parenteral feeding via gastrostomy, which improves measures of weight for height,[80] reduces constipation, vomiting, and sialorrhea (one of the most distressing sequelae of oromotor dysfunction), and tends to improve micronutrient status.[84] However, major complications are possible,[84,85] minor complications, especially infection, occur frequently,[84] the risk of reflux requiring fundoplication or medication is increased,[86] and it is not universally welcomed by caregivers who may believe that it removes an important opportunity for social interaction.[87]

Furthermore, the weight gained following gastrostomy in persons with moderate or severe CP who have low energy requirements is primarily as fat rather than fat-free mass[88]; this may be desirable for thermal protection,[89] but higher fat mass and gastrostomy feeding has been associated with a greater risk of bone fracture,[90] suggesting that the formulae used for parenteral feeding in persons with CP may need further refinement.

The vulnerability to bone fracture[91] is a result of the osteoporosis frequently seen in persons with severe CP.[92] Nutritional deficiencies and difficulty of achieving weight-bearing exercise are compounded by the likelihood of receiving little sun exposure and the possibility of drug exposure. Thus bone mineral acquisition is frequently insufficient for skeletal growth.[90]

MANAGEMENT

Cure, in the sense that the brain damage is repaired, is not currently an option, although stem cell therapy hovers on an uncertain horizon.[93] Parents find this difficult to accept and are vulnerable to extravagant claims of expensive and unproven therapies. For example, hyperbaric oxygen therapy professes the ability to rescue compromised neurons, but has not furnished any convincing evidence of effectiveness and may have undesirable side effects.[94]

With cure unavailable, the objective of CP management is to improve quality of life and prevent or minimize the secondary pathologies. Beyond this, the means by which quality of life can be improved depends on the clinical description of impairments, and the aspirations and inclinations of the person with CP and their caregivers. For those with mild impairments, optimal management typically involves normalization of appearance and of performance of activities of daily living, but for the most severely impaired primary goals are typically comfort and maximizing their potential for satisfying pastimes.

The traditional therapies for CP management of stretching, casting, and orthoses has broadened considerably in recent years, as outlined in a previous Seminar on CP.[95] Much research is being conducted to optimize protocols, measure efficacy, identify adverse effects, and identify the descriptions of CP most likely to benefit from each management protocol that includes the new therapies such as botulinum toxin A,[96] intrathecal baclofen,[97,98] selective dorsal rhizotomy,[99–101] and multilevel surgery.[102] Less invasive new techniques include constraint-induced therapy for asymmetrical motor impairments[103,104] and strength training.[105]

Management of the many problems associated with CP must be tailored to the individual and has become highly specialized, frequently requiring the input of many specialties. As the number and severity of impairments increase, such teams may include physiotherapists, occupational therapists, orthotists, developmental pediatricians, neurologists, radiologists, orthopedic surgeons, speech pathologists, alternative communication and IT specialists, psychologists, ophthalmologists, dentists, social workers, special educators, educational aides, and respite carers. These specialist services must be continuously coordinated to achieve maximum benefit, and the role of the general practitioner is particularly important when the person is transferring from pediatric to adult services.

PREVENTION

Rational prevention addresses causes. If CP is defined by motor impairment resulting from a cerebral abnormality, then the cerebral abnormality is the most proximal cause of the motor impairment. However, by the time the abnormality exists, it is too late to enact prevention. Preceding causes must be sought. Any factor that can interrupt cerebral development is potentially a proximal cause of the cerebral abnormality. Such factors include genetic conditions and teratogens (physical, infectious, metabolic, or toxic),[106] the effects on cerebral development varying with the gestational age of exposure, genetic susceptibility, and environmental factors.

In practice, prevention is often approached by addressing proximal causes as they become apparent: for example, inducing hypothermia following acute hypoxia,[107] exchange transfusion following severe hyperbilirubinemia, mechanical ventilation to prevent hypoxia in very prematurely born infants, or emergency cesarean section in the face of fetal distress. Pharmacologic neuroprotection is being intensively investigated, primarily in animal models relevant to CP in very preterm births.[108–110] Several human trials of maternally administered magnesium sulfate when very preterm birth is imminent have been systematically reviewed,[111] and are associated with a relative risk for CP of 0.68 (95% confidence interval [CI] 0.54–0.87). However, the reviewers' conclusion that "the neuroprotective role for antenatal magnesium sulfate therapy given to women at risk of preterm birth for the preterm fetus is now established" sits uneasily with their reported relative risks of 1.07 (CI 0.82–1.4) for major neurodisability, 0.94 (CI 0.78–1.12) for combined death or CP, and 1.00 (CI 0.91–1.11) for death or any neurologic impairment. If magnesium has no effect on these risks of combined poor outcomes, a reduced risk of CP suggests that the risks of other adverse outcomes must be increased.

These late strategies may help those reaching these unenviable situations, but are reactive rather than proactive. Earlier strategies are preferable. For example, recent animal work suggests that fetal vulnerability to hypoxia may be decreased by adding naturally occurring nutrients such as creatine[112] and melatonin[113] to the maternal diet by mid pregnancy. Strategies enacted only once pathology is apparent may, by enabling survival of the already compromised, equally well increase the number of CP as decrease it. This conundrum is no doubt the reason that, despite great advances in community health, and obstetric and neonatal technologies over the last 50 years, the rate of CP has not declined in parallel with rates of perinatal mortality.

To effectively reduce the proportion of persons with CP (ie, to prevent without simultaneously causing), distal causes must be addressed, factors that lie on potential causal paths before any pathology is present. Many distal factors are recognized and addressed by public health measures or standard medical care. Iodine is added to salt to avoid cretinism, foodstuffs are protected from contaminants such as mercury, girls are vaccinated against rubella, periconceptional folate is advised or added to basic foodstuffs to reduce the risk of neural tube defects including cerebral defects, Rh status of prospective parents is routinely investigated to allow recognition of Rhesus incompatibility and the need for anti-D treatment to avoid the possibility of Rh isoimmunization and kernicterus in future offspring, and the dimensions of the fetal head are compared with those of the maternal pelvis to gauge the likelihood of cephalopelvic disproportion and need for elective abdominal delivery. In the developed world these preventive activities, which may be enacted years before the pregnancy exists, are routine, and the factors they address seldom cause CP. If we take to its logical conclusion the idea that it is prophylaxis, not rescue, that is the most effective means of prevention, then we must consider as potentially preventable causes all genetic and environmental factors known to be associated with suboptimal pregnancy outcomes, of which CP is but one.

The lifestyle advice pertinent to optimizing pregnancy outcome is as follows. Enter the periconceptional period in optimum physical and nutritional condition, without chronic health problems and keeping alcohol intake low, in particular avoiding both binge drinking and drugs, whether prescribed or recreational. During pregnancy maintain optimal physical, dental, and nutritional condition, avoid exposure to infections, psychological stress, or physical trauma. And finally, desist in the face of repeated reproductive failure. These ideals are more easily attainable when pregnancy is planned and sufficient material and emotional resources are available. Advocating this advice in this context may seem an attempt to blame the woman for poor pregnancy outcomes. This is not the aim: a good pregnancy outcome can never be assured however much care is taken. However, the likelihood of a good pregnancy outcome can be greatly improved by the choices a woman makes over the timing of and self care in pregnancy; the worst choice may be to fail to choose.

The role of the medical profession is not only to apply standard medical care and encourage uptake of appropriate lifestyle advice, as outlined in this article, but to desist from enabling and encouraging reproduction (in parents) or survival (in neonates) of those who are patently unfit. Such advice is not what many prospective parents or clinicians want to hear, but it is the advice most likely to reduce the risk of CP.

SUMMARY

CP is not a diagnosis but an umbrella term for many clinical descriptions. These conditions, which by definition include impairments of movement or posture of cerebral origin, are neither curable nor fatal. Management strategies aiming to improve quality of life have developed considerably over the last two decades and are likely to increase longevity of the most severely impaired, half of whom already reach adulthood. However, the CP label can only be applied to survivors of an age at which motor impairment can exist, so early death is a competing outcome. There are many causal pathways to CP but, although those that are understood have been addressed, its frequency has not decreased over the past 50 years both despite and because of advances in obstetric, neonatal, and early childhood care as well as decreasing perinatal mortality.

Search Strategy and Selection Criteria

The information in this article is based on material in peer-reviewed medical journals, the Cochrane database of systematic reviews, conference proceedings of material not yet otherwise published, textbooks, and reports from registers and surveillance systems of CP. In selecting material when many references address the same topic preference has been given, in order, to more recent publications, systematic reviews, original observations, and reviews. Where possible, contributions representing different geographic areas have been selected, provided English language abstracts were available. The most recent publications were sought using the Medline database, entering *cerebral palsy* as a search term in combination with keyword(s) describing the associated concept: for example, <cerebral palsy> and <gastrostomy>.

ACKNOWLEDGMENTS

I thank Sarah Love for reading the manuscript and advice, Linda Watson for help with **Figs. 1** and **2** and running the Western Australian CP Register, and Professor H. Kerr Graham for permission to reprint **Fig. 3**.

REFERENCES

1. Bax MC. Terminology and classification of cerebral palsy. Dev Med Child Neurol 1964;6:295–7.
2. Mutch LW, Alberman E, Hagberg B, et al. Cerebral palsy epidemiology: where are we now and where are we going? Dev Med Child Neurol 1992;34:547–55.
3. Rosenbaum P, Dan B, Leviton A, et al. Proposed definition and classification of cerebral palsy, April 2005. Dev Med Child Neurol 2005;47:571–6.
4. Onions CT. The Shorter Oxford Dictionary. 3rd edition. Oxford: Clarendon Press; 1968. p. 473.
5. Taylor EJ. Dorland's illlustrated medical dictionary. 27th edition. Philadelphia: WB Saunders; 1988. p. 438.
6. Blair E, Love S. Commentary on the definition and classification of cerebral palsy. Dev Med Child Neurol 2005;47:510.
7. Stanley F, Blair E, Alberman E. 'What are the cerebral palsies?' Cerebral palsies: epidemiology and causal pathways. London: MacKeith Press; 2000. p. 8–13, Chapter 2.
8. Reid S, Lanigan A, Reddihough D. Post-neonatally acquired cerebral palsy in Victoria, Australia, 1970–1999. J Paediatr Child Health 2006;42(10):606–11.
9. Stanley F, Blair E, Alberman E. Post neonatally acquired cerebral palsy: incidence and antecedents. Cerebral Palsies: epidemiology and causal pathways. London: MacKeith Press; 2000. p. 124–37, Chapter 11.
10. Constantinou J, Adamson-Macedo E, Mirmiran M, et al. Movement, imaging and neurobehavioural assessment as predictors of cerebral palsy in preterm infants. J Perinatol 2007;27(4):225–9.
11. Nelson KB, Ellenberg JH. Children who 'outgrew' cerebral palsy. Pediatrics 1982;69:529–36.
12. Watson L, Blair E, Stanley F. Report of the Western Australian cerebral palsy register to birth year 1999. Perth (Western Australia): Telethon Institute for Child Health Research; 2006.
13. Smithers-Sheedy H, McIntyre S, Watson L, et al. Report of the international survey of cerebral palsy registers and surveillance systems. Sydney (Australia): CP Institute; 2009. Available at: http://www.cpinstitute.com.au/publications/index.html. Accessed July 19, 2010.
14. Badawi N, Watson L, Petterson B, et al. What constitutes cerebral palsy? Dev Med Child Neurol 1998;40:520–7.
15. SCPE. Surveillance of cerebral palsy in Europe: a collaboration of cerebral palsy surveys and registers. Dev Med Child Neurol 2000;42(12):816–24.
16. Gainsborough M, Surman G, Maestri G, et al. Validity and reliability of the guidelines of the Surveillance of Cerebral Palsy in Europe for the classification of cerebral palsy. Dev Med Child Neurol 2008;50(11):828–31.
17. Tu J, Willison D, Silver F, et al. Impracticality of informed consent in the registry of the Canadian Stroke Network. N Engl J Med 2004;350:1414–21.
18. Ingelfinger J, Drazen J. Registry research and medical privacy. N Engl J Med 2004;350(14):1452.
19. Littenberg B, MacLean C. Passive consent for clinical research in the age of HIPAA. J Gen Intern Med 2006;21(3):207–11.
20. Johnston M, Hagberg H. Sex and the pathogenesis of cerebral palsy. Dev Med Child Neurol 2007;49(1):74–8.
21. Aly H. Mechanical ventilation and cerebral palsy. Pediatrics 2005;115(6):1765–6.
22. McManus V, Guillem P, Surman G, et al. SCPE work, standardization and definition—an overview of the activities of SCPE: a collaboration of European CP registers. Zhongguo Dang Dai Er Ke Za Zhi 2006;8(4):261–5.
23. Stanley F, Blair E, Alberman E. 'The special case of multiple pregnancy'. Cerebral palsies: epidemiology and causal pathways. London: MacKeith Press; 2000. p. 109–37, Chapter 10.

24. Sher A, Petterson B, Blair E, et al. The risk of mortality or cerebral palsy in twins: a collaborative population-based study. Pediatr Res 2002;52: 671–81.

25. Topp M, Huusom L, Langhoff-Roos J, et al. Multiple birth and cerebral palsy in Europe: a multicenter study. Acta Obstet Gynecol Scand 2004;83(6): 548–53.

26. Little S, Ratcliffe J, Caughey A. Cost of transferring one through five embryos per in vitro fertilization cycle from various payor perspectives. Obstet Gynecol 2006;108(3 Pt 1):593–601.

27. Taylor C, de Groot J, Blair E, et al. The risk of cerebral palsy in survivors of multiple pregnancies with co-fetal loss or death. Am J Obstet Gynecol 2009;201(1):41.e1–6.

28. Blickstein I. Cerebral palsy in multifoetal pregnancies. Dev Med Child Neurol 2002;44(5):352–5.

29. Erkin G, Delialioglu S, Ozel S, et al. Risk factors and clinical profiles in Turkish children with cerebral palsy: analysis of 625 cases. Int J Rehabil Res 2008;31(1):89–91.

30. Sinha G, Corry P, Subesinghe D, et al. Prevalence and type of cerebral palsy in a British ethnic community: the role of consanguinity. Dev Med Child Neurol 1997;39(4):259–62.

31. Sundrum R, Logan S, Wallace A, et al. Cerebral palsy and socioeconomic status: a retrospective cohort study. Arch Dis Child 2005; 90(1):15–8.

32. Dolk H, Pattenden S, Johnson A. Cerebral palsy, low birthweight and socio-economic deprivation: inequalities in a major cause of childhood disability. Paediatr Perinat Epidemiol 2001;15:359–63.

33. Nelson K. Thrombophilias, perinatal stroke, and cerebral palsy. Clin Obstet Gynecol 2006;49(4): 875–84.

34. Blair E, Stanley FJ. When can cerebral palsy be prevented? The generation of causal hypotheses by multivariate analysis of a case-control study. Paediatr Perinat Epidemiol 1993;7:272–301.

35. Pharoah P, Cooke T, Rosenbloom L, et al. Effects of birth weight, gestational age, and maternal obstetric history on birth prevalence of cerebral palsy. Arch Dis Child 1987;62(10):1035–40.

36. Hong T, Paneth N. Maternal and infant thyroid disorders and cerebral palsy. Semin Perinatol 2008;32(6):438–45.

37. Blair E, deGroot J. Prediction or causation: the nature of the association between maternal preeclampsia and cerebral palsy [AusACPDM abstracts]. Dev Med Child Neurol 2008;50:32.

38. Maruyama Y, Sameshima H, Kamitomo M, et al. Fetal manifestations and poor outcomes of congenital cytomegalovirus infections: possible candidates for intrauterine antiviral treatments. J Obstet Gynaecol Res 2007;33(5):619–23.

39. Neufeld M, Frigon C, Graham A, et al. Maternal infection and risk of cerebral palsy in term and preterm infants. J Perinatol 2005;25(2): 108–13.

40. Stelmach T, Kallas E, Pisarev H, et al. Antenatal risk factors associated with unfavorable neurologic status in newborns and at 2 years of age. J Child Neurol 2004;19(2):116–22.

41. Costantine M, How H, Coppage K, et al. Does peripartum infection increase the incidence of cerebral palsy in extremely low birthweight infants? Am J Obstet Gynecol 2007;196(5):e6–8.

42. Wu Y, Escobar G, Grether J, et al. Chorioamnionitis and cerebral palsy in term and near-term infants. JAMA 2003;290(2):2677–84.

43. Jacobsson B, Ahlin K, Francis A, et al. Cerebral palsy and restricted growth status at birth: population-based case-control study. BJOG 2008; 115(10):1250–5.

44. Glinianaia S, Jarvis S, Topp M, et al. Intrauterine growth and cerebral palsy in twins: a European multicenter study. Twin Res Hum Genet 2006;9(3): 460–6.

45. Gibson C, MacLennan A, Hague W, et al. Associations between inherited thrombophilias, gestational age, and cerebral palsy. Am J Obstet Gynecol 2005;193(4):1437.

46. Garne E, Dolk H, Krageloh-Mann I, et al. Cerebral palsy and congenital malformations. Europ J Paediatr Neurol 2008;12:82–8.

47. Blair E, Al Asedy F, Badawi N, et al. Is cerebral palsy associated with birth defects other than cerebral defects? Dev Med Child Neurol 2007;49(4): 252–8.

48. Blair E, Stanley F. Etiologic pathways to spastic cerebral palsy. Paediatr Perinat Epidemiol 1993;7: 302–17.

49. Nelson K. Causative factors in cerebral palsy. Clin Obstet Gynecol 2008;51(4):749–62.

50. Kondo K. Congenital Minamata disease: warnings from Japan's experience. J Child Neurol 2000;15 (7):458–64.

51. Pharoah P, Connolly K, Hetzel B, et al. Maternal thyroid function and motor competence in the child. Dev Med Child Neurol 1981;23(1):76–82.

52. Ma T, Lian ZC, Qi SP, et al. Magnetic resonance imaging of brain and the neuromotor disorder in endemic cretinism. Ann Neurol 1993;34(1): 91–4.

53. Okereafor A, Allsop J, Counsell S, et al. Patterns of brain injury in neonates exposed to perinatal sentinel events. Pediatrics 2008;121(5):906–14.

54. Palisano R, Rosenbaum P, Walter S, et al. Gross motor function classification system for cerebral palsy. Dev Med Child Neurol 1997;39:214–23.

55. Eliasson A, Krumlinde-Sundholm L, Rosblad B, et al. The Manual Ability Classification System

(MACS) for children with cerebral palsy: scale development and evidence of validity and reliability. Dev Med Child Neurol 2006;48(7):549–54.

56. Cooley Hidecker M, Paneth N, Rosenbaum P, et al. Development of the Communication Functional Classification System (CFCS) for individuals with cerebral palsy. Dev Med Child Neurol 2009;51 (Suppl 2):48 [abstracts of the Third International Cerebral Palsy Conference].

57. Barty E, Caynes K. Development of the functional communication classification system. 3rd International Cerebral Palsy Conference. Sydney (Australia), February 19, 2009.

58. Carnahan K, Arner M, Hagglund G. Association between gross motor function (GMFCS) and manual ability (MACS) in children with cerebral palsy. A population-based study of 359 children. BMC Musculoskelet Disord 2007;8:50.

59. Eliasson A, Krumlinde-Sundholm L, Rosblad B, et al. Using the MACS to facilitate communication about manual abilities of children with cerebral palsy. Dev Med Child Neurol 2007;49(2):156–7.

60. Romain M, Benaim C, Allieu Y, et al. Assessment of hand after brain damage with the aim of functional surgery. Ann Chir Main Memb Super 1999;18(1): 28–37.

61. Scholtes V, Bech J, Beelen A, et al. Clinical assessment of spasticity in children with cerebral palsy: a critical review of available instruments. Dev Med Child Neurol 2006;48(1):64–73.

62. Gibson N, Love S, Blair E. Towards a better description of spastic cerebral palsy: use of the Australian Spasticity Assessment Scale and the Reliable Description of Cerebral Palsy form. Advanced Practitioner Workshop. 3rd International Cerebral Palsy Conference. Sydney (Australia), July 19, 2009.

63. Damiano D. Activity, activity, activity: rethinking our physical therapy approach to cerebral palsy. Phys Ther 2006;86(11):1534–40.

64. Korzenieswski S, Birbeck G, DeLano M, et al. A systematic review of neuroimaging for cerebral palsy. J Child Neurol 2008;23(2):216–27.

65. Krageloh-Mann I, Horber V. The role of magnetic resonance imaging in elucidating the pathogenesis of cerebral palsy: a systematic review. Dev Med Child Neurol 2007;49:144–51.

66. Robinson M, Peake L, Ditchfield M, et al. Magnetic resonance imaging findings in a population-based cohort of children with cerebral palsy. Dev Med Child Neurol 2008;51(1):39–45.

67. Govaert P, de Vries L. An atlas of neonatal brain sonography. London: MacKeith press; 1997.

68. Nanba Y, Matsui K, Aida N, et al. Magnetic Resonance Imaging Regional T1 abnormalities at term accurately predict motor outcome in preterm infants. Pediatrics 2007;120(1):e10–9.

69. Laptook A, O'Shea T, Shankaran S, et al. Adverse neurodevelopmental outcomes among extremely low birth weight infants with a normal head ultrasound: prevalence and antecedents. Pediatrics 2005;115(3):673–80.

70. Krageloh-Mann I. Imaging of early brain injury and cortical plasticity. Exp Neurol 2004;190(Suppl 1): S84–90.

71. Bax M, Tydeman C, Flodmark O. Clinical and MRI correlates of cerebral palsy: the European cerebral palsy study. JAMA 2006;296:1602–8.

72. Cooper J, Majnemer A, Rosenblatt B, et al. The determination of sensory deficits in children with hemiplegic cerebral palsy. J Child Neurol 1995; 10(4):300–9.

73. van Roon D, Steenbergen B, Meulenbroek R. Movement-accuracy control in tetraparetic cerebral palsy: effects of removing visual information of the moving limb. Motor Control 2005;9(4): 372–94.

74. Wingert J, Burton H, Sinclair R, et al. Joint-position sense and kinesthesia in cerebral palsy. Arch Phys Med Rehabil 2009;90(3):447–53.

75. Wingert J, Burton H, Sinclair R, et al. Tactile sensory abilities in cerebral palsy: deficits in roughness and object discrimination. Dev Med Child Neurol 2008;50(11):832–8.

76. Ueda Y, Yoshikawa T, Koizumi M, et al. Cervical laminoplasty combined with muscle release in patients with athetoid cerebral palsy. Spine 2005; 30(21):2420–3.

77. Durufle A, Petrilli S, Le Guiet J, et al. Cervical spondylotic myelopathy in athetoid cerebral palsy patients: about five cases. Joint Bone Spine. Revue du Rhumatisme 2005;72(3):270–4.

78. Blair E, Watson L, Badawi N, et al. Life expectancy among people with cerebral palsy in Western Australia. Dev Med Child Neurol 2001;43:508–15.

79. Wynter M, Gibson N, Kentish M, et al. Consensus statement on hip surveillance for children with cerebral palsy: Australian standards of care. 2008. Available at: http://www.cpaustralia.com.au/ ausacpdm/hip_surveillance/DOC1.pdf. Accessed July 19, 2009.

80. Day S, Strauss D, Vachon P, et al. Growth patterns in a population of children and adolescents with cerebral palsy. Dev Med Child Neurol 2007;49(3):167–71.

81. Feeley B, Gollapudi K, Otsuka N. Body mass index in ambulatory cerebral palsy patients. J Pediatr Orthop 2007;16(3 part B):165–9.

82. Soylu O, Unalp A, Uran N, et al. Effect of nutritional support in children with spastic quadriplegia. Pediatr Neurol 2008;39(5):330–4.

83. Campanozzi A, Capano G, Miele E, et al. Impact of malnutrition on gastrointestinal disorders and gross motor abilities in children with cerebral palsy. Brain Dev 2007;29(1):25–9.

84. Craig G, Carr L, Cass H, et al. Medical, surgical, and health outcomes of gastrostomy feeding. Dev Med Child Neurol 2006;48(5):353–60.

85. Sridhar A, Nichani S, Luyt D, et al. Candida peritonitis: a rare complication following early dislodgement of percutaneous endoscopic gastrostomy tube. J Paediatr Child Health 2006;42 (3):145–6.

86. Vernon-Roberts A, Sullivan P. Fundoplication versus post-operative medication for gastro-oesophageal reflux in children with neurological impairment undergoing gastrostomy. Cochrane Database Syst Rev 2007;1:CD006151.

87. Petersen M, Kedia S, Davis P, et al. Eating and feeding are not the same: caregivers' perceptions of gastrostomy feeding for children with cerebral palsy. Dev Med Child Neurol 2006; 48(9):713–7.

88. Sullivan P, Alder N, Bachlet A, et al. Gastrostomy feeding in cerebral palsy: too much of a good thing. Dev Med Child Neurol 2006;48(11):877–82.

89. Gisel E. Gastrostomy feeding in cerebral palsy: too much of a good thing. Dev Med Child Neurol 2006; 48(11):869.

90. Stevenson R, Conaway M, Barrington J, et al. Fracture rate in children with cerebral palsy. Pediatr Rehabil 2006;9(4):396–403.

91. Presedo A, Dabney K, Miller F. Fractures in patients with cerebral palsy. J Pediatr Orthop 2007;27(2): 147–53.

92. Henderson R, Kairalla J, Barrington J, et al. Longitudinal changes in bone density in children and adolescents with moderate to severe cerebral palsy. J Pediatr 2005;146(6):769–75.

93. Regenberg A, Mathews D, Blass D, et al. The role of animal models in evaluating reasonable safety and efficacy for human trials of cell-based interventions for neurologic conditions. J Cereb Blood Flow Metab 2009;29(1):1–9.

94. McDonagh M, Morgan D, Carson S, et al. Systematic review of hyperbaric oxygen therapy for cerebral palsy: the state of the evidence. Dev Med Child Neurol 2007;49:942–7.

95. Koman L, Paterson Smith B, Shilt J. Cerebral palsy. Lancet 2004;363:1619–31.

96. Gibson N, Graham H, Love S. Botulinum toxin A in the management of focal muscle overactivity in children with cerebral palsy. Disabil Rehabil 2007; 29(23):1813–22.

97. Kofler M, Quirbach E, Schauer R, et al. Limitations of intrathecal baclofen for spastic hemiparesis following stroke. Neurorehabil Neural Repair 2009;23:26–31.

98. Borowski A, Shah S, Littleton A, et al. Baclofen pump implantation and spinal fusion in children: techniques and complications. Spine 2008;33 (18):1995–2000.

99. Cole G, Farmer S, Roberts A, et al. Selective dorsal rhizotomy for children with cerebral palsy: the Oswestry experience. Arch Dis Child 2007;92(9): 781–5.

100. Li Z, Zhu J, Liu X. Deformity of lumbar spine after selective dorsal rhizotomy for spastic cerebral palsy. Microsurgery 2008;28(1):10–2.

101. Nordmark E, Josenby A, Lagergren J, et al. Long-term outcomes five years after selective dorsal rhizotomy. BMC Pediatr 2008;8:54.

102. Seniorou M, Thompson N, Harrington M, et al. Recovery of muscle strength following multi-level orthopaedic surgery in diplegic cerebral palsy. Gait Posture 2007;26(4):475–81.

103. Hoare B, Wasiak J, Imms C, et al. Constraint-induced movement therapy in the treatment of the upper limb in children with hemiplegic cerebral palsy. Cochrane Database Syst Rev 2007;2: CD004149.

104. Charles J, Gordon A. A repeated course of constraint-induced movement therapy results in further improvement. Dev Med Child Neurol 2007; 49(10):770–3.

105. Mockford M, Caulton J. Systematic review of progressive strength training in children and adolescents with cerebral palsy who are ambulatory. Pediatr Phys Ther 2008;20(4):318–33.

106. Moscoso G. Congenital structural defects of the brain. In: Levene M, Chervenak F, editors. Fetal and neonatal neurology and neurosurgery. 4th edition. Philadelphia (PA): Churchill Livingstone, Elsevier; 2009. p. 222–65, Chapter 13.

107. Schulzke S, Rao S, Patole S. A systematic review of cooling for neuroprotection in neonates with hypoxic ischemic encephalopathy—are we there yet? BMC Pediatr 2007;7:30.

108. Kumral A, Baskin H, Yesilirmak D, et al. Erythropoietin attenuates lipopolysaccharide-induced white matter injury in the neonatal rat brain. Neonatology 2007;92(4):269–78.

109. Gerstner B, Sifringer M, Dzietko M, et al. Estradiol attenuates hyperoxia-induced cell death in the developing white matter. Ann Neurol 2007;61(6): 562–73.

110. Shouman B, Fontaine R, Baud O, et al. Endocannabinoids potently protect the newborn brain against AMPA-kainate receptor-mediated excitotoxic damage. Br J Pharmacol 2006;148(4):442–51.

111. Doyle L, Crowther C, Middleton P, et al. Magnesium sulphate for women at risk of preterm birth for neuroprotection of the fetus. Cochrane Database Syst Rev 2009;1:CD004661.

112. Ireland Z, Dickinson H, Snow R, et al. Maternal creatine: does it reach the fetus and improve survival after an acute hypoxic episode in the spiny mouse (Acomys cahirinus)? Am J Obstet Gynecol 2008;431:e1–6.

113. Miller S, Yan E, Castillo-Melendez M, et al. Melatonin provides neuroprotection in the late-gestation fetal sheep brain in response to umbilical cord occlusion. Dev Neurosci 2005;27(2—4):200—10.

114. Andersen G, Irgens L, Haagaas I, et al. Cerebral palsy in Norway: prevalence, subtypes and severity. Eur J Paediatr Neurol 2008;12(1):4—13.

115. Himmelmann K, Hagberg G, Beckung E, et al. The changing panorama of cerebral palsy in Sweden. IX. Prevalence and origin in the birth-year period 1995—1998. Acta Paediatr 2005;94:287—94.

116. Smith L, Kelly K, Prkachin G, et al. The prevalence of cerebral palsy in British Columbia, 1991—1995. Can J Neurol Sci 2008;35(3):342—7.

117. Surman G, Newdick H, King A, et al. 4 Child: four counties database of cerebral palsy, vision loss, and hearing loss in children. Annual report 2008: including data for births 1984 to 2002. Oxford (UK): National Perinatal Epidemiology Unit; 2008.

118. Peek A, van Essen P, Gibson C, et al. 2007 Annual Report of the South Australian Cerebral Palsy Register. Adelaide (South Australia): Children, Youth and Women's Health Service; 2008.

119. Reid SM, Lanigan A, Walstab JE, et al. The Victorian Cerebral Palsy Register. Melbourne (Australia): Murdoch Childrens' Research Institute; 2005.

120. Yeargin-Allsopp M, Van Naarden Braun K, Doernberg N, et al. Prevalence of cerebral palsy in 8-year-old children in three areas of the United States in 2002: a multisite collaboration. Pediatrics 2008;121(3):547—54.

Classification Systems in Cerebral Palsy

Susan A. Rethlefsen, PT[a], Deirdre D. Ryan, MD[a,b], Robert M. Kay, MD[a,b],*

KEYWORDS

- Cerebral palsy • Classification • Impairment
- Activity limitation

The past decade has seen significant progress made in the evaluation of cerebral palsy (CP) and treatments for its sequelae. Because of advances in neonatal care and increased survival rates for preterm and low birth weight infants, efforts are being made to document the incidence and prevalence of CP through registries in Europe and Australia. Advances in orthopaedic care for children with CP have also been significant. Computerized gait analysis has led to refinements of orthopedic surgeries performed in these patients. Single event, multilevel surgery is now considered the standard of care in areas where gait analysis testing is available. New treatments have emerged, such as botulinum toxin injection and intrathecal baclofen, to treat spasticity and other types of hypertonia directly.

Because of increasing interest in conducting large-scale, multicenter investigations into the epidemiology of CP and its prevention and treatment, efforts have been made to establish a standard definition and classification systems for CP. In recent years there has also been increased focus on measurement of functional status of patients, and new classifications for gross and fine motor function have been developed.

The purpose of this article is to update the orthopaedic community on the current classification systems for patients with CP. This information will be of value to surgeons in determining patients' suitability for certain treatments and will also assist them in reviewing current literature in CP.

DEFINITION OF CEREBRAL PALSY

In 2007, the results of an International Workshop on Definition and Classification of CP were published.[1] The group included experts in the field of CP and developmental disorders from around the world. The purpose of the workshop was to update the existing definition and classification of CP to incorporate current knowledge about the disorder, and to improve communication among clinicians, researchers and epidemiologists. The following definition of CP was agreed upon:

> Cerebral palsy describes a group of permanent disorders of the development of movement and posture, causing activity limitation, that are attributed to non-progressive disturbances that occurred in the developing fetal or infant brain. The motor disorders of cerebral palsy are often accompanied by disturbances of sensation, perception, cognition, communication and behavior, by epilepsy, and by secondary musculoskeletal problems.[2]

This definition improves upon previous ones by emphasizing that CP involves a variety of disorders caused by various factors acting at different points in fetal development, and also highlights the importance of comorbidities that accompany the orthopaedic and neurologic manifestations. The definition excludes neurodevelopmental disabilities in which movement and posture are unaffected, as well as progressive disorders of the brain. The

None of the authors received funding support for the preparation of this manuscript.

[a] Childrens Orthopaedic Center, Childrens Hospital Los Angeles, 4650 Sunset Boulevard, MS 69, Los Angeles, CA 90027, USA

[b] Keck School of Medicine, University of Southern California, 1521 San Pablo Street, Los Angeles, CA 90033, USA

* Corresponding author. Childrens Orthopaedic Center, Childrens Hospital Los Angeles, 4650 Sunset Boulevard, MS 69, Los Angeles, CA 90027.

E-mail address: rkay@chla.usc.edu

Orthop Clin N Am 41 (2010) 457–467

doi:10.1016/j.ocl.2010.06.005

orthopedic.theclinics.com

definition does not specify an upper age limit for onset of disorders, but inclusion of the phrase "fetal or infant" implies that it refers to insults occurring before full development, before specific milestones, such as walking, would have been achieved.

There remains some disagreement about this definition, but it is generally accepted and being used. Current issues with it include the lack of definition of an upper limit for age at onset in postnatally acquired cases, the need for definition of a lower limit for severity of involvement for a case to be classified as CP, and the need for a decision regarding whether to categorize syndromes, genetic disorders, or brain abnormalities resulting in static encephalopathy as CP.

INTERNATIONAL CLASSIFICATION OF FUNCTIONING, DISABILITY, AND HEALTH

In 2001, the World Health Organization published the International Classification of Functioning, Disability, and Health (ICF) for member states to use to standardize health and disability data worldwide.[3] The ICF is increasingly being incorporated into research in developmental disabilities. The ICF describes disability as dysfunction at 1 or more of 3 levels: *impairment* of body structures (organs or limbs) or functions (physiologic or psychological), limitations in *activities* (execution of tasks or actions by the individual), and restriction of *participation* (involvement in life situations). Researchers frequently design studies addressing these various domains of disability. Currently, classification schemes exist for CP at both the impairment and activity limitation levels, and these are the focus of this article. No classification systems exist to date for restriction of participation.

CLASSIFICATION OF IMPAIRMENTS
Motor Abnormalities

It has been estimated that about 80% of children with CP have some type of movement disorder.[4] CP is most often classified as either spastic, dyskinetic, or ataxic.[5] Although spasticity is often the dominant disorder, many children with CP have mixed spasticity and dystonia. When more than 1 type of movement disorder is present in patients, experts recommend classifying patients by the predominant disorder, for epidemiologic purposes,[1] with listing of secondary disorders as well.[6] Secondary movement disorders should be noted because this may impact treatment decisions. In particular, the results of soft-tissue surgeries are often less predictable in children with movement disorders.

The most current and comprehensive set of classifications for motor disorders has been published by the Task Force on Childhood Motor Disorders.[7,8] The group is an interdisciplinary panel of experts in the field of movement disorders and cerebral palsy, including pediatric neurologists and neurosurgeons, orthopaedic surgeons, pediatricians, physical and occupational therapists, and other specialists. Their aims included establishment of definitions and classifications of motor disorders, with an ultimate goal of allowing improved communication among clinicians and researchers, and improving classification of patients for clinical and research purposes. To date, definitions have been established for hypertonic and hyperkinetic movement disorders, as well as negative motor signs in children.

Hypertonia

Hypertonia is defined as "abnormally increased resistance to externally imposed movement about a joint."[8] Hypertonicity can be caused by spasticity, dystonia, or rigidity (though rigidity is rare in children and not associated with cerebral palsy).

Spasticity

Spasticity is hypertonia in which resistance to passive movement increases with increasing velocity of movement (or exhibits a spastic catch), and "varies with direction of the movement, and/or rises rapidly above a threshold speed or joint angle."[8] Spasticity is often a component of upper motor neuron syndrome, along with hyperreflexia, clonus, reflex overflow, positive Babinski sign, and pyramidal distribution weakness (upper extremity extensors, lower extremity flexors). Spasticity is caused by a hyperactive stretch reflex mechanism and is amendable to treatments, such as botulinum toxin, baclofen, selective dorsal rhizotomy, and orthopaedic surgery, for resultant contractures or balancing of muscle/tendon forces about the joints.

Dystonia

Dystonia is defined as "a movement disorder in which involuntary sustained or intermittent muscle contractions cause twisting and repetitive movements, abnormal postures, or both."[8] When dystonic postures are such that they are present at rest and do not relax upon attempts at passive movement, they cause hypertonia. Dystonia can also be classified as hyperkinetic (see the following). Dystonic hypertonia is present in cases where the resistance to passive movement does not change with changes in speed of passive movement or joint angle (is present at low and high speeds with no spastic catch), may be associated with simultaneous agonist and antagonist contraction (equal resistance when the direction of passive movement is reversed), the limb tends to return to a fixed involuntary posture, and is triggered or worsened by voluntary movements at distant joints.[8] Dystonia is not associated with hyperreflexia and often disappears when the child is asleep. Because myelination is needed for development of dystonia, it typically occurs later in life than spasticity (around 5–10 years of age).[4]

It is postulated that a significant proportion of patients with cerebral palsy have a secondary component of dystonia, resulting in mixed hypertonia. Dystonia is associated with disruption of the basal ganglia and therefore is not improved by selective dorsal rhizotomy. In fact, what was previously considered recurrent spasticity after rhizotomy is now thought to be unrecognized dystonia.[4] It is generally accepted that tendon lengthening and transfer procedures are contraindicated in cases of dystonia, because of the risk for recurrence of deformity or development of reverse deformities. Although this is the conventional wisdom, evidence in the literature is limited. Occasionally, surgery may be required despite optimal medical management of the dystonia. This outcome is most commonly seen with deformities of the foot and ankle, particularly varus deformities, which may make shoe wear and bracing problematic. In such cases, surgery with split tendon transfers may be considered to address the varus foot. Whole tendon transfers should be avoided in children with dystonia. Dystonic hypertonia is responsive to botulinum toxin as well as intrathecal baclofen, which generally weaken overactive muscles or muscle groups. For patients in whom the primary movement disorder is hypertonic dystonia (vs spasticity), evaluation by a specialist in movement disorders is recommended before considering orthopaedic surgery for tendon lengthening or transfers. However, bony deformities in these patients, such as femoral anteversion, tibial torsion or bony foot deformities, are appropriate and beneficial when indicated.

Hyperkinetic Movements

Hyperkinetic movements are defined as "any unwanted excess movement"[9] that is performed voluntarily or involuntarily by the patient, and represent what have traditionally been referred to as extrapyramidal symptoms. The hyperkinetic movements most commonly seen in CP include dystonia, chorea, athetosis, and tremors.

Hyperkinetic dystonia is characterized by "abnormal postures that are superimposed upon or substitute for voluntary movements."[9] These are repeated postures that are unique to each patient, although some common patterns exist, such as foot inversion and wrist ulnar deviation. They can be of varying durations, and can be triggered by volitional movement. Chorea is defined as "an ongoing random-appearing sequence of one or more discrete involuntary movements or movement fragments."[9] It is similar to hyperkinetic dystonia except that it involves brief extraneous movements rather than postures, which imply maintenance for a length of time. Choreiform movements are also random, can appear continuous and jerky, and can be difficult for patients to relax. Athetosis is defined as "a slow, continuous, involuntary writhing movement that prevents maintenance of a stable posture,"[9] where discrete, repetitive movements or postures cannot be identified. It usually involves the hands or feet, and perioral muscles. Athetosis is not common as an isolated movement disorder in CP and is most often found in combination with chorea. The taskforce recommends that the term *dyskinetic CP* is used instead of *athetotic CP*, because athetosis is rare as an isolated finding, and when present is not often the primary movement disorder.[9]

Orthopaedic surgery in cases of predominantly hyperkinetic movement disorders associated with cerebral palsy is most often limited to bony procedures, because fixed contractures are rare because of the often nearly continuous movements of the extremities and joints. Such patients should be referred to a movement disorders specialist for management, because this type of movement disorder may be best managed through medications.

As noted, bony surgery is more commonly performed in such patients than is tendon surgery. Tendon lengthening in patients with hyperkinetic movement disorders are unreliable and may result in a reverse deformity compared with that seen preoperatively (eg, a posterior tibial tendon lengthening may result in a previously varus foot being positioned in valgus postoperatively). If tendon transfer surgery is contemplated, it should be remembered that split tendon transfers are more successful in patients with dystonia than are whole tendon transfers. Isolated osseous surgery has more reliable results in these patients, but casting should be minimized when possible because these patients often do not tolerate casts well and their dystonia may be exacerbated following cast removal.

Hypertonia in CP is most often rated using the Modified Ashworth Scale (MAS).[10] The Tardieu scale[11] is preferred by some clinicians and researchers, because it assesses resistance to both fast and slow stretches, the angle at which resistance is felt initially (R1), as well as the end of passively available range of motion (R2). Neither test is able to distinguish spasticity from hypertonic dystonia (or contracture, in the case of the MAS). There are no pure measures of spasticity available. Dystonia in children with CP (hypertonic and hyperkinetic) is assessed using the Barry-Albright Dystonia scale,[12] which was adapted for use in CP from the Fahn-Marsden Movement scale used in adults with primary dystonia. A new scale is being developed to quantify both spasticity and dystonia in the same patient, because this is a frequent occurrence, and determine the primary disorder (Hypertonia Assessment Tool-Discriminant).[13]

Negative Signs

Hypertonicity and dyskinetic movements constitute positive motor signs of increased activity. Negative signs include characteristics that are decreased or insufficient and include weakness (insufficient muscle activation), poor selective motor control (inability to activate a specific pattern of muscles in an isolated fashion), ataxia (inability to activate the correct pattern of muscles during a movement), and apraxia/developmental dyspraxia (inability to activate the correct pattern of muscles to perform a specific task, either because of loss of ability or lack of acquisition of the skill).[7] These problems often coexist with positive signs and can be more disabling than positive signs in some patients. Negative signs should be recognized because their presence may contribute to poor surgical outcomes. These problems are best addressed through physical and occupational therapy.

Topography or Limb Distribution

The traditional classifications of limb distribution for the hypertonic (primarily spastic) form of CP, hemiplegia, diplegia, and quadriplegia/tetraplegia (and occasionally triplegia), continue to be used clinically. However, these classifications have shown poor inter-rater reliability and have been the source of discrepancies in proportions of CP subtypes reported by registries in different countries.[14] Inconsistencies arise because of lack of definition of how much upper extremity impairment is needed to classify patients as quadriplegic versus diplegic. In addition, children with hemiplegia often have some motor signs on the contralateral side, which could put them in a category of asymmetric diplegia, quadriplegia, or triplegia. Some experts recommend abandonment of these labels[2,6] and advocate simplified classifications, such as unilateral or bilateral, with an indication

of upper and lower extremity function (such as Gross Motor Function Classification System level, or Manual Ability Classification System level) as is done in the Surveillance of Cerebral Palsy in Europe registry.[14] This change in classification is controversial, however, because there are suggestions in the literature of etiologic, radiological, and functional distinctions between diplegia and quadriplegia.[15–20] If the traditional terms (diplegia, quadriplegia, hemiplegia) are used, complete description of the motor impairments in all body regions (including the trunk and oropharynx) is recommended.[2] The term paraplegia is no longer used with respect to CP, because all children with diplegia have some level of impairment of fine motor upper extremity skills. If no upper extremity involvement is seen in a child with spasticity in the lower extremities there should be a suspicion of hereditary (familial) spastic paraparesis, tethered cord, or spinal cord tumor.[5,21] Some experts suggest a limb-by-limb description of motor impairment and tonal abnormalities seen in each limb, such as that used in the Australian CP register.[1] Their thought is that a description of the clinical presentation yields more valid and reliable information than placement of patients into categories, such as diplegia and quadriplegia.

CLASSIFICATION OF ACTIVITY LIMITATION
Gross Motor Function Classification System

In the past, patients' gross motor functional limitations were categorized as mild, moderate, and severe. Alternatively, some were characterized using the descriptors published by Hoffer and colleagues[22] for myelomeningocele (ie, household and community walkers). Although these descriptions conveyed information regarding the patients' ambulatory function, they were not standardized or validated. In 1997 a hallmark paper was published by Palisano and colleagues[23] that provided a new classification system for gross motor function in children with CP, the Gross Motor Function Classification System (GMFCS). This system rated patients' ambulatory function, including use of mobility aids and performance in sitting, standing, and walking activities. The original GMFCS had some limitations. These limitations included an upper age limit of 12 years (before adolescence) and the necessity of using a single rating to describe a child's ambulatory performance across different terrains and distances, resulting in a tendency of parents and therapists to rate a child based on their best capability rather than their typical performance when forced by the rating scale to choose a single category.[24] These issues were considered and addressed in an updated version of the scale.[25] The GMFCS-Expanded and Revised includes children up to 18 years of age. The descriptions of gross motor function were also revised to incorporate aspects of the framework of the ICH and recognizing that a child's environment and other factors may affect gross motor performance.

The GMFCS-ER provides a method for communicating about gross motor function, based on the use of mobility aids and performance in sitting, standing, and walking activities. It is intended to classify a patient's level of gross motor function based on his or her typical performance, rather than their best capability. It classifies gross motor function on a 5-point ordinal scale, with descriptions of skills provided for 5 age groups: less than 2 years of age, 2 to 4 years of age, 4 to 6 years of age, 6 to 12 years of age, and finally 12 to 18 years of age. In general, the levels are as follows (**Fig. 1**):

Level I: Walks without limitations
Level II: Walks with limitations
Level III: Walks using a hand-held mobility device
Level IV: Self-mobility with limitations; may use powered mobility
Level V: Transported in a manual wheelchair.

The validity and reliability of the GMFCS-ER have been demonstrated repeatedly in multiple studies.[26–29] Gross motor reference curves have been developed using GMFCS level data to allow clinicians to compare patients' status to that of children at the same age and GMFCS level, as well as to enable them to give patients and families a prognosis for gross motor progress over time.[30,31] The GMFCS has also been used to study and document the age at which peak gross motor function is achieved for each level (approximately 5 years of age for GMFCS levels I and II, 8 years of age for level III, and 7 years of age for levels IV and V), and to document the stability or decline in gross motor skills through adolescence (no decline for levels I and II, approximately 5%, 8% and 6 % decline in GMFM scores by 21 years of age for levels III, IV, and V, respectively).[30] Further, the GMFCS has been useful in categorizing patients for orthopaedic prognostic and experimental studies, both short and long term. Hip surveillance data in children with CP have shown that the incidence of hip dislocation increases linearly with GMFCS classification from level I (0% incidence) to level V (>90% incidence).[32] Patients at GMFCS levels IV and V have been shown to have greater acetabular dysplasia and hip subluxation than those at levels II and III.[33] Satisfaction

with the functional and cosmetic outcome of multi-level orthopaedic surgery has been shown to be higher among parents of patients classified at GMFCS level I than those whose children function at levels II and III.[34] Stability of GMFCS classification in patients over time has also been documented. McCormick and colleagues[27] demonstrated that the GMFCS level observed around 12 years of age is highly predictive of adult gross motor function. Children who are independent walkers at 12 years of age (GMFCS levels I and II) have an 88% chance of having a similar functional status as an adult and children who use a wheelchair as their primary mode of mobility have a 96% chance that they will continue to use the wheelchair into adulthood. Single-event multilevel surgery (SEMLS) can affect the stability of the GMFCS over time as patients at all levels, especially levels II, III and IV, have been shown to experience an improvement in GMFCS level after such surgery.[35] Although children functioning at GMFCS level IV can show improvement in ambulatory function after SEMLS, they have been found not to benefit from the addition of distal rectus femoris transfer to multilevel surgery.[36] All of this information is beneficial to orthopaedic surgeons, patients, family members, and caregivers in preparing, administering, and planning for long-term care.

Functional Mobility Scale

The Functional Mobility Scale (FMS) was designed by Graham and colleagues[24] as a measure of ambulatory performance in children with CP. It has been shown to be a better discriminator of differences in ambulatory function among children with CP than the Rancho Scale.[22] The FMS is the only existing functional scale that accounts for the fact that children may demonstrate different ambulatory abilities and use different assistive devices to walk various distances. Intended as an outcome measure, the FMS is also useful as a means of classifying ambulatory ability.

The FMS is administered via parent/patient interview and categorizes the assistance needed (none, canes, crutches, walker, wheelchair) for a child to walk 3 distances (5, 50, and 500 yards, or 5, 50, and 500 m). The distances are not specifically measured, but are used as estimates to represent household, school, and community ambulation. Ratings are given for each distance category: 1, uses wheelchair; 2, uses walker or frame; 3, uses crutches; 4, uses sticks (canes); 5, independent on level surfaces; 6, independent on all surfaces. A rating of *C* is given if the child crawls the designated distance, and an *N* is given if the

A GMFCS E & R between 6th and 12th birthday: Descriptors and illustrations

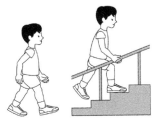

GMFCS Level I

Children walk at home, school, outdoors and in the community. They can climb stairs without the use of a railing. Children perform gross motor skills such as running and jumping, but speed, balance and coordination are limited

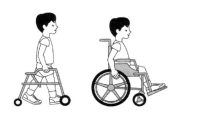

GMFCS Level II

Children walk in most settings and climb stairs holding onto a railing. They may experience difficulty walking long distances and balancing on uneven terrain, inclines, in crowded areas or confined spaces. Children may walk with physical assistance, a hand-held mobility device or used wheeled mobility over long distances. Children have only minimal ability to perform gross motor skills such as running and jumping.

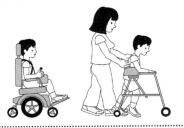

GMFCS Level III

Children walk using a hand-held mobility device in most indoor settings. They may climb stairs holding onto a railing with supervision or assistance. Children use wheeled mobility when traveling long distances and may self-propel for shorter distances.

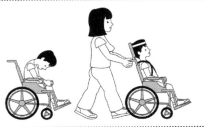

GMFCS Level IV

Children use methods of mobility that require physical assistance or powered mobility in most settings. They may walk for short distances at home with physical assistance or use powered mobility or a body support walker when positioned. At school, outdoors and in the community children are transported in a manual wheelchair or use powered mobility.

GMFCS Level V

Children are transported in a manual wheelchair in all settings. Children are limited in their ability to maintain antigravity head and trunk postures and control leg and arm movements.

GMFCS descriptors: Palisano et al. (1997) Dev Med Child Neurol 39:214-23
CanChild: www.canchild.ca

Illustrations copyright © Kerr Graham, Bill Reid and Adrienne Harvey,
The Royal Children's Hospital, Melbourne

Fig. 1. (*A*) GMFCS expanded and revised, for children aged 6 to 12 years. (*B*) GMFCS expanded and revised, for children aged 12 to 18 years. (*Courtesy of* Kerr Graham, MD, The Royal Children's Hospital, Melbourne, Australia.)

B GMFCS E & R between 12ᵗʰ and 18ᵗʰ birthday: Descriptors and illustrations

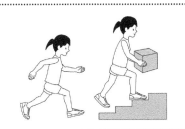

GMFCS Level I

Youth walk at home, school, outdoors and in the community. Youth are able to climb curbs and stairs without physical assistance or a railing. They perform gross motor skills such as running and jumping but speed, balance and coordination are limited.

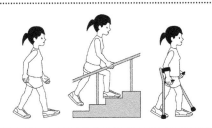

GMFCS Level II

Youth walk in most settings but environmental factors and personal choice influence mobility choices. At school or work they may require a hand held mobility device for safety and climb stairs holding onto a railing. Outdoors and in the community youth may use wheeled mobility when traveling long distances.

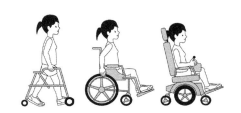

GMFCS Level III

Youth are capable of walking using a hand-held mobility device. Youth may climb stairs holding onto a railing with supervision or assistance. At school they may self-propel a manual wheelchair or use powered mobility. Outdoors and in the community youth are transported in a wheelchair or use powered mobility.

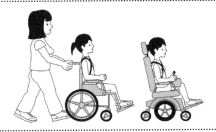

GMFCS Level IV

Youth use wheeled mobility in most settings. Physical assistance of 1-2 people is required for transfers. Indoors, youth may walk short distances with physical assistance, use wheeled mobility or a body support walker when positioned. They may operate a powered chair, otherwise are transported in a manual wheelchair.

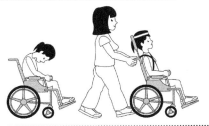

GMFCS Level V

Youth are transported in a manual wheelchair in all settings. Youth are limited in their ability to maintain antigravity head and trunk postures and control leg and arm movements. Self-mobility is severely limited, even with the use of assistive technology.

GMFCS descriptors: Palisano et al. (1997) Dev Med Child Neurol 39:214-23
CanChild: www.canchild.ca

Illustrations copyright © Kerr Graham, Bill Reid and Adrienne Harvey, The Royal Children's Hospital, Melbourne

Fig. 1. (*continued*)

child is unable to move through a given distance. A child who ambulates independently for all distances and on all types of surfaces would be given a rating of 6, 6, and 6. A child who ambulates independently on level surfaces in the home, uses crutches at school, and a wheelchair for shopping trips and family outings would be given a rating of 5, 3, and 1 (**Fig. 2**).

Like the GMFCS, the FMS assesses a child's average performance in daily life rather than their maximum capability. The FMS has been demonstrated to have good construct and concurrent

Rating

Independent on all surfaces:

Does not use any walking aids or need any help from another person when walking over all surfaces including uneven ground, curbs etc. and in a crowded environment.

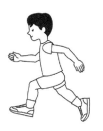

Rating **3**

Uses crutches:

Without help from another person.

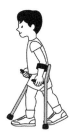

Rating **5**

Independent on level surfaces:

Does not use walking aids or need help from another person.* Requires a rail for stairs.

*If uses furniture, walls, fences, shop fronts for support, please use 4 as the appropriate description.

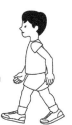

Rating **2**

Uses a walker or frame:

Without help from another person.

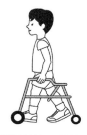

Rating **4**

Uses sticks (one or two):

Without help from another person.

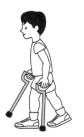

Rating **1**

Uses wheelchair:

May stand for transfers, may do some stepping supported by another person or using a walker/frame.

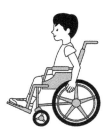

Walking distance	Rating: select the number (from 1–6) which best describes current function
5 metres (yards)	
50 metres (yards)	
500 metres (yards)	

Rating **C**   **Crawling:**

Child crawls for mobility at home (5m).

Rating **N**   **N = does not apply:**

For example child does not complete the distance (500 m).

Fig. 2. Functional Mobility Scale. (*Courtesy of* Kerr Graham, MD, The Royal Children's Hospital, Melbourne, Australia.)

validity, good inter-rater reliability (substantial agreement among therapists and orthopaedic surgeons), as well as showing sensitivity to change after surgery (positive and negative change).[24,37,38]

The FMS specifically addresses ambulation and, therefore, is not intended to substitute for the GMFCS, which assesses mobility on a more general level. The FMS should be used as a companion rating scale to the GMFCS.

Manual Ability Classification System

In 2006 a classification system similar to the GMFCS was developed for the upper extremity called The Manual Ability Classification System (MACS).[39] The MACS was designed to describe upper-extremity performance in activities of daily living for children with CP. As with the GMFCS-ER, the MACS takes into account the fact that upper-limb function is influenced by personal, environmental, and contextual factors. The MACS is not designed to describe best capacity or the function of individual upper extremities, such as comparing involved to uninvolved sides. It reports on performance of upper-limb tasks in daily living, regardless of how they are accomplished, and the collaboration of both hands together (bimanual tasks).

The MACS is also designed as a 5 category scale and the levels include (Full descriptions and distinctions between levels is available at: www.macs.nu):

   Level I: Handles objects easily and successfully
   Level II: Handles most objects but with somewhat reduced quality or speed of achievement
   Level III: Handles objects with difficulty; needs help to prepare or modify activities
   Level IV: Handles a limited selection of easily managed objects in adapted situations
   Level V: Does not handle objects and has severely limited ability to perform even simple actions.

The MACS is intended to apply to children of all ages and, therefore, does not include age bands. Raters are instructed to consider the child's performance doing age-appropriate tasks and using age-appropriate objects. The MACS has been demonstrated to be both reliable and valid.[39-41] Eliasson and colleagues demonstrated excellent reliability of MACS among children aged 4 to 18 years. Morris and colleagues found good reliability among children aged 6 to 12 years. Finally, Plasschaert and colleagues looked at reliability in children aged 1 to 5 years. Results showed moderate reliability among this age group with overall less reliability in children aged less than 2 years. Imms and colleagues[42] looked at stability of caregiver-reported MACS and GMFCS-ER. Levels were found to be generally stable over 12 months (67% for MACS and 79% for GMFCS). It is important to note that there are other hand classifications in the literature, but these all focus on specific aspects of grasping and not overall functional performance.[43-46]

Carnahan and colleagues[47] and Gunel and colleagues[48] looked at how closely associated the GMFCS-ER and MACS are when classifying children. Overall results showed that the 2 systems often show some discrepancies in children with CP. However, when looking at the 2 systems in relation to CP subtypes some associations were found. In diplegic CP, children were found to have a lower level (higher functioning) MACS score and higher level (lower functioning) GMFCS-ER. The opposite was found for hemiplegic CP; in these children manual ability was generally found to be more limited than ambulatory function. In general, the study found that there were differences in gross motor function and manual ability when looking at different CP subtypes. It is, therefore, essential to combine information on CP subtype with both the GMFCS and MACS systems when evaluating these children.[47,48]

It should be noted that neither the GMFCS-ER nor the MACS are intended to identify the cause of activity limitation (neurologic or musculoskeletal impairments, cognitive or attention deficits), but are simply intended to categorize a child's ability to function in daily life.

The development of both the GMFCS-ER and the MACS has revolutionized the way we describe the gross motor and manual abilities in CP patients. However, there is limited information in the literature on the communication skills in this patient population. In response to this weakness The Communication Function Classification System (CFCS) is currently under development by an international development and research team led by Michigan State University.[49] The CFCS is also a 5-level classification system that is being modeled after the GMFCS and MACS. The goal of this classification system is to be a quick and simple instrument easily used by a person familiar with patients. This system will help parents and clinicians understand how different communication environments, partners, and communication tasks affect the CFCS level, and will also assist in individual goal setting for communication.[49]

Although still evolving, the standardization of definitions and classifications has been an essential step forward for the CP community. Armed with these tools we can communicate more clearly about our patients and evaluate interventions more effectively. This progress has made conducting large-scale multicenter investigations more meaningful. As a result, we will continue to advance our collective understanding of the condition, further advance the care and improve the quality of life for our patients with CP.

REFERENCES

1. The definition and classification of cerebral palsy. Dev Med Child Neurol 2007;49:1.
2. Rosenbaum P, Paneth N, Leviton A, et al. A report: the definition and classification of cerebral palsy April 2006. Dev Med Child Neurol Suppl 2007;109:8.
3. World Health Organization. International Classification of Functioning, Disability and Health. Geneva: World Health Organization; 2001.
4. Delgado MR, Albright AL. Movement disorders in children: definitions, classifications, and grading systems. J Child Neurol 2003;18(Suppl 1):S1.
5. Horstmann H, Bleck E, editors. Orthopaedic management in cerebral palsy. 2nd edition. London: Mac Keith Press; 2007.
6. Bax M, Goldstein M, Rosenbaum P, et al. Proposed definition and classification of cerebral palsy, April 2005. Dev Med Child Neurol 2005;47:571.
7. Sanger TD, Chen D, Delgado MR, et al. Definition and classification of negative motor signs in childhood. Pediatrics 2006;118:2159.
8. Sanger TD, Delgado MR, Gaebler-Spira D, et al. Classification and definition of disorders causing hypertonia in childhood. Pediatrics 2003;111:e89.
9. Sanger TD, Chen D, Fehlings DL, et al. Definition and Classification of Hyperkinetic Movements in Childhood. Movement Disorders 2010. [Epub ahead of print).
10. Bohannon RW, Smith MB. Interrater reliability of a modified Ashworth scale of muscle spasticity. Phys Ther 1987;67:206.
11. Boyd RN, Graham HK. Objective measurement of clinical findings in the use of botulinum toxin type A for the management of children with cerebral palsy. Eur J Neurol 1999;6:S23.
12. Barry MJ, VanSwearingen JM, Albright AL, et al. Reliability and responsiveness of the Barry-Albright Dystonia Scale. Dev Med Child Neurol 1999;41:404.
13. Jethwa A, Mink J, Macarthur C, et al. Development of the Hypertonia Assessment Tool (HAT): a discriminative tool for hypertonia in children. Dev Med Child Neurol 2010;52:e83.
14. Surveillance of cerebral palsy in Europe. Surveillance of cerebral palsy in Europe: a collaboration of cerebral palsy surveys and registers. Surveillance of Cerebral Palsy in Europe (SCPE). Dev Med Child Neurol 2000;42:816.
15. Gorter JW, Rosenbaum PL, Hanna SE, et al. Limb distribution, motor impairment, and functional classification of cerebral palsy. Dev Med Child Neurol 2004;46:461.
16. Hoon AH Jr, Belsito KM, Nagae-Poetscher LM. Neuroimaging in spasticity and movement disorders. J Child Neurol 2003;18(Suppl 1):S25.
17. Robinson MN, Peake LJ, Ditchfield MR, et al. Magnetic resonance imaging findings in a population-based cohort of children with cerebral palsy. Dev Med Child Neurol 2009;51:39.
18. Shevell MI. The terms diplegia and quadriplegia should not be abandoned. Dev Med Child Neurol 2010;52:508–9.
19. Shevell MI, Dagenais L, Hall N. The relationship of cerebral palsy subtype and functional motor impairment: a population-based study. Dev Med Child Neurol 2009;51:872.
20. Shevell MI, Majnemer A, Morin I. Etiologic yield of cerebral palsy: a contemporary case series. Pediatr Neurol 2003;28:352.
21. Renshaw TS. Cerebral palsy. In: Raymond T, Morrissy SLW, editors, Lovell and Winter's pediatric orthopaedics, vol. 1. Philadelphia: Lippincott Williams & Wilkins; 2001. p. 563.
22. Hoffer MM, Feiwell E, Perry R, et al. Functional ambulation in patients with myelomeningocele. J Bone Joint Surg Am 1973;55:137.
23. Palisano R, Rosenbaum P, Walter S, et al. Development and reliability of a system to classify gross motor function in children with cerebral palsy. Dev Med Child Neurol 1997;39:214.
24. Graham HK, Harvey A, Rodda J, et al. The Functional Mobility Scale (FMS). J Pediatr Orthop 2004; 24:514.
25. Palisano R, Rosembaum P, Bartlett D, et al. GMFCS-E&R Gross Motor Function Classification System expanded and revised. Ontario (Canada): CanChild Centre for Childhood Disability Research; 2007.
26. Jahnsen R, Aamodt G, Rosenbaum P. Gross Motor Function Classification System used in adults with cerebral palsy: agreement of self-reported versus professional rating. Dev Med Child Neurol 2006;48:734.
27. McCormick A, Brien M, Plourde J, et al. Stability of the Gross Motor Function Classification System in adults with cerebral palsy. Dev Med Child Neurol 2007;49:265.
28. McDowell BC, Kerr C, Parkes J. Interobserver agreement of the Gross Motor Function Classification System in an ambulant population of children with cerebral palsy. Dev Med Child Neurol 2007;49:528.
29. Palisano RJ, Rosenbaum P, Bartlett D, et al. Content validity of the expanded and revised Gross Motor

Function Classification System. Dev Med Child Neurol 2008;50:744.

30. Hanna SE, Rosenbaum PL, Bartlett DJ, et al. Stability and decline in gross motor function among children and youth with cerebral palsy aged 2 to 21 years. Dev Med Child Neurol 2009;51:295.

31. Rosenbaum PL, Walter SD, Hanna SE, et al. Prognosis for gross motor function in cerebral palsy: creation of motor development curves. JAMA 2002;288:1357.

32. Soo B, Howard JJ, Boyd RN, et al. Hip displacement in cerebral palsy. J Bone Joint Surg Am 2006;88:121.

33. Gose S, Sakai T, Shibata T, et al. Morphometric analysis of acetabular dysplasia in cerebral palsy: three-dimensional CT study. J Pediatr Orthop 2009;29:896.

34. Lee SH, Chung CY, Park MS, et al. Parental satisfaction after single-event multilevel surgery in ambulatory children with cerebral palsy. J Pediatr Orthop 2009;29:398.

35. Godwin EM, Spero CR, Nof L, et al. The gross motor function classification system for cerebral palsy and single-event multilevel surgery: is there a relationship between level of function and intervention over time? J Pediatr Orthop 2009;29:910.

36. Rethlefsen SA, Kam G, Wren TA, et al. Predictors of outcome of distal rectus femoris transfer surgery in ambulatory children with cerebral palsy. J Pediatr Orthop B 2009;18:58.

37. Harvey A, Graham HK, Morris ME, et al. The Functional Mobility Scale: ability to detect change following single event multilevel surgery. Dev Med Child Neurol 2007;49:603.

38. Harvey AR, Morris ME, Graham HK, et al. Reliability of the functional mobility scale for children with cerebral palsy. Phys Occup Ther Pediatr 2010;30:139.

39. Eliasson AC, Krumlinde-Sundholm L, Rosblad B, et al. The Manual Ability Classification System (MACS) for children with cerebral palsy: scale development and evidence of validity and reliability. Dev Med Child Neurol 2006;48:549.

40. Morris C, Kurinczuk JJ, Fitzpatrick R, et al. Reliability of the manual ability classification system for children with cerebral palsy. Dev Med Child Neurol 2006;48:950.

41. Plasschaert VF, Ketelaar M, Nijnuis MG, et al. Classification of manual abilities in children with cerebral palsy under 5 years of age: how reliable is the Manual Ability Classification System? Clin Rehabil 2009;23:164.

42. Imms C, Carlin J, Eliasson AC. Stability of caregiver-reported manual ability and gross motor function classifications of cerebral palsy. Dev Med Child Neurol 2010;52:153–9.

43. Beckung E, Hagberg G. Neuroimpairments, activity limitations, and participation restrictions in children with cerebral palsy. Dev Med Child Neurol 2002;44:309.

44. House JH, Gwathmey FW, Fidler MO. A dynamic approach to the thumb-in palm deformity in cerebral palsy. J Bone Joint Surg Am 1981;63:216.

45. Krageloh-Mann I, Hagberg G, Meisner C, et al. Bilateral spastic cerebral palsy—a comparative study between south-west Germany and western Sweden. I: clinical patterns and disabilities. Dev Med Child Neurol 1993;35:1037.

46. Zancolli EA, Zancolli ER Jr. Surgical management of the hemiplegic spastic hand in cerebral palsy. Surg Clin North Am 1981;61:395.

47. Carnahan KD, Arner M, Hagglund G. Association between gross motor function (GMFCS) and manual ability (MACS) in children with cerebral palsy. A population-based study of 359 children. BMC Musculoskelet Disord 2007;8:50.

48. Gunel MK, Mutlu A, Tarsuslu T, et al. Relationship among the Manual Ability Classification System (MACS), the Gross Motor Function Classification System (GMFCS), and the functional status (Wee-FIM) in children with spastic cerebral palsy. Eur J Pediatr 2009;168:477.

49. Hidecker MJC, Paneth N, Rosembaum P, et al. Developing the communication function classification system (CFCS). Presented at the American Speech-Language-Hearing Association Convention, Chicago, 2008.

Examination of the Child with Cerebral Palsy

Tom F. Novacheck, MD*, Joyce P. Trost, PT, Sue Sohrweide, PT

KEYWORDS
- Children • Cerebral palsy • Examination

CLINICAL EVALUATION

To prepare treatment plans and accurately assess outcomes of treatment of children with cerebral palsy (CP), a balanced combination of medical history, detailed physical examination, functional assessment, imaging, observational gait analysis, computerized gait analysis, and assessment of patient and family goals must be interpreted.

THE MEDICAL HISTORY

The medical history should include a collection of information regarding birth history, developmental milestones, medical problems, surgical history, current physical therapy treatment, and current medication. Treatment plans depend on parent report of current functional walking level at home, school, and in the community, as well as other functional skills such as stair climbing, jumping, and running.

Birth history and other medical problems are important pieces of information for accurate diagnosis, future prognosis, treatment, and goal setting. Developmental milestones give information regarding the maturity of a skill such as walking and provide insight into the child's future capacity. When considering surgical treatment, it is important to obtain the operative reports of previous surgeries to accurately assess current deformities and compensations. For example, iatrogenic weakness of the soleus muscle caused by heel cord lengthening may require a different treatment plan than primary soleus weakness.

Besides the medical history, the reason for referral and current surgical or treatment considerations are helpful. Complaints of pain, and behavior or learning issues assist the clinician in performing a good evaluation.

FUNCTIONAL OUTCOME MEASURES

Current level of function can be assessed using tools such as the Functional Assessment Questionnaire (FAQ),[1] the Pediatric Orthopaedic Society of North America (Pediatric) Outcomes Data Collection Instruments (PODCI),[2] or the evaluative Functional Mobility Scale (FMS).[3] The FAQ is a validated 10-level parent report of ambulation. A child who is typically able to keep up with peers is scored at level 10; the scale decreases with decreasing ability for community ambulation. A companion FAQ-22 can be used to report other functional skills related to ambulation such as stair climbing, running, and encountering obstacles in the community such as curbs. The PODCI is also a validated parent report instrument designed to be used across ages and musculoskeletal disorders to assess functional health outcomes. It measures outcomes that can be affected by orthopedic treatment, and includes measures of upper and lower extremity motor skills, relief of pain, and restoration of activity. Correlations have been found between the FAQ, PODCI, and gait measures in children. When used in conjunction with gait data, they provide a more complete survey of change.[4] The FMS is an evaluative

James R Gage Center for Gait and Motion Analysis, Gillette Children's Specialty Healthcare, 200 East University Avenue, St Paul, MN 55101, USA
* Corresponding author.
E-mail address: novac001@umn.edu

Orthop Clin N Am 41 (2010) 469–488
doi:10.1016/j.ocl.2010.07.001

measure of functional mobility in children with CP aged 4 to 18 years.[5] It quantifies functional mobility at both the activity level and participation domains of the International Classification of Functioning, Disability and Health.[6] A unique feature of the FMS is reporting assistive device use in various environmental settings. The FMS has been shown to have adequate sensitivity to measure change after orthopedic intervention in children with CP.[5]

PHYSICAL EXAMINATION

The standard physical assessment form used in the motion analysis laboratory at Gillette Children's Specialty Healthcare provides a useful reference to a comprehensive physical examination (**Fig. 1**).

The physical examination can be separated into 7 broad categories:

1. Strength and selective motor control of isolated muscle groups
2. Degree and type of muscle tone
3. Degree of static muscle and joint contracture
4. Torsional and other bone deformities
5. Fixed and mobile foot deformities
6. Balance, equilibrium responses, and standing posture
7. Gait by observation.

Of course, physical examination is crucial, but its limitations in developing a plan for intervention must be recognized. The information collected during a physical examination is based on static responses, whereas functional activities, such as walking, are dynamic. Gait analysis data cannot be predicted by any combination of physical examination measurements either passive or active; however, there is a moderate correlation between time and distance parameters and strength and selectivity measures.[7–9] The independence of gait analysis and physical examination measures supports the notion that each provides information that is important in the delineation of problems of children with CP.[9] Numerous investigators have reported the lack of correlation between crouch gait and hamstring contracture identified by popliteal angle, for example. The method of assessment, the skill of the examiner, and the participation of the child can all affect the validity and reliability of the examination. The degree of tone can change with the position of the child, whether they are moving or at rest, the level of excitement or irritability, or the time or day of the assessment. Objective evaluation of muscle strength is difficult in small children and children with neurologic impairments.[8,10] In addition, motor control and the assessment of movement dysfunction are subjective and rely heavily on the experience and expertise of the examiner.

MUSCLE STRENGTH

Strength evaluation is necessary to assess appropriateness for interventions such as selective dorsal rhizotomy or lower extremity surgery. Children with CP are weak. Motor function and strength are directly related.[11,12] Manual muscle testing (MMT) using the Kendall scale is the typical method for measuring muscle strength in children with CP.[13] Isometric assessment with a dynamometer is becoming more common in the clinic, and is often used in research and outcome studies. Isokinetic evaluations are used when evaluating strength throughout the range of motion (ROM).

The 5-point Kendall scale provides an easy and quick way to assess a child for significant weakness or muscle imbalance, and requires only a table and standardized positioning. However; it does rely heavily on the examiner's judgment, experience, the amount of force generated by the examiner, and the accuracy of the positioning of the patient. Small yet clinically significant differences in strength may not be detected using this method. It is subjective and prone to examiner bias. However, under strict evaluation protocols, this method is useful.[14] For children who are less than the age of 5 years, and who cannot follow complex directions for maximal force production, the MMT method, as well as any other method of strength assessment, should be considered a screening tool at best.

Because of the wide variation that is seen with manual muscle assessment of isometric strength, the use of a hand-held dynamometry (HHD) has increased in the clinic and in research protocols to better quantify strength variation. The HHD approach has been shown to be a valid and reliable tool to measure isometric strength in patients with brain lesions[10,15] and in children with CP.[16] However, it has an upper limit, and exceeds that limit when used with stronger patients. Strength profiles for children with CP[17] and normative data for young children[18] have been published. Validity of this examination still depends on appropriate positioning, whether stabilization is used, and the experience of the tester. Normalization is required for body weight and lever length for strength comparisons.[18]

Isokinetic strength assessment is used to measure torque generated continuously through an arc of movement. The length of time required

Gillette Children's Specialty Healthcare
Physical Assessment

Name:
MR#:
DOB:

	MOTION		SELECTIVITY, STRENGTH	
	L	R	L	R
HIPS				
Flexion	_____	_____	_____	_____
Extension				
Thomas test	_____	_____		
knee 0			_____	_____
knee 90			_____	_____
Abduction				
hips extended	_____	_____	_____	_____
hips flexed	_____	_____		
Adduction			_____	_____
Ober test				
Internal rotation	_____	_____		
External rotation	_____	_____		
Anteversion	_____	_____		
KNEE				
Extension	_____	_____	_____	_____
Flexion				
prone	_____	_____	_____	_____
supine	_____	_____		
Popliteal angle				
unilateral	_____	_____		
bilateral	_____	_____		
HS shift	_____	_____		
Extensor lag	_____	_____		
Patella alta	_____	_____		
TIBIA				
TF angle	_____	_____		
BM axis	_____	_____		
2nd toe test	_____	_____		
ANKLE SUBTALAR				
Dorsiflexion				
knee 90	_____	_____		
knee 0	_____	_____		
Confusion test	_____	_____		
Plantarflexion	_____	_____	_____	_____
Anterior tibialis			_____	_____
Posterior tibialis			_____	_____
Peroneus longus			_____	_____
Peroneus brevis			_____	_____
Extensor hallucis longus			_____	_____
Flexor hallucis longus			_____	_____

STANDING POSTURE

BALANCE

COMMENTS

	FOOT POSITION	
	L	R
FOOT NON-WEIGHTBEARING		
Subtalar neutral	_____	_____
Hindfoot position	_____	_____
Hindfoot motion		
eversion	_____	_____
inversion	_____	_____
Arch	_____	_____
Midfoot motion	_____	_____
Forefoot position 1	_____	_____
Forefoot position 2	_____	_____
Bunion def.	_____	_____
1st MTP DF	_____	_____
FOOT WEIGHTBEARING		
Hindfoot position	_____	_____
Midfoot position	_____	_____
Forefoot position 1	_____	_____
Forefoot position 2	_____	_____

SPASTICITY (Ashworth Scale)		
Hip flexors	_____	_____
Adductors	_____	_____
Hamstrings	_____	_____
Rectus femoris	_____	_____
Plantarflexors	_____	_____
Posterior tibialis	_____	_____
Ankle clonus	_____	_____

Selectivity Grade Key	**Ashworth Scale**
0 - Only patterned movement observed.	1 - No increase in tone
	2 - Slight increase in tone
1 - Partially isolated movement observed.	3 - More marked increase in tone
2 - Completely isolated movement observed	4 - Considerable increase in tone
	5 - Affected part rigid

POSTURE / TRUNK		
Abdominal Strength		_____
Back Extensor Strength		_____
LIG LAXITY	_____	_____
LEG LENGTH	_____	_____

Fig. 1. The standard physical assessment form used in the James R Gage Center for Gait and Motion Analysis at Gillette Children's Specialty Healthcare.

for this assessment, the expense and lack of portability of the equipment, and the difficulties young children have complying with this test modality have limited the incorporation of isokinetic strength testing in the pediatric clinical setting.

SELECTIVE MOTOR CONTROL

Impaired ability to isolate and control movements confounds strength assessment and contributes to ambulatory and functional motor deficits. Assessment of selective motor control involves isolating movements on request, appropriate timing, and maximal voluntary contraction without overflow movement. A typical scale for muscle selectivity reports 3 grades of control: 0, no ability; 1, partial ability; and 2, complete ability to isolate movement. The detailed definitions and descriptions for the lower extremity muscles groups assist in accurately describing a patient's motor control and are always reported together with strength (**Table 1**).

During static physical examination, a child with hemiplegia may not be able to actively dorsiflex the ankle on the involved side without a mass flexion pattern including hip and knee flexion. On examination muscle strength of 3/5 (3 out of 5), with a selectivity grade of 0/2 (0 out of 2) is identified. While walking this child may have difficulty with clearance of their foot in early swing phase because of the inability to perform dorsiflexion with the hip in extension. However, in midswing, dorsiflexion with inversion could occur because of the child's inability to regulate the pull of the anterior tibialis and the extensor digitorum longus. In this situation, adequate dorsiflexion occurs, but the timing is late and the motion is not controlled. No surgical treatment would be able to address the problems of timing and balance. An orthotic may be the more appropriate recommendation.

MUSCLE TONE ASSESSMENT

Tone is the resistance to passive stretch while a person is attempting to maintain a relaxed state of muscle activity. Hypertonia has been defined as abnormally increased resistance to an externally imposed movement about a joint. It can be caused by spasticity, dystonia, rigidity, or a combination of these features.[19] Resting muscle tone can be influenced by the degree of cooperation, apprehension, or excitement present in the patient as well as the position during the assessment. Time spent playing or talking with the child before and during the examination often helps with the accuracy of the examination. Muscle tone assessment on different occasions by different practitioners may be necessary to accurately characterize the nature of the child's muscle tone. Standardization within a facility for testing positions and the use of a grading scale are imperative. Sanger and colleagues[19] recommend this process: start by palpating the muscle in question to determine if there is a muscle contracture at rest. Next, move the limb slowly to assess the available passive ROM. The limb can then be moved through the available range at different speeds to assess the presence or absence of a catch and how this catch varies with a variety of speeds. Next, change the direction of motion of the joint at various speeds and assess how the resistance (including timing) varies. Last, observe the limb/joint while asking the patient to move the same joint on the contralateral side. Observe and document any involuntary movement or a change in the resistance to movement on the side being assessed. By using a standard process for evaluation, the consistency and completeness of tone abnormality documentation improve.

Spastic (compared with dystonic) hypertonia causes an increase in the resistance felt at higher speeds of passive movement. Resistance to externally imposed movement rises rapidly above a speed threshold (spastic catch). The Ashworth scale,[20] modified Ashworth scale,[15,21,22] Tardieu scale,[23] and an isokinetic dynamometer in conjunction with surface electromyography[24,25] are methods used to assess severity of spastic hypertonia.

On the other hand, dystonic hypertonia shows an increase in muscle activity when at rest, has a tendency to return to a fixed posture, increases resistance with movement of the contralateral limb, and changes with a change in behavior or posture. There are also involuntary sustained or intermittent muscle contractions causing twisting and repetitive movements, abnormal postures, or both. The Hypertonia Assessment Tool (HAT)[26] is a tool developed to distinguish between spasticity, dystonia, and rigidity in the pediatric clinical setting (**Fig. 2**). The reliability and validity for spasticity and rigidity is good, but only moderate for dystonia and mixed tone. The Barry Albright Dystonia (BAD) scale, a 5-point ordinal scale, is another measure of generalized dystonia.[27] Mixed tone is often identified with a combination of both types of hypertonicity in the same patient. Mixed tone is more difficult to diagnosis and quantify than pure spasticity. However, in children with CP, it is important to assess the degree of mixed tone present, because the outcome of surgery may be less predictable.

ROM AND CONTRACTURE

Variation in ROM measurements between observers is common and frustrating. These errors are most likely the result of how much stretch is applied before recording the value for the range of movement. Should it be a little (when resistance is first felt) or a lot (to patient tolerance)? Cusick[28] states that the findings pertaining to the initial end point are more significant to functional ability than the stretched end-point findings.

Differentiation between static and dynamic deformity may be difficult in the nonanesthetized patient.[29] However, static examination of muscle length provides some insight into whether contractures are static or dynamic. Because of the velocity-dependent nature of spasticity, it is important that assessment of ROM is performed slowly. However, comparison of joint ROM with slow and rapid stretch can be useful in the evaluation of spasticity.[30] Dynamic contracture disappears under general anesthesia. Thus the ROM examination under general anesthesia can be used to help decide whether to inject botulinum toxin to address spasticity in a muscle or perform surgery to lengthen a contracture of the tendon.

Differentiation between contracted biarticular and monoarticular muscles is important. The Silverskiöld test (**Fig. 3**) assesses the difference between gastrocnemius and soleus contracture. The Duncan-Ely test (**Fig. 4**) differentiates between contracture of the monoarticular vasti and the biarticular rectus femoris. However, Perry and colleagues[31] have shown that when these tests are performed in conjunction with fine-wire electromyography, both the monoarticulator and the biarticular muscles crossing the joint contract. For example, in the nonanesthetized patient, the Duncan-Ely test induces contraction of not only the rectus femoris but also the iliopsoas, and the Silverskiöld test induces contraction of both the gastrocnemius and the soleus. However, under general anesthesia these biarticular muscle tests reliably differentiate the location of the contracture. Consequently, they should routinely be included as part of the presurgical examination under anesthesia.

Hip

The Thomas test is used to measure the degree of hip flexor tightness. It is performed with the patient in a supine position and the pelvis held such that the anterior superior iliac spine (ASIS) and the posterior superior iliac spine (PSIS) are aligned vertically. Defining the pelvic position consistently rather than using the flatten-the-lordosis method improves reliability. Because of the origin and insertion points, the cause of limited hip abduction ROM can be distinguished by measuring hip abduction in various positions of the hip and knee with the patient supine. The one-joint adductors (adductor longus, brevis, and magnus) are isolated with the knee flexed. In this position, the gracilis is relaxed. With the knee in full extension the length of the 2-joint gracilis is in a position of maximum stretch. If hip abduction is more limited when the knee is extended compared with the knee flexed, contracture of the gracilis is the cause. Controlling and stabilizing pelvic position is imperative for a correct measurement of hip ROM.

Knee

In children with CP, capsular contracture causes knee flexion contracture. It is imperative to differentiate between true knee joint contracture and hamstring contracture. Knee joint contracture is identified if knee extension is limited with the hip in extension (to relax the hamstrings) and the ankle relaxed in a position of equinus (to relax the gastrocnemius). Hamstring contracture is identified if knee extension is limited when the hip is flexed 90° (the popliteal angle). Normal values for popliteal angle are age and gender dependent, with boys tighter than girls and both tighter with increasing age, especially around the time of the adolescent growth spurt. Like the test for hip flexion contracture, it is important to control pelvic position (the line connecting the ASIS and PSIS vertical) when assessing hamstring length. In the patient's normal resting supine position, a hip contracture causes lumber lordosis and anterior pelvic tilting that shifts the origin of the hamstrings on the ischial tuberosity proximally. The contralateral hip is in full extension, whereas the ipsilateral hip is flexed to 90°. The measurement of the degrees lacking from full extension is recorded as the unilateral popliteal angle (**Fig. 5**A). The bilateral popliteal angle measurement is performed with the contralateral hip flexed until the ASIS and PSIS are aligned vertically (comparable with the test for hip flexion contracture described earlier) (see **Fig. 5**B). A significantly smaller popliteal angle with the pelvic position corrected is referred to as a hamstring shift. The value of the popliteal angle with a neutral pelvis is a measure of the true hamstring contracture and the value with the lordosis present is the functional hamstring contracture. The difference between the 2 represents the degree of hamstring shift.

Hamstring contracture is frequently implicated as a cause of crouch gait. However, increased anterior pelvic tilt is common in crouch gait caused

Table 1
Selective motor control grading scale description

Definitions of Selective Motor Control

Hip Flexion

Position: patient seated supported or unsupported with hips at a 90° angle, legs over the side of the table. Arms folded across chest or resting in lap (not on the able or hanging on to the edge)

2: hip flexion in a superior direction without evidence of adduction, medial or lateral rotation, or trunk extension

1: hip flexion associated with adduction, medial or lateral rotation, or trunk extension that is not obligatory but occurs in conjunction with the desired motion through at least a portion of the ROM

0: hip flexion that occurs only with obligatory knee flexion, ankle dorsiflexion, and adduction

Hip Extension (Hamstrings plus Gluteus Maximus)

Position: patient lying prone, head resting on pillow (prone on elbows not allowed). Knees in maximum possible extension. Pelvis stabilized as necessary

2: hip extension in a superior direction without evidence of medial or lateral rotation, trunk extension, or abduction

1: hip extension associated with medial or lateral rotation, trunk extension, or abduction that is not obligatory but occurs in conjunction with the desired motion through at least a. portion of the ROM

0: hip extension that occurs only with obligatory trunk extension, arm extension, or neck extension. May also include medial or lateral rotation, or abduction

Hip Extension (Gluteus Maximus)

Position: patient lying prone, head resting on pillow (prone on elbows not allowed). Knees in 90° or more flexion, hips in neutral extension, pelvis flat on table. Pelvis stabilized as necessary

2: hip extension in a superior direction without evidence of medial or lateral rotation, knee extension, or hip abduction

1: hip extension associated with knee extension, trunk extension, medial or lateral rotation, or abduction that is not obligatory but occurs in conjunction with the desired motion through at least a portion of the ROM

0: hip extension that occurs only with obligatory knee extension, trunk extension, medial or lateral rotation, or abduction

Hip Abduction

Position: side-lying, the hip in neutral or slight hip extension, neutral medial or lateral rotation, knee in maximum possible extension. Pelvis stabilized as necessary

2: hip abduction in a superior direction without evidence of medial or lateral rotation or hip flexion

1: hip abduction in a superior direction associated with hip flexion, or medial or lateral rotation that is not obligatory but occurs in conjunction with the desired motion through at least a portion of the ROM

0: hip abduction that occurs with obligatory hip flexion, or medial or lateral rotation

Hip Adduction

Position: side-lying body in straight line with legs, the hip in neutral or slight hip extension, neutral medial or lateral rotation, knee in maximum possible extension, opposite limb supported in alight abduction. Pelvis stabilized as necessary

2: hip adduction in a superior direction without evidence of hip flexion, medial or lateral rotation, or tilting/rotation of the pelvis

1: hip adduction in a superior direction associated with hip flexion, or medial or lateral rotation, pelvis tilting/rotation that is not obligatory but occurs in conjunction with the desired motion through at least a portion of the ROM

0: hip adduction that occurs with obligatory hip flexion, or medial or lateral rotation

Knee Extension

Position: patient seated supported or unsupported with hips at a 90° angle, knees at 90° angle resting over the side of the table. Thigh stabilized as necessary

2: knee extension in a superior direction, without evidence of hip or trunk extension, medial or lateral rotation of the thigh or hip flexion

(continued on next page)

Table 1
(*continued*)

Definitions of Selective Motor Control

1: knee extension associated with hip or trunk extension, hip flexion, or medial or lateral rotation of the thigh that is not obligatory but occurs in conjunction with the desired motion through at least a portion of the ROM

0: knee extension that occurs with obligatory hip or trunk extension, hip flexion, or medial or lateral rotation of the thigh

Knee Flexion

Position: patient lying prone, head resting on pillow (prone on elbows not allowed). Knees in maximum possible extension. Pelvis and thigh stabilized as necessary

2: knee flexion in a superior direction without evidence of hip flexion, medial or lateral thigh rotation, or tilting, rotation of the pelvis, or ankle plantarflexion

1: knee flexion associated with a pelvic rise, hip flexion, medial or lateral rotation of the thigh, or ankle plantarflexion that is not obligatory but occurs in conjunction with the desired motion through at least a portion of the ROM

0: knee flexion that occurs with obligatory hip flexion, pelvic tilting or rotation, medial or lateral rotation of the thigh or ankle plantarflexion

Ankle Dorsiflexion (Anterior Tibialis)

Position: patient seated supported or unsupported with hips at a 90° angle, knees in extension (flexion may be allowed to achieve a range of dorsiflexion). Lower leg supported. Thigh stabilized as necessary

2: ankle dorsiflexion and inversion without evidence of increased knee flexion, subtalar eversion, or extension of the great toe

1: ankle dorsiflexion and inversion associated with increased knee flexion, subtalar eversion, or extension of the great toe that is not obligatory but occurs in conjunction with the desired motion through at least a portion of the ROM

0: ankle dorsiflexion and inversion that occurs with obligatory knee flexion, subtalar eversion, or extension of the great toe

Ankle Plantarflexion (Soleus)

Position: patient lying prone, head resting on pillow (prone on elbows not allowed). Knees in 90° of flexion. Lower leg stabilized proximal to the ankle as necessary. Ankle in neutral plantarflexion/dorsiflexion position

2: ankle plantarflexion in a superior direction without evidence of knee extension, subtalar inversion, eversion, or toe flexion

1: ankle plantarflexion associated with knee extension, subtalar inversion, eversion, or toe flexion that is not obligatory but occurs in conjunction with the desired motion through at least a portion of the ROM

0: ankle plantarflexion that occurs with obligatory knee extension, subtalar inversion, eversion, or toe flexion

Ankle Plantarflexion (Gastrocnemius)

Position: patient lying prone, head resting on pillow (prone on elbows not allowed). Knees in maximum extension, foot projecting over the end of the table. Lower leg stabilized proximal to the ankle as necessary. Ankle in neutral plantarflexion/dorsiflexion position

2: ankle plantarflexion in a superior direction without evidence of subtalar inversion, eversion, or toe flexion

1: ankle plantarflexion associated with subtalar inversion, eversion, or toe flexion that is not obligatory but occurs in conjunction with the desired motion through at least a portion of the ROM

0: ankle plantarflexion that occurs with obligatory subtalar inversion, eversion, or toe flexion

Ankle Inversion (Posterior Tibialis)

Position: patient seated supported or unsupported with hips at a 90° angle, thigh in lateral rotation, knees in flexion with lower leg stabilized proximal to the ankle. Ankle in neutral plantar/dorsiflexion

2: inversion at the STJ with plantarflexion of the ankle without evidence of toe flexion

(*continued on next page*)

Table 1
(continued)

Definitions of Selective Motor Control

1: inversion at the STJ with plantarflexion of the ankle associated with toe flexion that is not obligatory but occurs in conjunction with the desired motion through at least a portion of the ROM

0: inversion at the STJ with plantarflexion of the ankle that occurs with obligatory and forceful toe flexion

Ankle Eversion (Peroneus Brevis plus Peroneus Longus)

Position: patient seated supported or unsupported with hips at a 90° angle, thigh in medial rotation, knees in flexion with lower leg stabilized proximal to the ankle. Ankle in neutral plantar/dorsiflexion

2: eversion at the STJ with plantarflexion of the ankle without evidence of toe flexion. If head of first metatarsal is depressed action of the peroneus longus is indicated

1: eversion at the STJ with plantarflexion of the ankle associated with toe flexion that is not obligatory but occurs in conjunction with the desired motion through at least a portion of the ROM

0: eversion at the STJ with plantarflexion of the ankle that occurs with obligatory and forceful toe flexion

Ankle Eversion (Peroneus Tertius)

Position: patient seated supported or unsupported with hips at a 90° angle, knees in flexion with lower leg stabilized proximal to the ankle. Ankle in neutral plantar/dorsiflexion

2: eversion at the STJ with dorsiflexion of the ankle and 2- to 5-toe extension

1: not applicable

0: not applicable (peroneus tertius and extensor digitorum longus are anatomically combined; the 2 muscles always act together)

Great Toe Extension (Extensor Hallucis Longus)

Position: patient seated supported or unsupported with hips at a 90° angle, knees in flexion with lower leg supported. Ankle in neutral plantar/dorsiflexion

2: extension of the metatarsophalangeal joint of the great toe without evidence of knee flexion or ankle dorsiflexion

1: extension of the metatarsophalangeal joint of the great toe associated with knee flexion or ankle dorsiflexion that is not obligatory but occurs in conjunction with the desired motion through at least a portion of the ROM

0: extension of the metatarsophalangeal joint of the great toe with obligatory knee flexion, or ankle dorsiflexion

Great Toe Flexion (Flexor Hallucis Longus)

Position: patient seated supported or unsupported with hips at a 90° angle, knees in maximum extension with lower leg supported. Ankle in neutral plantar/dorsiflexion

2: flexion of the metatarsophalangeal joint of the great toe without evidence of knee extension or ankle plantarflexion

1: flexion of the metatarsophalangeal joint of the great toe associated with knee extension or ankle plantarflexion that is not obligatory but occurs in conjunction with the desired motion through at least a portion of the ROM

0: flexion of the metatarsophalangeal joint of the great toe with obligatory knee extension, or ankle plantarflexion

From Gage JR, Schwartz MH, Koop SE, et al, editors. The identification and treatment of gait problems in cerebral palsy. London: Mac Keith Press; 2009. p. 187; with permission.

by CP. Like the supine examination for hamstring contracture described earlier, this produces a hamstring shift.[32–34] In this situation, hamstring length may be normal or even long, and hamstring lengthening surgery weakens hip extension and exacerbates the excessive hamstring length. Anterior pelvic tilt and lumbar lordosis may be worsened with variable improvement in crouch gait. Because of the relative length of the hamstring moment-arm at the hip and knee, Delp and colleagues[32] have estimated that for every 1° of excessive pelvic lordosis, there is a 2° increase in knee flexion. A hamstring shift greater than 20° usually indicates excessive anterior tilt

Hypertonia Assessment Tool
Clinical assessment of seven different features of hypertonia based on definitions of tone
for different body areas (Head/Neck is added)

Items in Order of Administration	Type of Hypertonia	Head/Neck		Upper Extremity				Lower Extremity			
				Left		Right		Left		Right	
		Yes	No	Yes	No	Yes	No	Yes	No	Yes	No
1. Increased involuntary movements or postures of the designated limb with tactile stimulus of a distant body part.	Dystonia										
2. Increased involuntary movements or postures with purposeful movement of a distant body part.	Dystonia										
3. Velocity dependent resistance to passive stretch.	Spasticity										
4. Presence of a spastic catch	Spasticity										
5. Equal resistance to passive stretch during bi-directional movement of a joint	Rigidity										
6. Increased tone with movement of a distant body part	Dystonia										
7. Maintenance of limb position after passive movement.	Rigidity										

Scoring: check if present or absent

Fig. 2. HAT is useful to determine the type of high muscle tone.

A

B

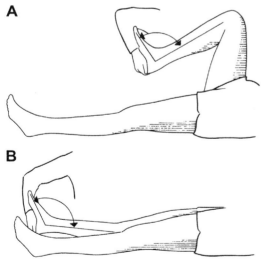

either from tight hip flexor musculature, weak abdominals, or weak hip extensors.[32] Normal popliteal angle measurements of a 5- to 18-year-old should be 0 to 49° for optimal functioning (mean 26°).[35] A 50° popliteal angle is considered a mild deviation. Because of the difficulty in establishing dynamic hamstring length on physical examination and the danger of iatrogenic problems with inappropriate surgery, static hamstring length from supine physical examination should be supplemented by estimates of hamstring length

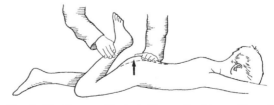

Fig. 3. The Silverskiöld test. (*A*) The Silverskiöld test differentiates tightness of the gastrocnemius and the soleus. In this test, the knee is flexed to 90°, the hind foot is positioned in varus, and maximal dorsiflexion obtained. (*B*) As the knee is extended, if the ankle moves toward plantarflexion, contracture of the gastrocnemius is present. (*From* Gage JR, Schwartz MH, Koop SE, et al, editors. The identification and treatment of gait problems in cerebral palsy. London: Mac Keith Press; 2009. p. 191; with permission.)

Fig. 4. The Duncan-Ely test. The patient is positioned prone. As the knee is flexed, a contracture of the rectus femoris causes the hip to flex because the rectus femoris is a hip flexor and knee extensor. (*From* Gage JR, Schwartz MH, Koop SE, et al, editors. The identification and treatment of gait problems in cerebral palsy. London: Mac Keith Press; 2009. p. 192; with permission.)

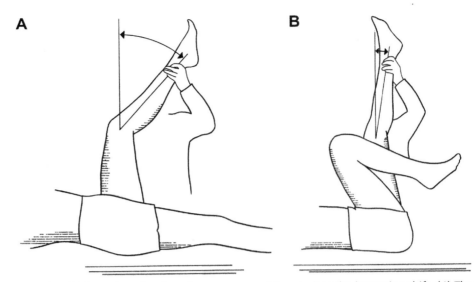

Fig. 5. Unilateral and bilateral popliteal angles are measured to calculate the hamstring shift. (*A*) The unilateral popliteal angle is measured with typical lordosis, contralateral hip extended, and the ipsilateral hip flexed to 90°. The number recorded is the degrees missing from full extension at the point of first resistance. (*B*) Bilateral popliteal angle is measured with the pelvic position corrected. The contralateral hip is flexed until the ASIS and PSIS are vertical (comparable with the test for hip flexion contracture). (*From* Gage JR, Schwartz MH, Koop SE, et al, editors. The identification and treatment of gait problems in cerebral palsy. London: Mac Keith Press; 2009. p. 193; with permission.)

obtained from gait analysis before consideration of hamstring lengthening surgery.

BONE DEFORMITY
Femoral Anteversion

Femoral anteversion refers to the relationship between the axis of the femoral neck and the femoral condyles in the transverse plane. This alignment can be estimated in the prone position by rotating the hip internally and externally until the greater trochanter is felt to be maximally prominent laterally. In this position, the neck of the femur is horizontal (**Fig. 6**). When the knee is flexed 90°, the tibia is typically perpendicular to the posterior aspect of the femoral condyles. Femoral anteversion is reported as the difference between the tibia and the vertical. Average normal adult values are 10° for men and 15° for women. Femoral anteversion at birth is 45°. If growth and development are typical, most infantile anteversion remodels between 1 and 4 years of age, reaching adult normal values by age 8 years.

Tibial Torsion

Tibial torsion is more difficult to measure accurately regardless of experience. Three methods of clinical assessment are used. Thigh-foot angle may be most reliable because it is most commonly used (**Fig. 7**). However, hind- and midfoot mobility

is necessary to properly align the foot in line with the talus primarily because it is difficult to standardize foot alignment, and foot deformities are common in children with CP. Through knee joint transverse plane rotation can also be inadvertently introduced. The bimalleolar axis method can be used particularly in cases of rigid foot deformity because alignment and position of the foot does not affect the measurement, but correct alignment of the knee joint and accurate identification of the axis of the malleoli is challenging (**Fig. 8**). The second-toe test is a third method. Developed at Gillette Children's Specialty Healthcare, this test is favored by the authors because the starting position is with the knee in extension, the position of interest during ambulation and standing, unlike the thigh-foot angle and because the axis of the tibia is easier to visualize than the bimalleolar axis (**Fig. 9**). The second-toe test allows visualization of the foot progression angle with the knee extended. It eliminates the rotational component of knee movement, but requires that the foot be placed in subtalar neutral alignment. Therefore, in children with equinus contracture and/or severe varus or valgus foot deformities, this test cannot be performed accurately. Despite the absence of tibia torsion, the presence of a true knee valgus increases the measurement of the second-toe test by the amount of true valgus that is present. Given the significant effect of even minor degrees

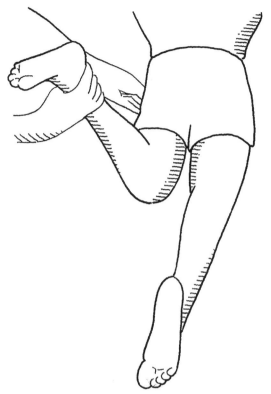

Fig. 6. Femoral anteversion by palpation of maximum trochanteric prominence. In the prone position with the knee flexed 90°, rotate the hip internally and externally until the greater trochanter is maximally prominent laterally. Femoral anteversion is the difference between the tibia and the vertical. (*From* Gage JR, Schwartz MH, Koop SE, et al, editors. The identification and treatment of gait problems in cerebral palsy. London: Mac Keith Press; 2009. p. 195; with permission.)

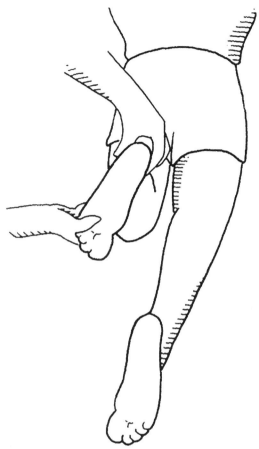

Fig. 7. The thigh-foot angle. The patient is positioned prone. Flex the knee to 90°, position the hindfoot vertically, and dorsiflex the ankle to 90° with the foot in subtalar neutral position. Place the proximal arm of the goniometer along posterior axis of femur and the distal arm along the bisector of the hindfoot and the point between the second and third metatarsal heads. (*From* Gage JR, Schwartz MH, Koop SE, et al, editors. The identification and treatment of gait problems in cerebral palsy. London: Mac Keith Press; 2009. p. 196; with permission.)

of tibial torsion on lever arm dysfunction, these measures may not be accurate and reliable enough to guide the amount of surgical correction. Therefore, other methods of detection and measurement of tibial torsion are necessary. At Gillette Children's Specialty Healthcare, we have also been relying on patient-specific data from motion analysis using functional model calibration (the difference between the functional knee and bi-malleolar axes).[36] Some centers rely on computed tomography scan measurement of tibial torsion.

Patella Alta

Patella alta is common in children with CP and is probably contributed to by the chronic excessive knee extensor forces of rectus femoris spasticity and crouch gait. These same forces may lead to inferior pole sleeve avulsion fractures. To screen

for patella alta, the patient is positioned supine with the knees extended. The top of the patella is then palpated. The superior pole of the patella is typically one finger width proximal to the adductor tubercle. Patella alta may contribute to patellofemoral instability, pain, and subluxation. Patella alta can also be associated with terminal knee extensor dysfunction (quadriceps insufficiency) measured by extensor lag. Extensor lag is measured with the patient positioned supine (to relax the hamstrings), and the leg flexed at the knee over the end of the examination table. The child is asked to actively extend the knee as

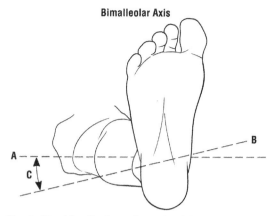

Bimalleolar Axis

Fig. 8. The bimalleolar axis angle. (A) With the knee fully extended in the supine position rotate the thigh segment until the medial and lateral femoral condyles are horizontal. (B) Mark the midpoints of the medial and lateral malleolus. (C) Using a goniometer or angle finder, measure the angle between the bimalleolar axis and the condylar axis. (*From* Gage JR, Schwartz MH, Koop SE, et al, editors. The identification and treatment of gait problems in cerebral palsy. London: Mac Keith Press; 2009. p. 197; with permission.)

much as possible. The extensor lag is recorded as the difference between the active range and the passive ROM. Patellar position can be measured with a lateral radiograph of the knee taken in full extension.

Foot

Pronation and supination are terms used to describe the triplanar motions in the foot and ankle. These 2 motions are pure rotations about an oblique axis, resulting in the same end position as 3 separate rotations in the cardinal planes.[37] Although inconsistently used, the terms pronation and supination should be used only in reference to the triplane motions of the foot and ankle, because they provide a consistent and logical description of the motion that is anatomically available.

Despite the complexity of foot anatomy and biomechanics, evaluating the foot and understanding its function in both the nonweight-bearing and weight-bearing position is essential. The foot must function as both a mobile adaptor and a rigid lever at different points in the gait cycle.

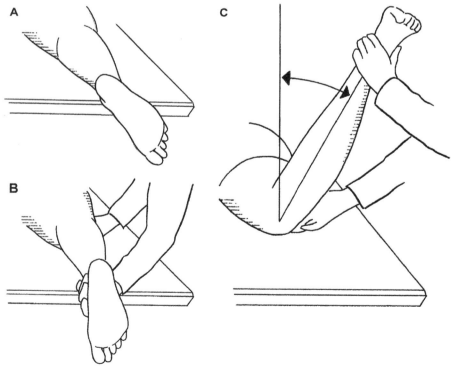

Fig. 9. The second-toe test. (*A*) An external tibial torsion leads to an outwardly pointed foot when the patient is relaxed in the prone position with the knee fully extended. (*B*) Rotate the leg to position the second toe pointing directly toward the floor (in this case requiring internal hip rotation). (*C*) Hold the thigh in this position (preventing internal or external hip rotation) as the knee is flexed. Measure the angle from vertical. (*From* Gage JR, Schwartz MH, Koop SE, et al, editors. The identification and treatment of gait problems in cerebral palsy. London: Mac Keith Press; 2009. p. 197; with permission.)

Correctly identifying structural abnormalities in the nonweight-bearing position and the compensations that occur as a result of these abnormalities in weight bearing is essential to determining interventions to improve foot position and the function of the entire lower extremity.

Because every foot has its own neutral subtalar joint (STJ) position, the use of the nonweight-bearing STJ neutral (STJN) position provides consistency in positioning the foot in order to assess and identify patient-specific structural abnormalities and their resultant compensations in weight bearing. Root and colleagues[38] originally defined STJN as the position from which the STJ can be maximally pronated and supinated and, therefore, the position from which the STJ can function optimally. It is the position of the STJ where it is neither pronated nor supinated. In addition, determining STJN and then naming positions of the rearfoot and forefoot in relation to the next most proximal segment is consistent with the orthopedic naming of deformities in relation to the adjacent, proximal segment. This strategy allows the evaluator a starting point from which to describe compensations/deviations in the foot that may (or may not) occur when going from the nonweight-bearing to the weight-bearing position.

STJN is found through palpation at the articulation between the head of the talus and the navicular. Congruency of the talonavicular joint is the position of the foot at which neither the medial nor lateral head of the talus protrudes and the examiner feels symmetry of the navicular on the head of the talus. From this starting point, the patient's rearfoot and forefoot relationships are evaluated. Further details regarding the method of finding STJN during physical examination have been published.[39]

Evaluation of the rearfoot position in STJN

Once the foot has been placed in the STJN position, rearfoot position in relationship to the lower one-third of the leg is assessed (**Fig. 10**). By visualizing the relationship of the bisector of the calcaneus relative to the bisector of the lower one-third of the leg, the rearfoot alignment can be described. If this relationship is linear, the rearfoot position is said to be vertical. If the orientation of the rearfoot with respect to the lower one-third of the leg is inverted, this position is known as a varus position of the rearfoot. If the line bisecting the calcaneus is everted in relation to the lower one-third of the leg, this position is referred to as a valgus position of the rearfoot.

Evaluation of the forefoot position in STJN

Once the rearfoot position has been determined, forefoot to rearfoot relationship can be evaluated in each of the 3 cardinal planes. While maintaining STJN, forefoot position in the frontal plane can be described by assessing the angle between a line that is perpendicular to the bisection of the posterior calcaneus (replicating the plane of the calcaneal condyles) and the plane of the metatarsal heads. In this position, if the plane of the metatarsal heads is in the same plane as the line that

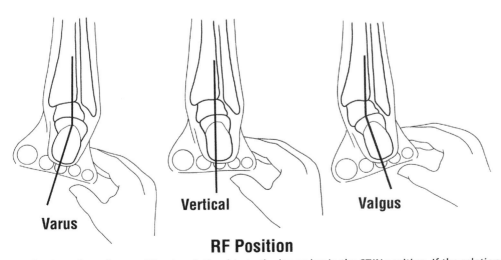

Varus   **Vertical**   **Valgus**

RF Position

Fig. 10. Evaluation of rearfoot position in relationship to the lower leg in the STJN position. If the relationship is linear, the rearfoot position is described as being vertical (most common). If inverted, the rearfoot is said to be in a varus position, and if everted, the rearfoot is said to be in a valgus position (rare). (*From* Gage JR, Schwartz MH, Koop SE, et al, editors. The identification and treatment of gait problems in cerebral palsy. London: Mac Keith Press; 2009. p. 214; with permission.)

is perpendicular to the bisection of the calcaneus, the forefoot position is described as being neutral (**Fig. 11**). If the plane of the forefoot in relationship to the rearfoot shows the medial side of the foot to be higher than the lateral side (forefoot inverted) this position is described as forefoot varus deformity (**Fig. 12**). If the opposite is seen (ie, the lateral border of the foot is higher than the medial border [forefoot everted]), this position is described as being a forefoot valgus deformity (**Fig. 13**). Typically, 2 types of forefoot valgus deformities exist. The first shows that all of the metatarsal heads are everted and is referred to as a total forefoot valgus. The second is caused by plantarflexion of the first ray (first cuneiform plus first MT), whereas the 2 to 5 metatarsal heads lie in the appropriate plane. The relationship of the forefoot to the rearfoot must also be assessed in the sagittal plane. If the examiner visualizes a plane representing the ground surface applied to the plantar surface of the calcaneus, the plantar surface of the metatarsal heads should also lie on this plane. If the plane of the metatarsals sits below that of the calcaneus, the forefoot would be described as being plantarflexed in relation to the rearfoot, often referred to as a forefoot equinus deformity. In the transverse plane, the typical relationship between the forefoot and rearfoot requires the forefoot to have the same longitudinal direction as the rearfoot. Deviations of the forefoot in the transverse plane toward the midline are referred to as adduction, and away from the midline as abduction.

Compensations

Compensation is a change in the structural alignment or position of the foot to neutralize the effect of an abnormal force, resulting in a deviation in structural alignment or position of another part.[40] When structural deformities are present in the foot and ankle, as described earlier, the foot has the ability to compensate for these deformities. Most often, these compensations occur through the motion of the subtalar and the midtarsal joint. Over time, abnormal compensations can lead to tissue stress and pain, as well as create lever arm dysfunction, which negatively affects gait and posture.

Forefoot varus

The foot with a structural forefoot varus has an inverted orientation of the forefoot to the rearfoot when placed in the nonweight-bearing STJN position. To compensate for this deformity during gait, this foot type typically shows an abnormal amount of pronation during midstance, because, when the medial calcaneal condyle has reached the ground in midstance, the forefoot, rather than being in

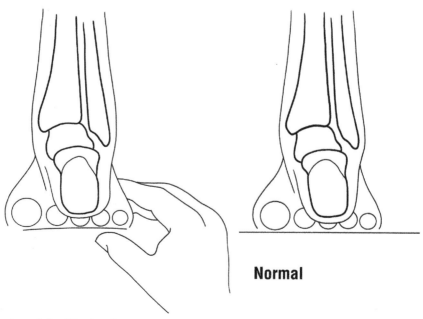

Normal

Fig. 11. Evaluation of the STJN forefoot position in the frontal plane. If the plane of the metatarsal heads lies in the same plane as a line that is perpendicular to the bisection of the calcaneus, the forefoot position is described as neutral. No compensation is required in the weight-bearing position. (*From* Gage JR, Schwartz MH, Koop SE, et al, editors. The identification and treatment of gait problems in cerebral palsy. London: Mac Keith Press; 2009. p. 215; with permission.)

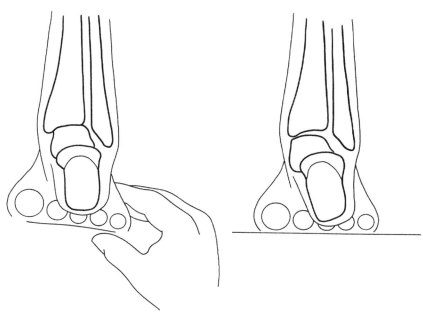

Fig. 12. Evaluation of the STJN forefoot position in the frontal plane. If the plane of the metatarsal heads, in relationship to the rearfoot, shows the medial side to be higher than the lateral side (forefoot inverted), the forefoot is described as being in a varus position. In weight bearing, the typical compensation for a forefoot varus deformity is abnormal pronation. (*From* Gage JR, Schwartz MH, Koop SE, et al, editors. The identification and treatment of gait problems in cerebral palsy. London: Mac Keith Press; 2009. p. 216; with permission.)

contact with the floor, shows an orientation where the medial border of the foot is elevated from the ground surface. To assist with the medial border reaching the ground, the STJ (if pain and motion allow) continues pronating as the midstance phase of gait begins (see **Fig. 12**). This excessive pronation is an abnormal compensation, and is manifested as eversion of the calcaneus, abduction of the forefoot, and lowering of the medial longitudinal arch. This compensated foot position leads to internal malrotation of the entire lower extremity as the talus plantarflexes and deviates medially. The clinician must appreciate the influence that the forefoot deformity has on the position of not only the rearfoot but the entire lower extremity, and address treatment accordingly. Placing a wedge under the medial forefoot may correct the compensated position of the rearfoot, confirming that the rearfoot position is flexible and being driven by the forefoot deformity. If correction of the rearfoot is not seen, a fixed rearfoot deformity may be present. However, hypermobility of the midfoot and diminished motor control and strength can limit the amount of correction seen with this maneuver.

Forefoot valgus

The foot with a structural forefoot valgus has an everted orientation of the forefoot in relation to

the rearfoot when placed in the nonweight-bearing STJN position. A typical compensation for this foot deformity may be abnormal supination during midstance. As with the forefoot varus deformity, when the medial calcaneal condyle has reached the ground in midstance, the forefoot is not plantigrade. However, with this foot deformity the lateral border of the foot is elevated from the ground surface. To get the lateral border of the foot on the ground, the STJ (if pain and motion allow) supinates (see **Fig. 13**B and D). This supination occurs at a time in the gait cycle when the foot should be pronating, and is characterized by inversion of the calcaneus, adduction of the forefoot, and an increase in the height of the medial longitudinal arch. This abnormal compensation can be seen when a total forefoot valgus deformity is present, or with a rigid plantarflexed first ray. If a plantarflexed first ray is present, it is important to assess its mobility, because the ability or inability of the first ray to dorsiflex can greatly affect the way the foot functions in weight bearing. If the plantarflexed first ray is mobile, meaning that the first ray can be easily dorsiflexed to the level of the other metatarsal heads, this most likely has little effect on overall foot position in weight bearing. If first ray mobility is limited, that is, it cannot be dorsiflexed to the level of the other metatarsal heads, the

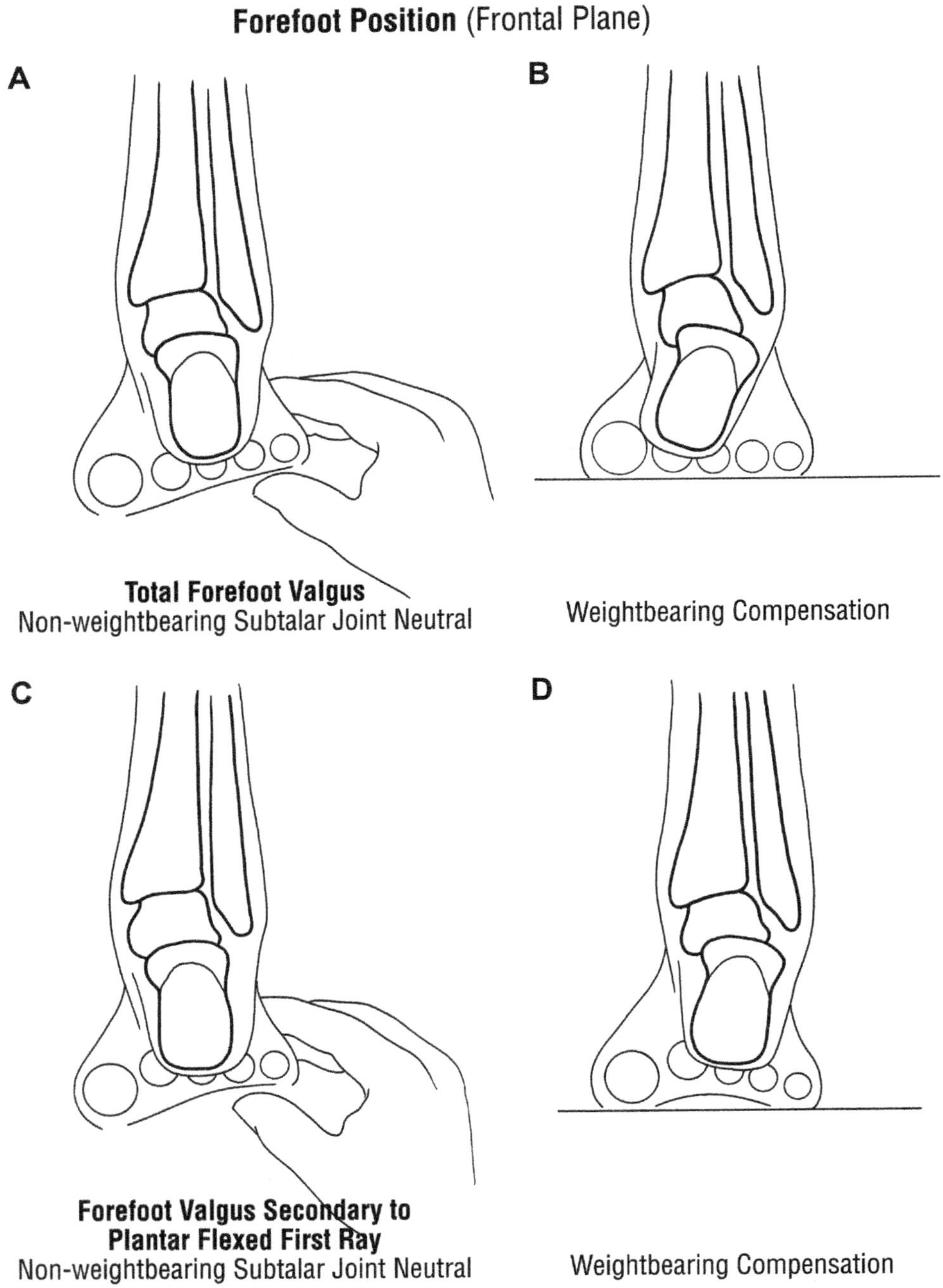

Forefoot Position (Frontal Plane)

A

B

Total Forefoot Valgus
Non-weightbearing Subtalar Joint Neutral

Weightbearing Compensation

C

D

**Forefoot Valgus Secondary to
Plantar Flexed First Ray**
Non-weightbearing Subtalar Joint Neutral

Weightbearing Compensation

Fig. 13. Evaluation of the STJN forefoot position in the frontal plane. If the plane of the metatarsal heads, in relationship to the rearfoot, shows the lateral side to be higher than the medial (forefoot everted), the forefoot is described as being in a valgus position. This position may be secondary to a total forefoot valgus (*A*), or a plantar-flexed first ray (*C*). A typical compensation for a forefoot valgus deformity is abnormal supination (*B* and *D*).

weight-bearing foot functions differently from the foot with a mobile plantarflexed first ray. If, on the other hand, the plantarflexed first ray is rigid, assessment of rearfoot mobility is also necessary. If the hindfoot is flexible and the forefoot valgus deformity fixed, then correction of the forefoot secondarily causes correction of the rearfoot. If the hindfoot is not flexible, then correction of the forefoot cannot produce rearfoot correction.[41] The Coleman block test is a simple test to help determine the driving force behind the rearfoot position. To perform the test, the lateral border of the forefoot is placed on a block, varying from 0.5 to 2.5 cm, and the medial forefoot allowed to settle to the floor. If the rearfoot corrects with this test, then treatment should address only the forefoot. If the rearfoot does not correct, then treatment needs to address a combination of the forefoot and rearfoot. Similarly, use of lateral forefoot wedging can be used to assess the role the forefoot plays in the position of the rearfoot when a total forefoot valgus deformity is present.

Forefoot equinus

Forefoot equinus is a position of plantarflexion of the forefoot compared with the rearfoot. If adequate dorsiflexion ROM is available at the ankle joint, no other compensation is required for this forefoot deformity. If ankle joint dorsiflexion is insufficient, compensation has to occur through the oblique axis of the midtarsal joint, because that is the only other source of dorsiflexion ROM in the foot and ankle complex. For this to occur, the STJ must be pronated to allow the needed mobility of the midtarsal joint. As with other abnormal compensations, this inappropriate timing and/or range of pronation may cause difficulty with pain and/or gait abnormalities.

Developmental trends

It is essential that those of us who deal with the pediatric patient appreciate normal and abnormal developmental parameters for the various stages of growth. In general, a newborn shows increased varus positioning of both the forefoot and rearfoot, metatarsus adductus, and excessive ROM in the subtalar and ankle joints. There is little clinical evidence of a medial longitudinal arch until age 4 to 5 years. By 7 to 8 years of age, the child's foot should have developed the adult values of 0 to 2° of rearfoot and forefoot varus, 5 to 15° of metatarsus adductus, and significantly less ROM through the ankle and STJs.[42] Clinical evaluation of the foot must be directly related to the child's age to determine if the deformity or problem is significant or not.

Leg Length

Good assessment of limb length inequality can by complicated by scoliosis, hip subluxation, pelvic obliquity, unilateral contracture of the hip adductors or abductors, or knee flexion contracture. In the absence of an asymmetric hip or knee contractures, limb length can be measured clinically in supine using the inferior border of the ASIS and the distal aspect of the medial malleolus, or

standing using blocks to equalize the ASIS or the iliac crest height. Radiographic assessment is necessary if too many compounding factors are present.

POSTURE AND BALANCE

Assessment of posterior, anterior, and medial-lateral equilibrium responses should not be neglected when planning treatment. Many children with CP have delayed or deficient posterior equilibrium responses. Assessment of posture, including trunk, pelvis, and lower extremity posture in static standing and during walking in the sagittal and coronal planes often gives insight to areas of weakness, poor motor control, and the compensation strategies that the child is using to circumvent them.

GAIT BY OBSERVATION

Observational gait analysis consists of observing a patient without the use of formal gait analysis equipment. Experience and use of a systematic method can improve the ability to identify primary and compensatory gait deviations. Various forms and scales have been developed to assist the observer in organizing the analysis as well as for reporting the observations.[43–45] The Observational Gait Scale,[46] and the Edinburgh Visual Gait Score[45] are validated scales for outcome measurement but may not fully describe what the clinician is seeing. Krebs and colleagues[47] reported that observational gait analysis is more consistent with a single observer. They further observed that viewing a video of a patient walking is more consistent than viewing the patient live with repeated walks. Finally, if slow motion video is used, these investigators found that the consistency of observation improved markedly.

Beginning with the feet, here are several questions to consider while observing gait:

1. What is the position of the foot at the end of terminal swing? Is the foot neutral or is it in a varus or valgus position?
2. Is the ankle in a neutral position or equinus?
3. Which portion of the foot contacts the floor first?
4. What is the foot progression angle during stance and swing with respect to both the line of progression and the alignment of the knee?
5. Is the foot plantigrade in stance?
6. Does the forefoot maintain its alignment with the hindfoot, and is the arch maintained?
7. At which point in the cycle does any deviation in the foot occur?

8. Does the foot go through the normal sequence of rockers, or is there premature plantarflexion in midstance, or prolonged dorsiflexion in terminal stance?
9. What are the positions of the toes in stance and swing? Is there toe clawing that is occurring in stance, or hyperextension of the first metatarsophalangeal joint in swing?

At the knee the following should be noted:

1. What are the positions of the knee in terminal swing and at initial contact?
2. Is the normal loading response (slight flexion followed by extension in early stance as the limb is loaded) present?
3. Does the knee come to full extension at any point in stance? If so, when?
4. Does the knee hyperextend, or is the extension controlled?
5. What is the maximum knee flexion in swing? When does it occur?
6. Is the knee aligned with the foot?
7. Is the shank aligned with the thigh?
8. Is there a varus or valgus motion during loading?

Gait by observation is more difficult proximally. The mass of the trunk, and the soft tissue around the hips and pelvis frequently obscure these joint motions. Because selective motor control tends to be better in the proximal and worse in the distal muscles, compensatory motions for distal gait problems often occur proximally via hip or trunk motion. However, without computerized gait analysis, it is difficult to determine whether the abnormal movements are compensations, or primary deviations. When observing the trunk, pelvis, and hips, note:

1. Is the thigh (knee) aligned to the line of progression at initial contact? If not is the malrotation internal or external?
2. Does the hip extend fully in terminal stance?
3. Is hip abduction (circumduction) or adduction (scissoring) excessive in swing?
4. Is pelvic position normal or is it excessively anterior or posterior?
5. Is pelvic malrotation or obliquity present?
6. What are the trunk movements in each plane? Are these appropriate?
7. Are the abnormal motions likely to be primary or compensatory?
8. How are the arms moving during gait? Are they moving symmetrically and reciprocally or are they postured?
9. Does the child elevate his/her arms to assist with balance?

And finally, some general questions to be considered in a gait-by-observation analysis:

1. Is the stride length adequate and are the step lengths symmetric?
2. Does the walking pattern seem to be efficient or is there excessive body motion or other indications of excessive energy consumption?
3. What influence do assistive devices or orthotics have on the child's walking pattern?

REFERENCES

1. Novacheck TF, Stout JL, Tervo R. Reliability and validity of the Gillette Functional Assessment Questionnaire as an outcome measure in children with walking disabilities. J Pediatr Orthop 2000;20:75–81.
2. Daltroy LH, Liang MH, Fossel AH, et al. The POSNA pediatric musculoskeletal functional health questionnaire: report on reliability, validity, and sensitivity to change. Pediatric Outcomes Instrument Development Group. Pediatric Orthopaedic Society of North America. J Pediatr Orthop 1998;18:561–71.
3. Graham HK, Harvey A, Rodda J, et al. The Functional Mobility Scale (FMS). J Pediatr Orthop 2004;24:514–20.
4. Tervo RC, Azuma S, Stout J, et al. Correlation between physical functioning and gait measures in children with cerebral palsy. Dev Med Child Neurol 2002;44:185–90.
5. Harvey A, Graham HK, Morris ME, et al. The Functional Mobility Scale: ability to detect change following single event multilevel surgery. Dev Med Child Neurol 2007;49:603–7.
6. Rosenbaum P, Stewart D. The World Health Organization International Classification of Functioning, Disability, and Health: a model to guide clinical thinking, practice and research in the field of cerebral palsy. Semin Pediatr Neurol 2004;11:5–10.
7. Damiano DL, Abel MF. Functional outcomes of strength training in spastic cerebral palsy. Arch Phys Med Rehabil 1998;79:119–25.
8. Damiano DL, Dodd K, Taylor NF. Should we be testing and training muscle strength in cerebral palsy? Dev Med Child Neurol 2002a;44:68–72.
9. Desloovere K, Molenaers G, Feys H, et al. Do dynamic and static clinical measurements correlate with gait analysis parameters in children with cerebral palsy? Gait Posture 2006;24:302–13.
10. Bohannon RW. Is the measurement of muscle strength appropriate in patients with brain lesions? A special communication. Phys Ther 1989;69:225–36.
11. Damiano DL, Vaughan CL, Abel MF. Muscle response to heavy resistance exercise in children

with spastic cerebral palsy. Dev Med Child Neurol 1995;37:731–9.

12. Kramer JF, MacPhail HE. Relationships among measures of walking efficiency, gross motor ability, and isokinetic strength in adolescents with cerebral palsy. Pediatr Phys Ther 1994;6:3–8.

13. Kendall HO, Kendall FP, Wadsworth GE, editors. Muscle testing and function. 2nd edition. London: Williams and Wilkins; 1971.

14. Wadsworth CT, Krishnan R, Sear M, et al. Intrarater reliability of manual muscle testing and hand-held dynametric muscle testing. Phys Ther 1987;67: 1342–7.

15. Bohannon RW, Smith MB. Interrater reliability of a modified Ashworth scale of muscle spasticity. Phys Ther 1987;67:206–7.

16. Berry ET, Giuliani CA, Damiano DL. Intrasession and intersession reliability of handheld dynamometry in children with cerebral palsy. Pediatr Phys Ther 2004;16:191–8.

17. Wiley ME, Damiano DL. Lower-extremity strength profiles in spastic cerebral palsy. Dev Med Child Neurol 1998;40:100–7.

18. Macfarlane TS, Larson CA, Stiller C. Lower extremity muscle strength in 6- to 8-year-old children using hand-held dynamometry. Pediatr Phys Ther 2008; 20:128–36.

19. Sanger TD, Delgado MR, Gaebler-Spira D, et al. Classification and definition of disorders causing hypertonia in childhood. Pediatrics 2003;111: 89–97.

20. Lee KC, Carson L, Kinnin E, et al. The Ashworth Scale: a reliable and reproducible method of measuring spasticity. J Neurol Rehabil 1989;3: 205–9.

21. Gregson JM, Leathley M, Moore AP, et al. Reliability of the Tone Assessment Scale and the modified Ashworth scale as clinical tools for assessing poststroke spasticity. Arch Phys Med Rehabil 1999;80:1013–6.

22. Clopton N, Dutton J, Featherston T, et al. Interrater and intrarater reliability of the Modified Ashworth Scale in children with hypertonia. Pediatr Phys Ther 2005;17:268–73.

23. Haugh AB, Pandyan AD, Johnson GR. A systematic review of the Tardieu Scale for the measurement of spasticity. Disabil Rehabil 2006;28:899–907.

24. Damiano DL, Quinlivan JM, Owen BF, et al. What does the Ashworth scale really measure and are instrumented measures more valid and precise? Dev Med Child Neurol 2002b;44:112–8.

25. Engsberg JR, Olree KS, Ross SA, et al. Quantitative clinical measure of spasticity in children with cerebral palsy. Arch Phys Med Rehabil 1996;77:594–9.

26. Jethwa A, Mink J, MacArthur C, et al. Development of the Hypertonia Assessment Tool (HAT): a discriminative tool for hypertonia in children. Dev Med Child Neurol 2010;52:e83–7.

27. Barry MJ, VanSwearingen JM, Albright AL. Reliability and responsiveness of the Barry-Albright Dystonia Scale. Dev Med Child Neurol 1999;41: 404–11.

28. Cusick BD, editor. Progressive casting & splinting. Tucson (AZ): Therapy Skill Builders; 1990.

29. Perry J, Hoffer MM, Giovan P, et al. Gait analysis of the triceps surae in cerebral palsy. A preoperative and postoperative clinical and electromyographic study. J Bone Joint Surg Am 1974;56:511–20.

30. Boyd RN, Graham HK. Objective measurement of clinical findings in the use of botulinum toxin type A for the management of children with cerebral palsy. Eur J Neurol 1999;6:s23.

31. Perry J, Hoffer MM, Antonelli D, et al. Electromyography before and after surgery for hip deformity in children with cerebral palsy. A comparison of clinical and electromyographic findings. J Bone Joint Surg Am 1976;58:201–8.

32. Delp SL, Arnold AS, Speers RA, et al. Hamstrings and psoas lengths during normal and crouch gait: implications for muscle-tendon surgery. J Orthop Res 1996;14:144–51.

33. Hoffinger SA, Rab GT, Abou-Ghaida H. Hamstrings in cerebral palsy crouch gait. J Pediatr Orthop 1993;13:722–6.

34. Schutte LM, Hayden SW, Gage JR. Lengths of hamstrings and psoas muscles during crouch gait: effects of femoral anteversion. J Orthop Res 1997; 15:615–21.

35. Katz K, Rosenthal A, Yosipovitch Z. Normal ranges of popliteal angle in children. J Pediatr Orthop 1992;12:229–31.

36. Schwartz MH, Rozumalski A. A new method for estimating joint parameters from motion data. J Biomech 2005;38:107–16.

37. Oatis C. Biomechanics of the foot and ankle under static conditions. Phys Ther 1988;68(12):1815.

38. Root ML, Orien WP, Weed JH. Clinical biomechanics: normal and abnormal function of the foot. Los Angeles (CA): Clinical Biomechanics Corp; 1977. [Chapter 1].

39. Sohrweide. Foot biomechanics & pathology. Chapter 3.2:205–221. In: Gage JR, Schwartz MH, Koop SE, et al, editors. Identification and treatment of gait problems in cerebral palsy. London: Mac Keith Press; 2009.

40. Gray H. The lower extremity. In: Pick T, Howden R, editors. Gray's anatomy. 35th edition. Philadelphia: Courage Books; 1974. p. 203.

41. Coleman SS, Chestnut WJ. A simple test for hindfoot flexibility in the cavovarus foot. Clin Orthop 1977; 123:60–2.

42. Gray G, Tiberio D, Witmer M, editors. When the feet hit the ground everything changes. Neutral subtalar position. Toledo (OH): The American Physical Rehabilitation Network; 1984.

43. Perry J. Gait analysis: normal and pathological function. Thorofare (NJ): Slack Inc; 1992.
44. Brown CR, Hillman SJ, Richardson AM, et al. Reliability and validity of the Visual Gait Assessment Scale for children with hemiplegic cerebral palsy when used by experienced and inexperienced observers. Gait Posture 2008;27:648–52.
45. Wren TA, Do KP, Hara R, et al. Gillette Gait Index as a gait analysis summary measure: comparison with qualitative visual assessments of overall gait. J Pediatr Orthop 2007;27:765–8.
46. Mackey AH, Lobb GL, Walt SE, et al. Reliability and validity of the observational gait scale in children with spastic diplegia. Dev Med Child Neurol 2003; 45:4–11.
47. Krebs DE, Edelstein JE, Fishman S. Reliability of observational kinematic gait analysis. Phys Ther 1985;65:1027–33.

The Role of Gait Analysis in Treating Gait Abnormalities in Cerebral Palsy

Frank M. Chang, MD[a,b,c,]*, Jason T. Rhodes, MD, MS[a,c],
Katherine M. Flynn, BA[c,d], James J. Carollo, PhD, PE[c,d,e]

KEYWORDS

- Instrumented gait analysis • Cerebral palsy
- Jump knee gait • Equinus gait • Crouch gait
- Stiff knee gait • Malicious malrotation

Most of us take walking for granted. Individuals with cerebral palsy (CP) cannot. CP is the most common pediatric neurologic disorder, with an incidence of 3.6 per 1000 live births.[1] There are approximately 9000 newly diagnosed cases annually with a total of 765,000 cases in the United States alone. The pathologic condition that leads to CP produces a central nervous system injury that adversely affects the gait of these individuals. Gait abnormalities are primarily caused by spasticity or abnormal muscle tone, diminished motor control, and impaired balance. Throughout an individual's growth, gait abnormalities are compounded by progressively developing skeletal deformities, soft tissue contractures of the musculotendinous units and capsular structures, and dynamic deformities caused by abnormal unbalanced muscle forces. As the patient matures, soft tissue contractures, muscle weakness, pain, and compensatory mechanisms result in continued gait abnormalities throughout their lifetime if not treated.[2]

The current trend in the treatment of individuals with CP is to perform a thorough evaluation including a complete patient history from birth to present, a comprehensive physical examination, appropriate radiographs, consultation with other medical specialists, and analysis of gait. Thoughtful consideration of all this information leads to a better understanding of the deformities and pathologies affecting an individual's characteristic gait at the current stage of development. Once the primary deformities are recognized, the orthopedic surgeon can assimilate this data to formulate a treatment plan with a combination of surgical and nonsurgical interventions. If orthopedic surgery is planned, single-event multilevel surgery (SEMLS) is preferred to performing multiple procedures spread over time. Mercer Rang described this as the birthday syndrome, reflecting a yearly (or every other year) series of hospital admissions, recovery, postoperative therapy, and missed school days.[3] Graham and colleagues[4] have shown improved outcomes

[a] Department of Orthopedic Surgery, University of Colorado Denver, 12631 East 17th Avenue, Academic Office 1, Room 2513, Mail Stop F-493, Aurora, CO 80045, USA
[b] Department of Physical Medicine and Rehabilitation, University of Colorado Denver, Mail Stop F-493, 12631 East 17th Avenue, Academic Office 1, Room 2513, Aurora, CO 80045, USA
[c] Center for Gait and Movement Analysis (CGMA), The Children's Hospital, B476, 13123 East 16th Avenue, Aurora, CO 80045, USA
[d] Musculoskeletal Research Center, The Children's Hospital, B476, 13123 East 16th Avenue, Aurora, CO 80045, USA
[e] Department of Bioengineering, University of Colorado School of Medicine, Aurora, CO, USA
* Corresponding author. Department of Physical Medicine and Rehabilitation, University of Colorado Denver, Mail Stop F-493, 12631 East 17th Avenue, Academic Office 1, Room 2513, Aurora, CO 80045.
E-mail address: Chang.Frank@tchden.org

Orthop Clin N Am 41 (2010) 489–506
doi:10.1016/j.ocl.2010.06.009

using the SEMLS approach, and it is becoming the standard of care for children with CP.

In the twenty-first century, no discussion of gait analysis in individuals with CP would be complete without incorporating the tools and techniques of instrumented gait analysis (IGA). As a diagnostic test, IGA has the unique capability of accurately measuring and providing information that is critical for distinguishing complex gait abnormalities. Knowing the 3-dimensional position of the pelvis, hip, femur, knee, tibia, ankle, and foot at any moment of the gait cycle assists the clinician in recognizing typical pathologic gait patterns. Integrating this information with dynamic electromyography (D-EMG) increases understanding of the pathologic gait patterns and deduces possible treatment options. IGA provides the objective information to assist the orthopedic surgeon in the decision-making process of treatment for these individuals with CP. IGA also measures outcomes during the growing life of the child with CP and helps the clinical provider understand the changing medical needs of the mature adult with the disease.[5]

Information provided by IGA enhances the understanding of gait abnormality by providing real-time objective data that cannot be appreciated visually or measured on a static physical examination. Using advanced technology to improve understanding in this way is similar to localization of a tumor and its surrounding anatomic structures using magnetic resonance imaging rather than relying solely on a 2- or 3-view radiograph when planning a malignant tumor surgical resection or reconstruction procedure.

In addition to the visual gait analysis and static physical examination traditionally used by the orthopedic surgeon to make treatment decisions, the orthopedic surgeon can now take advantage of the latest technology to accurately measure gait pathologies. IGA is not a substitute for clinical judgment and experience, and should be used to enhance clinical decision-making and provide evidence to support a particular treatment plan. The combination of systematic clinical assessment and measurements from IGA provides the basis for an orthopedic surgeon to develop the best treatment plan for a specific child or adult with CP, and represents the strongest outcomes-based approach to address the ambulatory needs of this challenging population.

The central nervous system pathology in CP is extremely variable, but common patterns can be determined. The complexity of the human brain and the interconnections of the various pathways results in complex gait deviations that are a mixture of the individual patterns depending on the exact location of the brain injury or dysfunction. Discussion of all the abnormal gait patterns would be extremely lengthy, so the authors have chosen to present clinical gait patterns that are the most prevalent in individuals with CP. The common gait patterns presented here have been previously described in the literature[2,6–8] and include jump knee gait, toe-toe gait pattern in which apparent equinus versus true equinus must be distinguished, crouch knee gait, stiff knee gait, and finally rotational abnormalities affecting gait. Before describing these specific gait patterns in depth, the authors provide some important background information related to classification of gait patterns and also introduce some of the fundamental principles of gait analysis.

FUNCTIONAL CLASSIFICATION IN CP

As mentioned in the previous section, the walking ability of individuals with CP is as varied as the possible sites of injury to the developing brain, and ranges from the highly functional community ambulators to individuals who are completely nonambulatory and who rely on other assisted methods of mobility. Some have a single-gait abnormality whereas others are more severely affected with multiple deformities, with each deformity interacting with the other resulting in an extremely complex gait pattern. Classification of gait and motor function is challenging because there are many different ways to approach classification, and no 2 individuals with CP are alike. To have a common frame of reference and to promote communication among caregivers, a validated classification scheme known as the Gross Motor Function Classification System (GMFCS) has been used to describe children with CP. Description of GMFCS is well documented in the literature, including the differences associated with age.[9] The GMFCS consists of 5 grades of motor function linked to decreasing levels of ambulatory independence. Level I children walk without assistance in most environments and can run and jump; however, speed, balance, and coordination are limited. Level II children walk in most settings and can climb stairs holding a railing, but may experience difficulty walking long distances or balancing on uneven terrain, and can rarely run or jump. Children at GMFCS level III use handheld assistive devices to walk, and rely on manual wheeled mobility for longer distances. At level IV, walking requires physical assistance; even for short distances and wheeled mobility, using a power wheelchair is required in most settings. At level V, children with CP are nonambulatory and require considerable assistance for most activities, are generally transported in a manual wheelchair, and are limited in their ability to maintain head and trunk postures. Further refinements and details have been established based on the child's age.[9] Although there are other functional classification schemes, the GMFCS is the most widely used, and is especially important when determining goals of treatment and comparing treatment outcomes for children with CP.

GAIT ANALYSIS FUNDAMENTALS

Before describing common gait patterns seen in individuals with CP, it is important to briefly discuss the foundation on which modern clinical gait analysis is based. An understanding of normal gait principles and terminology is basic to being able to communicate abstract concepts related to gait dysfunction. An overview of the gait measurements in common use provides a framework for identifying the causes of an underlying gait problem and a strategy for choosing between different interventions. It is not within the scope of this article to replace the excellent reference material already available on this subject.[5,8,10–12] However, an introduction to the major concepts is warranted to understand the procedures used in gait analysis described in the remainder of this article.

Normal Gait Cycle

The principal goal of locomotion is to propel the body forward. As bipeds, the most natural and efficient way to accomplish this task is to alternate the base of support from one leg to the other while minimizing unnecessary body movements. Typically developing individuals produce a repeatable gait pattern that is both cyclical and symmetric.[13] Because of the cyclic nature of bipedalism, it is useful to consider gait as a repeatable progression with specific events occurring in sequence during each repetition of the cycle. **Fig. 1** illustrates one complete gait cycle, or stride, and includes the time periods and temporal events relative to the shaded ipsilateral side and associated with foot-floor contact, which necessarily arise from changing the support limb. Temporal events are specific moments in time that divide the gait cycle into periods of specific duration, and are identified by the skeletal figures along the top of **Fig. 1**. Typically, the gait cycle begins when one foot makes contact with the walking surface (initial contact) and ends when that same foot makes contact again. Using such a convention allows a stride to be time normalized, whereby a specific stride location is expressed as a percentage of the total cycle time or stride period. This approach facilitates comparing subjects with different stride lengths, stride periods, and walking speeds on the same scale. The temporal event of foot-off separates

Critical Events in Each Phase of Gait

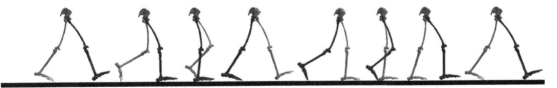

Periods	Stance Period					Swing Period		
Tasks	Weight Acceptance		Single Limb Support		Swing Limb Advancement			
Phases	Initial Contact (0%)	Loading Response (0-10%)	Mid Stance (10-30%)	Terminal Stance (30-50%)	Pre Swing (50-60%)	Initial Swing (60-75%)	Mid Swing (75%-87%)	Terminal Swing (87-100%)
Temporal Events	Initial Contact	B: Initial Contact E: Opposite Foot-off	B: Opposite Foot-Off E: Heel-off (body leads foot)	B: Heel-off (body leads foot) E: Opposite initial contact	B: Opposite initial contact E: Foot-off	B: Foot-off E: Feet adjacent (knee extends)	B: Feet adjacent (knee extends) E: Tibia Vertical	B: Tibia vertical E: Initial contact
Critical Events	• Heel first initial contact	• Hip stability • Controlled knee flexion for shock absorption • Controlled ankle PF	• Controlled tibial advancement	• Controlled ankle DF with heel rise • Trailing limb posture	• Passive knee flexion to 40° • Rapid ankle PF	• Max knee flexion (>60°)	• Max hip flexion (30°) • DF to neutral	• Knee extension to neutral

Fig. 1. Critical events of gait as described by Jacquelin Perry. (*Data from* Perry J. Gait analysis: normal and pathologic function. Thorofare (NJ): Slack; 1992.)

the gait cycle into stance and swing periods. In general, stance period occurs from 0% to 60% of the total gait cycle and swing period occurs from 60% to 100%, as seen in **Fig. 1**. In individuals with CP, the duration of the initial and final double limb support periods is often different and may vary on a step-to-step basis. The duration of each time period of the gait cycle, the step frequency (cadence), the distance traveled by each foot with each step (step length), and the average walking velocity are collectively known as temporal-spatial parameters, and if measured accurately, they can provide considerable insight into how the child and adult with CP have adapted to their physical limitations while still striving to walk independently.

Normal Gait Patterns

The need to alternate one's base of support and the existence of a repeatable gait cycle forces the segments of the lower limbs to adopt typical patterns of movement at each joint. Graphs of these patterns showing joint angles at different times in the gait cycle are collectively known as gait or motion kinematics. This term refers to the biomechanical description of the limb segments' motion as if they were a mechanical linkage aligned with the body's anatomic axes. **Fig. 2** shows normal kinematics for a group of typically developing 13-year-old children for the trunk, pelvis, hip, knee, and ankle in the sagittal, coronal, and transverse planes. For lower extremity kinematics, the pelvis marks the top of the kinematic chain and is referred to a fixed coordinate system, while each joint down the chain is (by convention) the angle of the distal segment relative to the more proximal segment. At the end of the chain, foot progression angle is again referred to the fixed coordinate system and is equivalent to the amount of toe-out or toe-in relative to the line of progression. The trunk can be referred either to the pelvis (see **Fig. 2**) or to the laboratory-fixed coordination system. Once oriented to the format of these kinematic graphs, common patterns of joint motion during normal gait are easily recognized. The largest and most easily observed angular displacements occur in the sagittal plane, whereas smaller, less obvious movements are seen in the coronal and transverse plane. The sagittal plane graph at the hip shows a single wave from flexion to extension during stance period and back to full flexion again in midswing, corresponding to the reciprocal motion at the hip necessary for limb advancement. At the knee joint, in the sagittal plane, the first wave is a smaller knee flexion peak occurring during weight acceptance to

account for shock absorption at the knee. The second wave is a larger knee flexion peak occurring in midswing to functionally shorten the leg during limb advancement to allow the foot to clear the walking surface. The sagittal plane ankle curve displays the "3 rockers" described by Perry.[14] The first (heel rocker) is associated with controlled plantar flexion (PF) to lower the foot to the floor during weight acceptance. The second (ankle rocker) is associated with controlled tibial advancement and increasing dorsiflexion during mid and terminal stance as the body center of mass advances over the stationary foot. The third (toe rocker) is associated with rapid ankle PF for propulsion during the second double support phase (preswing) and is the source of one of the two primary power generators during normal gait. The ankle sagittal plane curve shows the requirement for dorsiflexion to be near neutral for successful foot clearance during swing period. The remaining planes of motion described in the normal kinematic graphs also show characteristic movements that have been well documented elsewhere.[5,13,15,16] Having a quantitative description of the normal, 3-dimensional orientation of the pelvis and foot and the angular displacement of the joints of the lower limbs during a typical gait cycle provides a precise reference to compare with measurements obtained from the child and adult with CP. This comparison allows for detection of subtle deviations from normal, and provides a framework for a systematic analysis strategy that is the basis for describing many techniques and observations in the remainder of this article.

In addition to temporal-spatial parameters and 3-dimensional kinematics, there are also quantitative references for the following during normal walking of typically developing individuals: the forces of motion (kinetics),[17] the timing and activity level of the muscles (D-EMG),[18] foot plantar pressure, oxygen consumption, and more global measures of overall gait performance such as the gait deviation index.[19] The authors introduce some of these measures because they are needed in the remaining sections to clarify the gait patterns commonly seen in individuals with CP and how IGA can provide objective evidence of gait function to plan an appropriate course of treatment.

FUNCTIONAL GAIT PATTERNS IN CP

Every individual with CP presents a unique combination of impairment severity, compensatory movements, and overall ambulatory ability. Experienced clinicians who regularly treat CP attest that most patients display one or more distinct walking patterns. Describing and classifying the

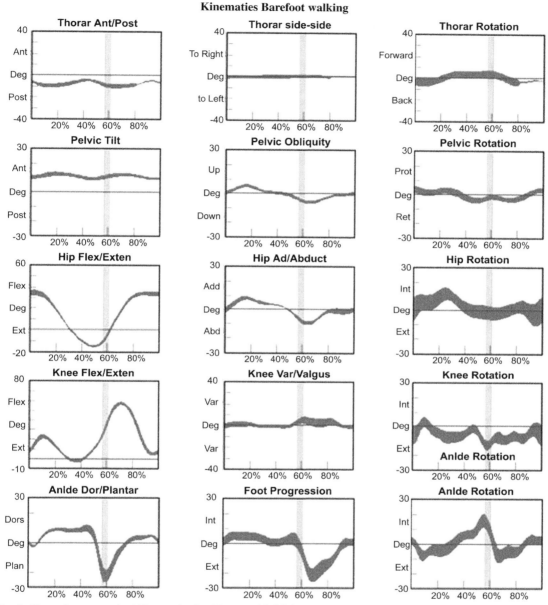

Fig. 2. Normal age-matched kinematics for 13-year-old children. Kinematics includes coronal, sagittal, and transverse planes. Vertical axis shows the degrees of motion. Horizontal axis shows the percentage gait cycle. The vertical gray bar represents toe-off. Graphs show 1 standard deviation.

gait patterns seen in this population provides a common starting point for further assessment and a connection to other patients with similar gait dysfunction at their current developmental stage. The ability of IGA to precisely measure gait function at the individual joint level lends itself to identifying these functional patterns, and gives much of the information needed to select appropriate treatments. The remaining sections describe the primary gait patterns seen in

individuals with CP and a description of how gait analysis can be used by the orthopedist to manage their treatment.

JUMP KNEE GAIT

Jump knee gait is defined primarily from sagittal plane kinematics, with dynamic changes easily identified using IGA. Jump knee gait is characterized by increased hip and knee flexion, with slight dorsiflexion at initial contact followed by rapid knee extension (KE) and ankle PF during loading response and midstance. These characteristic dynamic findings seen at the ankle begin with forefoot initial contact followed by stretch on the ankle plantar flexor gastrocnemius-soleus complex musculature. On achieving ultimate stretch, the plantar flexors contract rapidly as a stretch response to the commonly spastic triceps surae muscles. The rapid PF of the ankle causes heel rise and prevents the development of a second rocker at the ankle. The resultant proximal joint reactions include rapid knee and hip extension as the plantar flexors contract, giving the clinical appearance of the patient jumping up from one foot to the next. This combination of ankle PF and KE induced by foot position and/or calf spasticity is driven by a shift in the external ground reaction force (GRF) from behind the knee at initial contact and early loading response to a position anterior to the knee joint axis in midstance (**Fig. 3**). This shift in the GRF produces a force couple or external KE joint moment, commonly called the PF and KE couple, which prevents knee joint collapse without active quadriceps activity.

During swing period there is increased knee flexion in mid to terminal swing, leading to the increased flexion seen during initial contact and loading response. This occurrence is believed to be caused by near normal quadriceps and gastrocnemius-soleus strength with some spasticity of the hamstring muscles and hip flexors.[20] Other kinematic changes that are seen with jump knee gait include increased hip flexion throughout the gait cycle in the sagittal plane and increased hip adduction in the frontal plane due to hip adductor contracture and spasticity.

Jump knee gait can be identified in patients with spastic diplegia, hemiplegia, or quadriplegia. It is most often seen in patients with diplegia and hemiplegia and in patients with GMFCS levels II and III. Jump knee gait is not seen in GMFCS level V patients and is rare in patients classified as level IV. It is most commonly seen in younger patients learning to ambulate, and frequently changes as the patient gains weight and gait matures.

EQUINUS AND THE IMPORTANT DISTINCTION BETWEEN TRUE AND APPARENT

Equinus deformity is common in individuals with CP and is characterized by excessive PF of the calcaneus relative to the tibia. The simplest form includes normal bony alignment of the midfoot and forefoot, leading to an overall plantar flexed position of the entire foot. More complex deformities such as equinoplanovalgus and equinocavovarus occur when excessive PF of the hindfoot is accompanied by an abnormal midfoot and forefoot alignment.[21,22] In children with CP, equinus generally results from a dynamic imbalance between the muscles of the lower leg due to spasticity, poor motor control, and/or impaired balance function. This imbalance disrupts the normal ankle motion during walking, often producing a forefoot initial contact that persists throughout the stance period and may result in the emergence of a toe-toe gait.

Although the gastrocnemius and soleus are obvious contributors to this deformity, care should be taken before making either of these plantar flexors the target of surgical intervention. Specifically, special attention should be paid to the subtle difference between 2 distinct gait patterns that can produce the appearance of equinus and toe-toe gait but require completely different interventions. Rodda and Graham[23] have referred to these 2 patterns as true equinus and apparent equinus. In a true equinus gait pattern, calf spasticity or fixed ankle equinus contracture is dominant, resulting in excess ankle PF with hips and knees either extended or displaying relatively little deviation from normal over the gait cycle. With equinus, PF and KE coupling similar to that in the mid to terminal stance phases of jump knee gait is seen, and may result in knee recurvatum with increased hamstring length and gradual stretch of the posterior knee capsule. This pattern is most often seen in younger children with diplegia soon after they begin to walk, and rarely persists throughout childhood unless a fixed ankle contracture develops.

By contrast, apparent equinus is dominated by increased hip and knee flexion throughout the stance period with a relatively normal range of motion at the ankle. Observation reveals that the child is still walking on his or her toes and appears to be in equinus, but in fact the forefoot's initial contact is the result of the significant knee flexion that is present at the moment of weight acceptance.[24] As previously discussed, this pattern is characteristic of the early stance phase of jump knee gait but can also evolve from a previous true equinus that may have been present when the child was younger. As these children grow older and heavier, they lose much of their original equinus because of weakened plantar flexors, development of foot deformity, and/or the development of an ineffective PF and KE couple, and now have a pattern dominated by increased hip and knee flexion, especially at terminal swing and the initial double support period. For the child with apparent equinus, any procedure that further weakens the calf and allows the tibia to advance earlier and

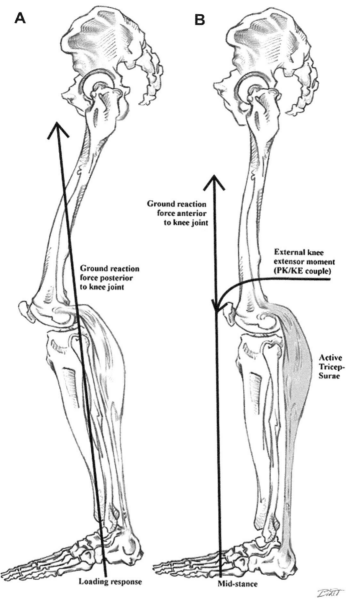

A

B

Ground reaction
force anterior
to knee joint

External knee
extensor moment
(PK/KE couple)

Ground reaction
force posterior
to knee joint

Active
Tricep-
Surae

Loading response   Mid-stance

Fig. 3. (*A, B*) PF and KE couple. During midstance, the forward movement of the tibia is constrained by calf musculature, shifting the GRF in front of the knee joint. This motion produces an external knee extension moment that improves knee stability and knee extension at terminal stance, and is referred to as the PF and KE couple. (*Courtesy of* Mike Binet, DPT, Aurora, CO, USA.)

more rapidly during loading response and midstance threatens to produce a crouch gait pattern that inevitably leads to significant functional impairment.[20] For this reason, Goldstein and Harper[25] have stated that failure to recognize apparent equinus is the most common error in observational gait analysis, and is of more than purely academic importance.

While it is sometimes challenging to distinguish between true equinus and apparent equinus using simple observation alone, using techniques from IGA make this task relatively straightforward. **Fig. 4**B and **Fig. 5**B show a still image of the right side midstance bilateral knee and ankle sagittal plane kinematics for 2 subjects with a toe-toe gait pattern. The subject in **Fig. 4**A has apparent

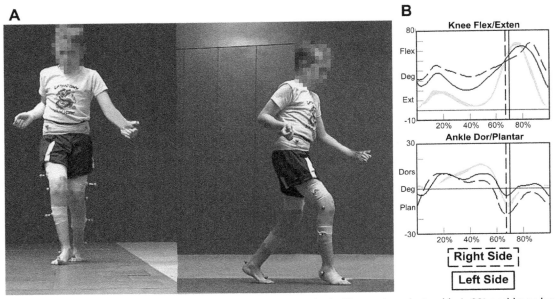

Fig. 4. Apparent equinus versus True equinus. Note: apparent looks like equinus, but ankle is 90° and knee has excessive flexion. (*A*) Initial contact shows ankle still in mild equinus. As weight is accepted, the child's ankle remains adequately dorsiflexed during the stance seen on the sagittal knee graph in *B*. Heel contact is late because of the excessive knee flexion. (*B*) Sagittal knee and ankle curves demonstrating apparent equinus. Note the excessive knee flexion throughout the stance phase causing delayed heel contact despite adequate ankle dorsiflexion.

equinus and the subject in **Fig. 5**A has true equinus. Comparing the ankle curves between the 2 subjects clearly shows that the subject with true equinus has excess PF starting in midstance and continuing for the rest of the gait cycle, whereas the subject with apparent equinus has a near normal ankle range of motion with an average value across the cycle of approximately zero. Notice that both ankle curves do not match the normal reference, because both subjects have a toe-toe gait

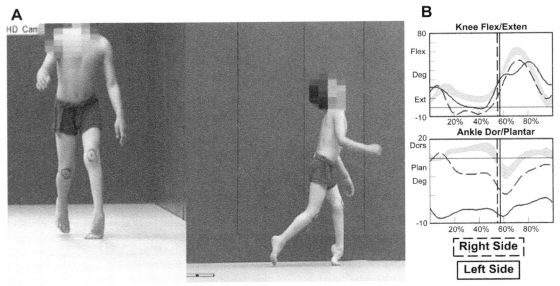

Fig. 5. (*A*) True equinus. (*B*) True equinus. Excessive equinus on sagittal ankle graphs with near normal knee flexion.

pattern. Comparing the knee kinematic curves, the subject with true equinus has a more normal knee range of motion with full KE at terminal stance, whereas the subject with apparent equinus has increased knee flexion throughout the stance period, most prominent on the right side. This comparison clearly illustrates the quantitative differences between these 2 similar gait patterns using just the sagittal plane kinematic curves, and demonstrates how IGA can facilitate identification of what Goldstein has described as the most common error in observational gait analysis.

Once these gait patterns are identified using kinematic evidence, a smaller group of possible interventions becomes apparent, and the most appropriate treatment can be determined after considering all the clinical findings. In younger children with CP displaying true equinus mediated predominately by calf spasticity, botulinum toxin can be very effective in improving stability in stance and allowing additional time for the children to develop a more mature gait pattern. Because the tibia is not advancing prematurely, a more stable base of support and improved rotational stability can be provided using a hinged ankle foot orthosis (AFO). If the patient's true equinus persists to the age of 7 to 8 years or if there is clear indication of contracture on physical examination, intramuscular lengthening of the gastrocnemius may be warranted. For the child with apparent equinus, botulinum toxin injections and/or intramuscular lengthenings of the plantar flexors should be avoided to prevent any further weakening. Instead, interventions should be directed at more proximal levels, where the hamstrings and iliopsoas may benefit from spasticity treatment or musculotendinous lengthening, and any bony malalignments can be corrected using appropriate osteotomies during an SEMLS procedure. To reduce the chance of further degradation of the gait pattern, solid or ground reaction AFOs can be used to force the GRF vector toward the front of the knee joint to restore the PF and KE couple and encourage improved KE following surgery. When comparing treatment options for individuals with CP with an equinus gait, it is essential to recognize that performing a tendo-Achilles lengthening in an individual with apparent equinus can directly result in a crouch gait postoperatively.

CROUCH GAIT

Crouch gait is defined as increased hip and knee flexion with excessive ankle dorsiflexion (calcaneus) seen throughout the gait pattern in the sagittal plane (**Fig. 6**).[26] Crouch gait can be caused by dynamic muscle contraction, spasticity, lever arm dysfunction, bony deformity, and/or fixed joint contractures.[27,28] Crouch gait is generally seen in weaker patients with diplegia; however, the same deformities can also be seen in patients with mild quadriplegia and hemiplegia.

Crouch gait pattern is rarely seen in early ages. If persistent fixed flexion deformities of the knee and hip develop over time as the patient continues to mature and ambulate, they will do so with a crouch deformity.[26] Crouch pattern is generally seen in GMFCS levels II, III, and IV. It is not usually seen in level I patients because the involved extremity is usually more affected in the distal aspects of the leg including the foot, ankle, and mild changes at the knee. Level IV patients often have a crouch gait but they are generally not independent ambulators, so correction may not significantly change gait or overall function. In crouch gait, the sagittal projection of the body's center of mass falls behind the already flexed knee joint, providing an increasingly larger deforming force as the child grows and increases his or her mass (**Fig. 7**). This growth places an even larger demand on the knee extensors, resulting in further knee flexion and an apparent worsening of all 3 aspects of the crouch gait deformity. The dynamic excessive soft tissue flexion deformities at the knee and hip eventually become fixed contractures. This anomaly also leads to development of patella alta and overlengthening of the extensor mechanism, which consequently decreases the KE force. The weakened quadriceps mechanism and progressive worsening of the knee flexion deformity cause issues at the patella related to the patella alta, including KE lag, anterior knee pain, and at times patellar avulsion fractures.[28]

The hip flexion contracture is caused by contracture and/or spasticity of the hip flexors, with most of the effect produced by the psoas and biarticular rectus femoris (RF) muscle combined with hip extensor weakness. The knee deformity is thought to be caused at first by hamstring contracture and/or spasticity, in conjunction with weakness and/or increased length of the knee extensors.[28] The excessive ankle dorsiflexion is caused by uncontrolled tibial advancement during second rocker, from a weak or overlengthened gastrocnemius-soleus complex. This development is usually iatrogenic, resulting from a previously overlengthened and weak gastrocnemius and/or soleus that was performed to address an equinus or jump knee gait pattern.[27,28]

STIFF KNEE GAIT

Stiff knee gait is one of the most common gait patterns that limit gait performance in children

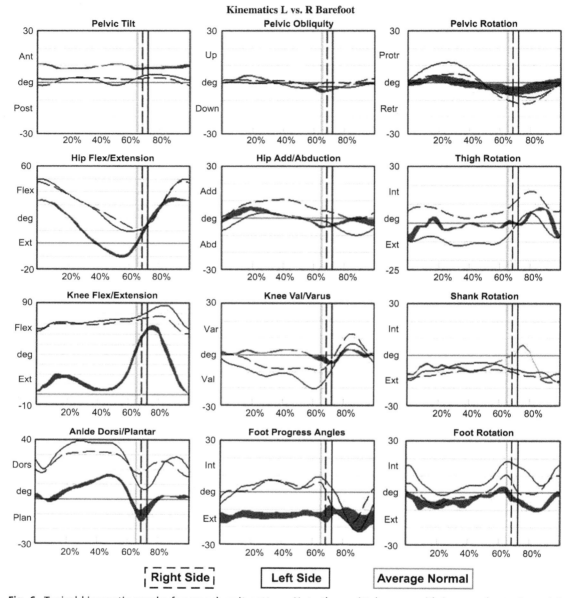

Fig. 6. Typical kinematic graphs for crouch gait pattern. Note the sagittal curves with increased anterior pelvic tilt, excessive hip flexion, constant knee flexion with no dynamic range, and excessive ankle dorsiflexion.

with CP, seen in 80% of the cases in a recent study.[29] Stiff knee gait was first described by Silf-verskiold in 1923, who found that spasticity of the RF muscle can obstruct initiation of knee flexion. Sutherland and Davids[2] later confirmed this description by gait analysis in 1983. In individuals with spastic CP and a stiff knee gait, the restriction of knee flexion due to the RF muscle occurs throughout the entire swing period,[8,30] seen as reduced dynamic range of knee flexion during swing period in the sagittal plane kinematic graph.

Patients with a stiff knee gait fail to achieve the critical gait events during swing period due to restriction of knee flexion. A stiff knee gait pattern is defined as a decrease in the magnitude of peak knee flexion of less than 45°, decreased dynamic range of knee flexion during swing period of the gait cycle, and delayed peak knee flexion.[2] The restriction of swing phase knee flexion makes foot clearance and the task of limb advancement difficult, and can result in tripping, falling, or the need to use energy-inefficient compensatory

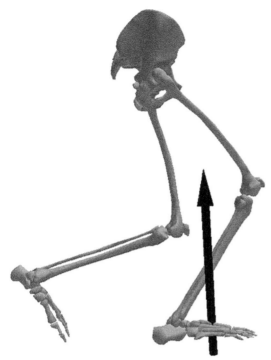

Fig. 7. Crouch gait pattern: ground reaction force, represented by black arrow, is posterior to knee joint axis encouraging knee flexion. Note excessive ankle dorsiflexion and hip flexion.

movements.[31] Compensatory mechanisms to improve clearance on the side displaying a stiff knee pattern include circumduction of the involved leg, external rotation of the foot, pelvic elevation, and a trunk lean away from the involved side. Compensations on the contralateral, less affected side include vaulting, seen as early heel rise in loading response and midstance to aid foot clearance on the affected side and decreased knee flexion at initial and midswing as required for foot clearance. These changes are clearly seen on sagittal plane kinematic graphs and are noticeably resolved when the stiff knee gait abnormality is corrected (**Fig. 8**A and B).

The cause of stiff knee gait is debated but is believed to be caused by a shortened biarticular RF muscle with inappropriate activity during swing period and low knee flexion velocities at toe-off.[1,8,31–40] Abnormal firing of the RF muscle during swing period can only be confirmed with IGA providing D-EMG during ambulation. Miller and colleagues[36] have described 3 distinct RF D-EMG patterns, 2 associated with stiff knee gait: (1) normal RF timing, which is not associated with a stiff knee gait, (2) abnormal predominant swing phase RF activity, and (3) constant

RF activity throughout the gait cycle (**Fig. 9**). Physical examination frequently yields a positive dynamic or fixed Duncan-Ely test; this is helpful to identify potential candidates for RF transfer but does not predict which patients with stiff knee gait will have positive outcomes postoperatively.[33,37]

ROTATIONAL ABNORMALITIES

Rotational abnormalities of the lower extremities such as femoral anteversion or tibial torsion are commonly seen in patients with CP.[29] Rotational deformities of the skeleton continue to progress until skeletal maturity. The severity of the deformities correlates with GMFCS levels; the more severe rotational deformities are seen in the higher GMFCS levels. IGA, coupled with the knowledge of the altered natural history of torsional deformities of the lower extremities in individuals with CP, can help the individual and clinician make the best decision-optimizing intervention that minimizes the impact of surgical treatment and maximizes the long-term benefits.[29,41] The treatment philosophy has evolved over the years toward more bony surgical intervention. Before any treatment decisions are made, it is absolutely mandatory that the treating clinician fully understand the deformities.

IGA accurately measures pelvic rotation and foot progression angles in 3 dimensions, essentially characterizing the beginning and end of the lower extremity kinematic chain. By convention, both are measured relative to a global laboratory coordinate system, with the limb segments in between measured relative to the more proximal segment. Static skeletal rotational deformities of the femur, tibia, and foot, combined with dynamic deformities caused by muscle imbalance, cause the rotational malalignments frequently present in individuals with CP. Dynamic position of the pelvis, femur, and tibia is difficult, if not impossible, to visualize with the naked eye but can be clearly and accurately measured with the use of IGA.[15]

Lever Arm Disease

Family members may express concern at the appearance of in- or out-toeing, but rotational malalignment of the legs is much more than just a cosmetic deformity. Malrotation of the lower extremities results in "lever arm disease," a term coined by Gage.[42] In simple terms, the presence of skeletal deformity results in decreased efficiency, requiring more work and effort for the muscles to provide the propulsion energy to move the body forward during gait. Malrotation of the pelvis, femur, tibia, or foot results in lever arm

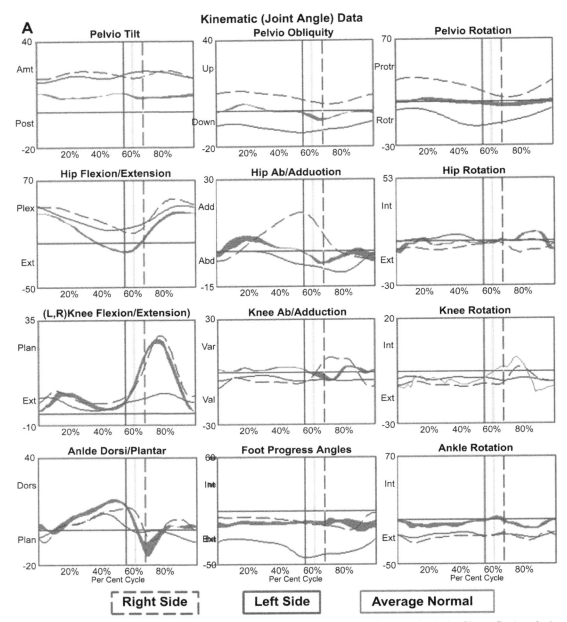

Fig. 8. (A) Typical kinematic graph of hemiplegic stiff knee gait. Most significant is the lack of knee flexion during swing, as seen on the sagittal knee graph. (B) Postoperative changes of improved stiff knee gait pattern. Note the improvement in all sagittal plane kinematics, and improved hip abduction and foot progression.

disease, with the severity directly proportional to the severity of the malrotation. When the foot is malrotated, the PF force is proportionately decreased (Fig. 10) due to the decreased moment arm of the foot. This weakness results in decreased push-off during midstance and a decreased PF and KE couple, increasing the risk of the patient acquiring a crouch gait pattern. The most severe malrotation is femoral anteversion coupled with

external tibial torsion, known as "malignant malalignment." This phenomenon not only affects the efficiency of gait but also is a frequent contributing factor to anterior knee pain in this population.[43]

Pelvic Rotation

The transverse orientation of the pelvis should on average be perpendicular to the line of

KINEMATIC DATA

B

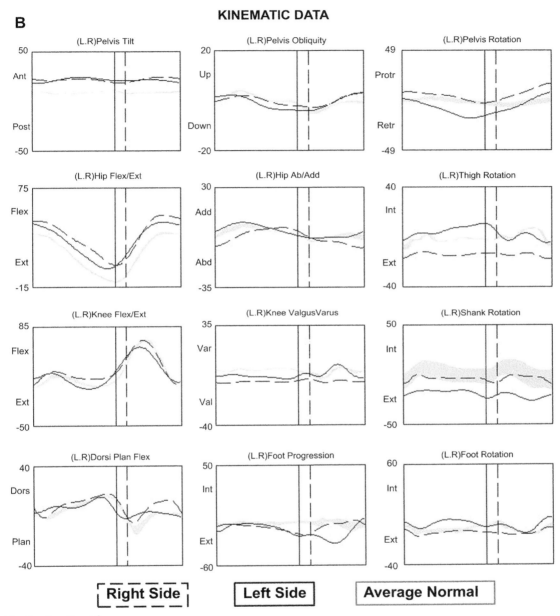

Fig. 8. (*continued*)

progression with the pubic symphysis anterior and the sacrum posterior. Any deviation of this alignment is referred to as pelvic rotation. Pelvic rotation is common in individuals with CP, especially if the tone is asymmetric from side to side, hemiplegia being a classic example. Typically, the stronger side is protracted (anterior) and the weaker side retracted (posterior). Although many start with the feet when analyzing malrotation, pelvic rotation is key to the rotational alignment of the lower extremities. The precise quantification of pelvic rotation is important in understanding the rotational abnormalities, and is difficult to accurately measure without IGA. When the pelvis is rotated to the line of progression (**Fig. 11**), both lower extremities are rotated in the same direction. The foot on the protracted side demonstrates increased internal rotation and the foot of the retracted side is more externally rotated. Abnormal pelvic rotation can be improved but

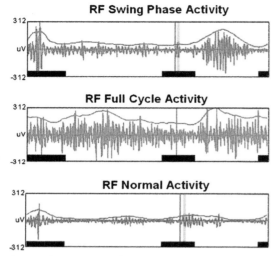

RF Swing Phase Activity

RF Full Cycle Activity

RF Normal Activity

Fig. 9. Three types of RF electromyography (EMG) patterns described by Miller. (*Top*) Swing phase activity, inappropriate burst of rectus femoris activity during swing phase. (*Middle*) full cycle activity, rectus femoris constantly firing during the entire gait cycle. (*Bottom*) normal RF activity. The black bars under the EMG indicate timing when the normal RF fires during the gait cycle. (*Data from* Miller F, Cardoso Dias R, Lipton GE, et al. The effect of rectus EMG patterns on the outcome of rectus femoris transfers. J Pediatr Orthop 1997;17(5):603–7.)

not completely corrected by correcting lower extremity malalignments, with both a femoral derotational osteotomy and soft tissue balancing procedures.[44,45]

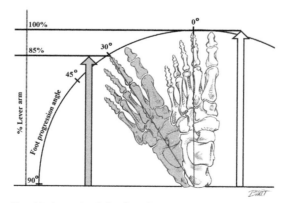

Fig. 10. Length of the foot lever arm decreases as the foot progression angle (FPA) increases. Light foot on right: FPA 0° and lever arm equals 100%. Dark foot on left: FPA 30° and lever arm decreases to about 85%, decreasing pushoff force. Figure is not quite accurate, because the actual lever arm is from the center of the ankle joint to the center of the second metatarsal head. (*Courtesy of* Mike Binet, DPT, Aurora, CO, USA.)

Femoral Rotation

Femoral rotation can be either internally or externally rotated. It is defined by the angle of the femoral head and neck in relation to the femoral shaft in the coronal plane. The gold standard for measurement is with a computed tomography scan that compares femoral neck alignment with the femoral condyles. If the distal femur is internally rotated relative to the proximal femur, this is femoral anteversion. If the distal segment is externally rotated, this is femoral retroversion. The natural history of the developing femur begins with natural physiologic anteversion of greater than 40° at birth, which gradually decreases to the normal 15° adult alignment by age 16 years.[46] This natural decrease is diminished and reversed in children with CP. At skeletal maturity, 64% of individuals with CP have persistent in-toeing. Wren and colleagues[29] have identified this as the fourth most common gait deformity. Femoral anteversion is the most common cause for in-toeing in individuals with CP, and dynamic femoral position is most accurately measured with IGA. Muscle activity, such as spastic hip rotators or medial hamstring spasticity, can also cause abnormal dynamic rotation at the hip, affecting femoral rotational alignment.[47] Correction of femoral anteversion should be done close to skeletal maturity to avoid recurrent deformity. If done earlier, combined with other procedures in an SEMLS event, the family should be counseled on the possible recurrence.

Tibial Torsion

Both excessive internal and external rotations of the tibia are common in individuals with CP. The natural history for tibial rotation is also altered. The tibia continues to remodel with increased external rotation until skeletal maturity occurs in children with spastic CP.[29] The abnormal internal forces of muscle imbalance, coupled with the external forces of gravity and friction from foot drag secondary to inadequate clearance, produce further abnormal forces affecting the tibial and foot alignment, resulting in excessive internal or external rotation of the tibia and foot. Typically, the tibia and foot deformities occur in the same direction, such as external tibial torsion coupled with planovalgus foot deformity or internal tibial torsion coupled with an equinovarus foot. Excessive tibial rotation also decreases the ankle PF moment arm and knee and hip extension power, thus increasing the risk for a crouched gait pattern.[48] Treatment and timing are similar to the femur. The authors' preference is for rotation

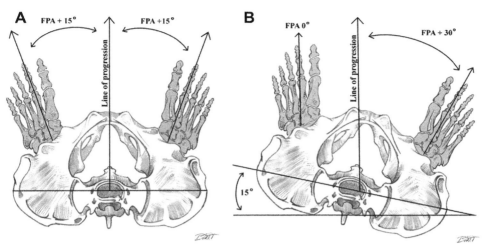

Fig. 11. Pelvic rotation affects foot progression angle (FPA). (*A*) Pelvis straight, symmetric bilateral FPA of 15°; (*B*) same pelvis, foot relationship with 15° of pelvic rotation alter the FPA of both feet. (*Courtesy of* Mike Binet, DPT, Aurora, CO, USA.)

osteotomy of the distal metaphysis using a locking plate.

Foot Rotation

Foot rotational alignment is typically measured relative to global laboratory coordinates, similarly to how in-toeing or out-toeing is seen relative to the line of progression in a clinical evaluation. Although the foot progression angle and line of progression can be estimated visually in typical walking, the more erratic gait often seen in CP leads to wide variation of foot rotation over the gait cycle, making it difficult to arrive at a single estimate of foot position using visual means alone. IGA provides great assistance here, because the accurate measurement can be averaged over the gait cycle to provide a better estimate of overall foot progression. Foot models continue to improve, evolving from a single rigid body to multiple segmented models. Foot alignment is measured by both kinematics and foot plantar pressure measurement (pedobarograph). Kinematic measurement provides a direct measurement of foot progression angle, and the pedobarograph arrives at roughly the same measure by averaging the distribution of pressures to arrive at an estimate of foot orientation relative to the direction of progression. Foot alignment is complex, because it involves bone and joint deformities within the foot in addition to the external rotational muscle forces from the anterior and posterior tibialis muscles and the long and short peroneal muscles.

Ounpuu and colleagues[17] and Gage[49] have described the kinetic effects of rotational

abnormalities and how these can clinically affect gait. Decreased moment arms resulting in decreased power, secondary to lever arm disease, as well as decreased muscle power can be measured with IGA kinetic measurements. Comparing the physical examination findings with dynamic gait measurements also reveals the effects of any muscle imbalance. For example, spasticity of the hip internal rotators results in more internal rotation of the thigh during gait than expected by the femoral anteversion measured on physical examination.

Once the rotational abnormalities are identified and objectively measured, a decision can be made as to whether surgical rotation will improve gait function. GMFCS levels should always be considered to determine whether the proposed treatments will actually affect functional level, implying the lowest functional levels. GMFCS levels IV to V may not be significantly improved by rotational realignment. Femoral rotation is easily corrected with a proximal or distal rotational osteotomy of the femur, which can be combined with a proximal varus femoral rotational osteotomy if there is concomitant neuromuscular hip dysplasia. Differentiating between posterior tibialis and anterior tibialis overpull causing forefoot internal rotation, adductus, and supination are aided by IGA using the respective D-EMGs to answer the question of which individual muscle or both muscles are contributing to the deformity.

ROLE OF IGA

The understanding of normal and pathologic gait has matured over the past 40 years, greatly enhanced by the development of IGA. Understanding the pathologic gait in an individual with CP is challenging. Several recognizable patterns have been defined, and the recognition of these patterns can greatly assist the clinician in the decision process for intervention; IGA can greatly assist the clinician in recognizing these patterns. Recognizing these primary gait deformities and how they affect overall function assists the clinician in making the best possible decision for improved outcomes.

With the advancement of motion capture and movement analysis technology, the diagnostic test of IGA has become the standard of care in most major centers around the world to objectively measure and diagnose the primary gait abnormalities in CP, assisting clinicians to determine an overall treatment protocol.[7,50-53] IGA has been used in direct clinical care for more than 40 years, providing accurate measurements of the diverse gait patterns observed. IGA is a diagnostic test that accurately measures the alterations in normal gait while a patient is walking (see **Fig. 1**). There is no alternative way of measuring and accurately obtaining the information gained from IGA, which is crucial for the understanding of complex gait abnormalities. Measurements such as the actual position of the pelvis, hip, femur, knee, tibia, ankle, and foot at any given moment, correlated with the real-time firing of the muscles, enhance our understanding of pathologic gait. Interpretation of the data allows the clinician to identify the primary gait abnormalities and differentiate them from the compensatory deformities, whether the gait abnormalities are simple or very complex. IGA provides objective information to help determine the appropriate treatment interventions to maximize the gait performance of the patient.

Most individuals with CP exhibit a combination or mixture of these patterns, which makes IGA even more important to accurately measure the gait while understanding the parameters of the individual patterns of gait in each person so as to individualize each patient's treatment.

SUMMARY

The advancement of IGA provides 2 obvious benefits. First, it enhances our ability to understand the pathologic condition beyond what we can observe and second, it provides dynamic information while the patient is ambulating. IGA has become the standard of care for diagnosing pathologic gait in CP. All gait deviations from normal can be accurately, objectively, and reproducibly determined with IGA. It is important to quantify the deformities causing the pathologic gait. IGA accomplishes this

by measuring and comparing the patient's gait to normal age-matched controls. Interpretation of the objective quantitative data allows the clinician to identify the primary gait abnormalities and differentiate them from the compensatory deformities, whether the gait abnormalities are simple or very complex. Diagnostic IGA provides the objective information to assist the orthopedic surgeon in determining the appropriate treatment interventions to maximize the gait performance of the individual with CP.

ACKNOWLEDGMENTS

The authors would like to acknowledge the talents and efforts of Michael Binet, PT, for his contribution of illustrations.

REFERENCES

1. Reinbolt JA, Fox MD, Arnold AS, et al. Importance of preswing rectus femoris activity in stiff-knee gait. J Biomech 2008;41(11):2362–9.
2. Sutherland DH, Davids JR. Common gait abnormalities of the knee in cerebral palsy. Clin Orthop Relat Res 1993;288:139–47.
3. Saraph V, Zwick EB, Zwick G, et al. Multilevel surgery in spastic diplegia: evaluation by physical examination and gait analysis in 25 children. J Pediatr Orthop 2002;22(2):150–7.
4. Graham HK, Harvey A. Assessment of mobility after multi-level surgery for cerebral palsy. J Bone Joint Surg Br 2007;89(8):993–4.
5. Gage JR. The identification and treatment of gait problems in cerebral palsy. London: Mac Keith Press: Distributed by Wiley-Blackwell; 2009.
6. Davids JR, Foti T, Dabelstein J, et al. Voluntary (normal) versus obligatory (cerebral palsy) toe-walking in children: a kinematic, kinetic, and electromyographic analysis. J Pediatr Orthop 1999;19(4): 461–9.
7. Gage JR, Novacheck TF. An update on the treatment of gait problems in cerebral palsy. J Pediatr Orthop B 2001;10(4):265–74.
8. Perry J. Distal rectus femoris transfer. Dev Med Child Neurol 1987;29(2):153–8.
9. Palisano R, Rosenbaum P, Walter S, et al. Development and reliability of a system to classify gross motor function in children with cerebral palsy. Dev Med Child Neurol 1997;39(4):214–23.
10. Kirtley C, Whittle MW, Jefferson RJ. Influence of walking speed on gait parameters. J Biomed Eng 1985;7(4):282–8.
11. Whittle MW, Jefferson RJ. Functional biomechanical assessment of the Oxford Meniscal Knee. J Arthroplasty 1989;4(3):231–43.

12. Alexander MA, Matthews DJ. Pediatric rehabilitation: principles and practice. New York: Demos Medical; 2010.
13. Carollo JJ, Matthews D. Strategies for clinical motion analysis based on functional decomposition of the gait cycle. Phys Med Rehabil Clin N Am 2002;13(4): 949–77.
14. Perry J. Kinesiology of lower extremity bracing. Clin Orthop Relat Res 1974;102:18–31.
15. Perry J. Gait analysis: normal and pathological function. Thorofare (NJ): SLACK; 1992.
16. Whittle MW. Gait analysis: an introduction. Oxford (UK): Butterworth-Heinemann; 2007.
17. Ounpuu S, Gage JR, Davis RB. Three-dimensional lower extremity joint kinetics in normal pediatric gait. J Pediatr Orthop 1991;11(3):341–9.
18. Perry J, Bontrager EL, Bogey RA, et al. The Rancho EMG analyzer: a computerized system for gait analysis. J Biomed Eng 1993;15(6):487–96.
19. Schwartz MH, Rozumalski A. The Gait Deviation Index: a new comprehensive index of gait pathology. Gait Posture 2008;28(3):351–7.
20. Sutherland DH, Cooper L. The pathomechanics of progressive crouch gait in spastic diplegia. Orthop Clin North Am 1978;9(1):143–54.
21. Davids JR, Foti T, Dabelstein J, et al. Objective assessment of dyskinesia in children with cerebral palsy. J Pediatr Orthop 1999;19(2):211–4.
22. Davids JR, Rowan F, Davis RB. Indications for orthoses to improve gait in children with cerebral palsy. J Am Acad Orthop Surg 2007;15(3): 178–88.
23. Rodda J, Graham HK. Classification of gait patterns in spastic hemiplegia and spastic diplegia: a basis for a management algorithm. Eur J Neurol 2001;8 (Suppl 5):98–108.
24. Epps CH, Bowen JR. Complications in pediatric orthopaedic surgery. Philadelphia: Lippincott; 1995.
25. Goldstein M, Harper DC. Management of cerebral palsy: equinus gait. Dev Med Child Neurol 2001;43(8): 563–9.
26. Rodda JM, Graham HK, Nattrass GR, et al. Correction of severe crouch gait in patients with spastic diplegia with use of multilevel orthopaedic surgery. J Bone Joint Surg Am 2006;88(12):2653–64.
27. Gage WH, Winter DA, Frank JS, et al. Kinematic and kinetic validity of the inverted pendulum model in quiet standing. Gait Posture 2004;19 (2):124–32.
28. Novacheck TF, Gage JR. Orthopedic management of spasticity in cerebral palsy. Childs Nerv Syst 2007;23(9):1015–31.
29. Wren TA, Rethlefsen S, Kay RM. Prevalence of specific gait abnormalities in children with cerebral palsy: influence of cerebral palsy subtype, age, and previous surgery. J Pediatr Orthop 2005;25(1): 79–83.
30. Waters RL, Garland DE, Perry J, et al. Stiff-legged gait in hemiplegia: surgical correction. J Bone Joint Surg Am 1979;61(6A):927–33.
31. Goldberg SR, Ounpuu S, Delp SL. The importance of swing-phase initial conditions in stiff-knee gait. J Biomech 2003;36(8):1111–6.
32. Granata KP, Abel MF, Damiano DL. Joint angular velocity in spastic gait and the influence of muscle-tendon lengthening. J Bone Joint Surg Am 2000;82(2):174–86.
33. Muthusamy K, Seidl AJ, Friesen RM, et al. Rectus femoris transfer in children with cerebral palsy: evaluation of transfer site and preoperative indicators. J Pediatr Orthop 2008;28(6):674–8.
34. Sutherland DH, Santi M, Abel MF. Treatment of stiff-knee gait in cerebral palsy: a comparison by gait analysis of distal rectus femoris transfer versus proximal rectus release. J Pediatr Orthop 1990;10(4):433–41.
35. Asakawa DS, Blemker SS, Gold GE, et al. Dynamic magnetic resonance imaging of muscle function after surgery. Skeletal Radiol 2006;35(12):885–6.
36. Miller F, Cardoso Dias R, Lipton GE, et al. The effect of rectus EMG patterns on the outcome of rectus femoris transfers. J Pediatr Orthop 1997; 17(5):603–7.
37. Chambers H, Lauer A, Kaufman K, et al. Prediction of outcome after rectus femoris surgery in cerebral palsy: the role of cocontraction of the rectus femoris and vastus lateralis. J Pediatr Orthop 1998;18(6):703–11.
38. Ounpuu S, Muik E, Davis RB 3rd, et al. Rectus femoris surgery in children with cerebral palsy. Part I: the effect of rectus femoris transfer location on knee motion. J Pediatr Orthop 1993;13(3):325–30.
39. Ounpuu S, Muik E, Davis RB 3rd, et al. Rectus femoris surgery in children with cerebral palsy. Part II: a comparison between the effect of transfer and release of the distal rectus femoris on knee motion. J Pediatr Orthop 1993;13(3):331–5.
40. Fox MD, Reinbolt JA, Ounpuu S, et al. Mechanisms of improved knee flexion after rectus femoris transfer surgery. J Biomech 2009;42(5):614–9.
41. Wren TA, Woolf K, Kay RM. How closely do surgeons follow gait analysis recommendations and why? J Pediatr Orthop B 2005;14(3):202–5.
42. Gage JR. Gait analysis. An essential tool in the treatment of cerebral palsy. Clin Orthop Relat Res 1993; 288:126–34.
43. Senaran H, Holden C, Dabney KW, et al. Anterior knee pain in children with cerebral palsy. J Pediatr Orthop 2007;27(1):12–6.
44. Kay RM, Rethlefsen S, Reed M, et al. Changes in pelvic rotation after soft tissue and bony surgery in ambulatory children with cerebral palsy. J Pediatr Orthop 2004;24(3):278–82.
45. Chung CY, Lee SH, Choi IH, et al. Residual pelvic rotation after single-event multilevel surgery in

spastic hemiplegia. J Bone Joint Surg Br 2008;90 (9):1234–8.

46. Shands AR Jr, Steele MK. Torsion of the femur; a follow-up report on the use of the Dunlap method for its determination. J Bone Joint Surg Am 1958;40(4):803–16.

47. Lovejoy SA, Tylkowski C, Oeffinger D, et al. The effects of hamstring lengthening on hip rotation. J Pediatr Orthop 2007;27(2):142–6.

48. Hicks J, Arnold A, Anderson F, et al. The effect of excessive tibial torsion on the capacity of muscles to extend the hip and knee during single-limb stance. Gait Posture 2007;26(4):546–52.

49. Gage JR. The clinical use of kinetics for evaluation of pathologic gait in cerebral palsy. Instr Course Lect 1995;44:507–15.

50. Cook RE, Schneider I, Hazlewood ME, et al. Gait analysis alters decision-making in cerebral palsy. J Pediatr Orthop 2003;23(3):292–5.

51. Fabry G, Liu XC, Molenaers G. Gait pattern in patients with spastic diplegic cerebral palsy who underwent staged operations. J Pediatr Orthop B 1999;8(1):33–8.

52. DeLuca PA, Davis RB 3rd, Ounpuu S, et al. Alterations in surgical decision making in patients with cerebral palsy based on three-dimensional gait analysis. J Pediatr Orthop 1997;17(5):608–14.

53. Chang FM, Seidl AJ, Muthusamy K, et al. Effectiveness of instrumented gait analysis in children with cerebral palsy—comparison of outcomes. J Pediatr Orthop 2006;26(5):612–6.

Assessment and Treatment of Movement Disorders in Children with Cerebral Palsy

Laura L. Deon, MD[a], Deborah Gaebler-Spira, MD[a,b],*

KEYWORDS

- Spasticity • Dystonia • Pediatric • Cerebral palsy
- Treatment • Management

Cerebral palsy is the most common motor disability in childhood. The management of children with cerebral palsy ideally involves a team of professionals, including physical therapists, occupational therapists, physiatrists, developmental pediatricians, and an orthopedic surgeon with clearly identified areas of expertise. The pediatric orthopedic surgeon manages contractures and alignment. Cerebral palsy was first described in 1843 by an orthopedic surgeon named William John Little.[1] Since then, pediatric orthopedic surgeons have contributed to prognosis, management, and development of new treatments that promote improved function in the population with cerebral palsy.

Orthopedic care depends on the appreciation and identification of muscle tone abnormalities on the overlay of the growth and development of the child. Abnormal muscle tone is a diagnostic feature of cerebral palsy. Abnormal tone includes hypotonia and hypertonia. Frequently, both exist in the child. Hypertonia is the most frequent tone abnormality appreciated in the extremities of children with cerebral palsy.

Hypertonia is caused by the upper motor neuron syndrome. The cascade of problems or impairments associated with the upper motor neuron syndrome is divided into negative and positive symptoms (**Fig. 1**). Hypertonia is one of the positive symptoms and plays an integral role in the formation of deformities in growing children with cerebral palsy (**Fig. 2**). Although it is not known to what extent hypertonia plays a role in the process of deformity or functional limitations, it is a major factor in reducing range of motion and inhibiting growth of muscle, which disadvantages alignment. Hypertonia and, in particular, spasticity act as a brake on the musculoskeletal system, which increases the work of walking, which in turn inhibits function.[2]

This article reviews hypertonia and provides information on discriminating between spasticity, dystonia, and rigidity. Medication and neurosurgical options for management of hypertonia are presented and compared. The orthopedic surgeon cares for the whole child and should become familiar with commonly used tone management strategies.

DISCRIMINATING BETWEEN HYPERTONIC SYNDROMES

Hypertonia is defined as abnormally increased resistance to externally imposed movement about

[a] Pediatric Physical Medicine and Rehabilitation, Rehabilitation Institute of Chicago at Northwestern University, 345 East Superior Street, Chicago, IL 60611, USA
[b] Cerebral Palsy Program, Rehabilitation Institute of Chicago at Northwestern University, 345 East Superior Street, Chicago, IL 60611, USA
* Corresponding author. Pediatric Physical Medicine and Rehabilitation, Rehabilitation Institute of Chicago at Northwestern University, 345 East Superior Street, Chicago, IL 60611.
E-mail address: dgaebler@ric.org

Orthop Clin N Am 41 (2010) 507–517
doi:10.1016/j.ocl.2010.06.001
0030-5898/10/$ – see front matter © 2010 Elsevier Inc. All rights reserved.

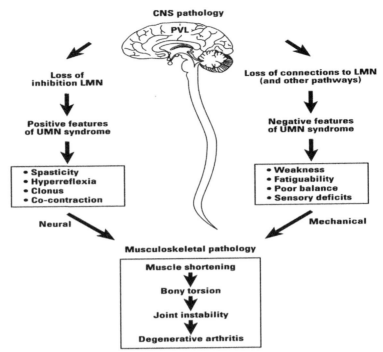

Fig. 1. The neuromusculoskeletal pathology in cerebral palsy. In motor terms, cerebral palsy results in an upper motor neuron lesion, which in this diagram is considered to have a series of positive and negative features that interact to produce the familiar musculoskeletal pathologic condition. (*Courtesy of* H. Kerr Graham, MD, The Royal Children's Hospital, Melbourne, Australia.

a joint perceived by the examiner. Hypertonia may be caused by spasticity, dystonia, and rigidity, alone or in combination.[3] It is important to be able to distinguish between these syndromes because each one is its own entity and may require different types of treatments. A US National Institutes of Health–sponsored Taskforce on Childhood Motor Disorders convened to propose a set of consensus

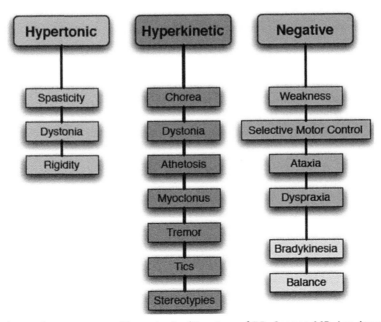

Fig. 2. Positive and negative symptoms of hypertonia. (*Courtesy of* T.D. Sanger, MD, Los Angeles, CA.)

definitions in 2003 to facilitate communication of clinical findings between colleagues, to aid in the selection of patients for inclusion in research trials, to assist with prediction of clinical outcomes, and to aid in clinical decision making for appropriate treatments.[4]

Definition of Spasticity

Spasticity is the most common tone abnormality in children with cerebral palsy. However, not all tight or hypertonic muscles are spastic. The consensus-based definition formulated by the taskforce is as follows[4]: "Spasticity is a velocity-dependent resistance of a muscle to stretch. It is defined as having one or both of the following signs: (1) resistance to externally imposed movement increases with increasing speed of stretch and varies with the direction of joint movement, and/or (2) resistance to externally imposed movement rises rapidly above a threshold speed or joint angle." Spasticity can vary depending on several factors such as the patient's level of activity, level of alertness, emotional state, and discomfort. On examination, upper motor neuron signs such as hyperreflexia, clonus, and Babinski response are commonly present. Spasticity is a result of injury to the central nervous system that produces an upper motor neuron lesion. Secondary consequences of the injury occur all the way to the muscle fiber. Fibers may have increased variability in size, and in some cases there is an increase in the number of type I muscle fibers and a deficiency of type IIb muscle fibers.[5] Spasticity is thought to be the most common tone abnormality in children with cerebral palsy, and it is certainly seen as a common consequence of injury to the white matter of the brain, such as periventricular leukomalacia caused by the stretching of the pyramidal tracts from intraventricular hemorrhage.[6] However, many children have additional dynamic hypertonia, which is attributable to other disorders such as the crossed extensor reflex, causing scissoring that contributes to decreased function. Children with damage only to the corticospinal tracts are more likely to have pure spasticity. Typically these children have periventricular leukomalacia as premature infants and have a typical spastic diplegic pattern of spasticity where legs are more involved than arms, fair to good trunk control, and learning disabilites more than intellectual disabilities.

Definition of Dystonia

Careful examination of children with cerebral palsy discloses mixed tone abnormalities. As spasticity treatments have evolved, such as the selective posterior rhizotomy, it is apparent that dystonia underlies some of the more complicated clinical pictures and impacts prognosis. A child with evidence of increased tone on examination that is not improving with standard anti-spasticity treatments may also be suffering from an underlying dystonia. The consensus-based definition formulated by the Taskforce on Childhood Motor Disorders is as follows[4]: "Dystonia in childhood is a movement disorder in which involuntary sustained or intermittent muscle contractions cause twisting and repetitive movements, abnormal postures, or both." Dystonia can cause hypertonia if there is dystonic muscle contraction opposing passive movement of the limb being tested by the examiner,[4] which is referred to as dystonic hypertonia. Dystonia can also be classified in relation to the region of the body that is affected. Focal dystonias affect a single body part, segmental dystonias affect contiguous body parts, and multifocal dystonias affect 2 or more noncontiguous body parts.[3,7] On examination, dystonia can be observed while the patient is at rest or is sometimes triggered by a voluntary task.[8] The physiology behind dystonia involves cocontraction of antagonist muscles, overflow of electromyographic activity onto uninvolved muscles during voluntary movement, and involuntary activation of muscles during passive shortening,[9] which may be the result of damage to deeper structures of the brain, including the basal ganglia, which acts as a feedback loop for cortical activity.[10] Children with damage to the basal ganglia or its connecting pathways may present with dystonia or mixed tone abnormalities such as spasticity with an underlying dystonia. Typically these children have more complex etiologies such as hypoxic ischemic encephalopathy, equal involvement of upper and lower extremities, fair to poor trunk control, and are more likely to have intellectual disability. On careful examination, many children with cerebral palsy will have dystonia.

Definition of Rigidity

Rigidity is defined as a condition in which any joint is unable to be moved. However, the consensus definition describes rigidity as cases in which all of the following are true[3]: "(1) the resistance to externally imposed joint movement is present at very low speeds of movement, does not depend on imposed speed, and does not exhibit a speed or angle threshold; (2) simultaneous co-contraction of agonists and antagonists may occur, and this is reflected in an immediate resistance to a reversal of direction of movement about a joint; (3) the limb does not tend to return toward a particular fixed posture or extreme joint angle; and (4) voluntary activity in distant muscle groups does not lead to involuntary movements about the rigid joints, although rigidity may worsen."

OTHER HYPERKINETIC MOVEMENT DISORDERS

Some other hyperkinetic movement disorders include chorea, myoclonus, restless legs syndrome, tics, and tremors. These hyperkinetic disorders are usually involuntary, but they occasionally occur voluntarily as part of a compulsion. Chorea refers to involuntary, irregular, purposeless, nonrhythmic, abrupt, rapid, unsustained movements that seem to flow from one body part to another. Myoclonus is a sudden, brief, shock-like jerk caused by a muscle contraction or relaxation. Restless legs syndrome refers to the phenomenon that describes an unpleasant crawling sensation in the legs while at rest. Tics are abnormal movements (motor tics) or sounds (phonic tics). Tremor is an oscillatory, usually rhythmic and regular, movement affecting one or more body parts.[11]

THE IMPORTANCE OF DISTINGUISHING BETWEEN HYPERTONIA AND OTHER HYPERKINETIC DISORDERS

It is important to distinguish between hypertonia and hyperkinetic movement disorders because they are treated differently. In addition, results of surgical treatment vary depending on the type of tone abnormality. Anticipating or predicting outcomes improves with accurate identification of the tone abnormality. Tone management is essential before and after orthopedic surgery to ensure best results. Postoperative comfort and care, with a focus on pain control and tone management, are essential for a positive functional outcome.

HOW SPASTICITY AND DYSTONIA ARE MEASURED

Clinical grading scales for either spasticity or muscle tone have primarily been used to assess spasticity. Scales used for the clinical assessment of spasticity are categorized according to their assessment technique and quantification.[12]

The Ashworth Scale is named after the person who first described the principle of muscle tone assessment by scoring on a 5-point scale the resistance encountered in a specific muscle group by passively moving a limb at one specified velocity through its range of motion. This scale is known as the original Ashworth Scale.[12,13] The Ashworth Scale has 3 modifications, all sharing the same principle. The first modification was made by the addition of an intermediate score, making it a 6-point scale: the Modified Ashworth Scale—Bohannon.[12,14] A second modification combined the Ashworth Scale and the Modified Ashworth Scale—Bohannon and added grading for the severity of spasticity: the Modified Ashworth Scale—Peacock.[12,15] A third modification, the New York University Tone Scale, combined the Ashworth Scale with range of motion at a fast velocity stretch.[12]

The Tardieu Scale is derived from the principle of spasticity assessment by joint angle measurement at different velocities of muscle stretch. When hypertonia is measured using the Tardieu Scale, spasticity is clinically assessed by passive movement of the joints at 3 specified velocities. The intensity and duration of the muscle reaction to the stretch are rated on a 5-point scale with the joint angle at which this muscle reaction is first felt.[12,16] Later, the scale was simplified to the Modified Tardieu Scale, which defines the moment of "catch," seen in the range of motion of a particular joint angle at a fast passive stretch.[17]

There are other ways to clinically measure spasticity, but the Modified Ashworth Scale and the Tardieu Scale are the 2 most popular methods.

The Barry-Albright Dystonia Scale allows one to quantify dystonia. This scale is a 5-point, criterion-based, ordinal scale designed to assess dystonia in 8 regions of the body: eyes, mouth, neck, trunk, and the 4 extremities. Dystonia is graded as none (score 0), slight (1), mild (2), moderate (3), or severe (4). Individual scores for each region are added for a total score. Each region has specific descriptors for scoring, but the following general rules apply: slight dystonia is present less than 10% of the time, mild dystonia does not interfere with function or care, moderate dystonia is characterized as interfering with a functional activity, and severe dystonia prevents the performance of the activity.[18] It is important to use a scale that is consistent and complementary to the orthopedic examination. Dynamic problems seen on the functional examination, such as scissoring, may be combined problems of spasticity and an underlying movement disorder.

TREATMENTS THAT TARGET SPASTICITY

There are many ways to treat spasticity. Carefully defining the goal of treatment is as important as the treatment itself. The goals should be explored and discussed in the context of the child's function with the family and the team. Management of spasticity or hypertonia is divided into global or whole body involvement and focal problems, which may affect 1 joint level of 1 extremity.

Choosing a medication over a more complicated surgical procedure should maximize the function or improve the child's general care and comfort and minimize the side effects or complications. The treatment should also suit the patient, the family, and the available community resources and capabilities.

Physical Treatment Methods

Hypertonia and decreased selective motor control contribute to decreased frequency and variety of voluntary movements.[19] With the decreased frequency and variety of movements, patients are at risk for contractures, which can be treated and often prevented with proper care. Passive stretching is commonly used to treat increased tone. There is some limited evidence that passive stretching can increase range of motion and reduce spasticity in children with cerebral palsy, which is especially true in cases in which sustained stretching is used.[20] Sustained stretching is easily achieved through bracing or serial casting.

Oral Medications for Spasticity Management

Spasticity can also be treated with oral medications. Benzodiazepines such as diazepam, as well as baclofen, dantrolene sodium, and tizanidine, have been quite popular.

The benzodiazepines facilitate transmission at the γ-aminobutyric acid type A (GABA$_A$) receptors, one of the principal types of inhibitory synapses in the central nervous system. This transmission results in increased inhibition and reduced monosynaptic and polysynaptic reflexes.[21] Benzodiazepines are able to act supraspinally and at the spinal cord and have been shown to reduce generalized spasticity, hyperreflexia, and muscle spasms.[22,23] Diazepam is one of the oldest pharmacologic treatments for spasticity, and it is still used today.[21] Diazepam has been shown to improve sleep and decrease anxiety and is an excellent agent for patients who have poor sleep accompanied by nighttime spasms.[24,25] Because sedation is one of the most common side effects, dosing usually starts with nighttime administration and tapers up to 2 to 3 doses per day in those who can tolerate it. Pediatric doses range from 0.12 to 0.8 mg/kg/d. For adults, dosing is from 2 to 10 mg administered twice or thrice daily. It is important to remember that there is a risk for tolerance and/or dependence with the use of diazepam. Diazepam should never be stopped abruptly in patients who have been taking the medicine for an extended period because of the risk of withdrawal. Withdrawal symptoms may include agitation, irritability,

tremor, muscle fasciculation, nausea, hyperpyrexia, and seizures.[21]

Baclofen is a structural analogue of GABA. Baclofen binds to the GABA$_B$ receptors, which occur both pre- and postsynaptically. The net effect is inhibition of monosynaptic and polysynaptic spinal reflexes.[21] Baclofen also reduces the release of excitatory neurotransmitters and substance P when it binds to the GABA$_B$ receptors. Baclofen primarily acts at the spinal cord level, so it is an excellent treatment for those with spasticity of spinal cord origin and is also used in children with cerebral palsy.[26,27] Baclofen has been shown to reduce spasms, clonus, and resistance to stretch, and in some cases it has demonstrated an anxiolytic effect.[21] Baclofen can often cause sedation, so dosing usually begins with nighttime administration and usually tapers up to 3 to 4 doses daily. Pediatric dosing for baclofen starts between 2.5 and 10 mg/d and can increase to 40 mg/d divided into 3 or 4 doses. For adults, dosing starts at 20 mg/d and can increase to 80 mg/d divided into 3 or 4 doses. Much like the benzodiazepines, care should be taken when stopping this medication. In patients who have been on baclofen for an extended period, withdrawal syndromes can sometimes occur. Symptoms of withdrawal may include intensified spasticity with increased spasms, hallucinations, confusion, seizures, and hyperpyrexia.[21,28]

Dantrolene is unique in that it actually acts at the site of the skeletal muscle as opposed to other oral agents, which act on the neurotransmitter systems. Dantrolene inhibits release of calcium from the sarcoplasmic reticulum during muscle contraction.[29] Dantrolene is generally preferred in hemiplegia, traumatic brain injury, or cerebral palsy, but it is also used as a secondary agent in some patients with spinal cord injury. This drug has been known to reduce clonus and muscle spasms resulting from innocuous stimuli.[21] Dantrolene is mildly sedating and may cause malaise, nausea, vomiting, dizziness, diarrhea, and paresthesia.[30] The most important side effect is hepatotoxicity. Although hepatotoxicity is rare, liver function tests should be performed before beginning a regimen of dantrolene sodium and monitored periodically. The drug should be tapered or discontinued if elevations in levels of enzyme are noted because most cases are reversible on prompt discontinuation.[31] The regimen for pediatric dosing of dantrolene is 6 to 8 mg/kg/d divided into 2 to 4 doses per day. The starting dose is usually 0.5 mg/kg/d for 7 days, and then the dosage is gradually increased week by week. The regimen for dosing in adults is 100 mg divided into 2 to 4 doses per day, but dosing usually begins at 25 mg/d and tapers up every week thereafter.

Tizanidine has also been used in the treatment of spasticity. Tizanidine is an α_2-adrenergic agonist that acts on receptors in the brain and spinal cord.[24,29] This drug causes a decrease in tone through the hyperpolarization of motoneurons.[25] α_2-adrenergic agonists may also have an antinociceptive effect, which may contribute to their ability to decrease tone.[32] Some common side effects include sedation, dizziness, nausea, hypotension, and dry mouth. Hepatotoxicity is also a concern when prescribing tizanidine because it is extensively metabolized by the liver. Liver function tests should be performed before initiation of tizanidine and periodically during treatment.[29] Pediatric dosing for tizanidine has not been defined, but most practitioners start at 2 mg at bedtime and taper the dosage up to 24 to 32 mg divided into 3 to 4 doses given throughout the day. Adult dosing starts at 4 mg and may taper up to 8 mg given 3 to 4 times daily (**Table 1**).

Intramuscular Medications

Neuromuscular blockade/chemodenervation is another way by which hypertonia can be treated quite effectively. Injections of phenol and ethyl alcohol have been used for several decades, and in the recent years the use of botulinum toxin has become popular.

Both phenol and alcohol have been used for the treatment of spasticity. To localize the nerve that needs to be injected, electrical stimulation is used. Electrical stimulation can be painful, so sedation or anesthesia is usually necessary, especially in children. The agent is injected perineurally, where it promotes denervation via axonal degeneration. The effect is not permanent, with functional reinnervation occurring over months to years.[33] Adverse effects of both agents include a significant risk of dysesthesia when targeting a mixed nerve, which may persist after the procedure is complete.[33,34] Other complications may include muscle necrosis or vascular complications. Phenol and ethyl alcohol are excellent cost-effective choices for patients with powerful muscles that are inadequately treated by the recommended amounts of botulinum toxin. Both types of injections require a skilled clinician.[34]

The introduction of botulinum toxin for the relief of focal muscle overactivity has resulted in a major advancement in the treatment of spasticity.[34] Botulinum toxin is an exotoxin produced by *Clostridium botulinum*, the bacterium that is responsible for tetanus. The site of action for botulinum toxin is at the neuromuscular junction. A protease cleaves one or more vesicle fusion

Table 1
Oral medications for hypertonia

Medication	Mechanism of Action	Side Effects	Pediatric Dosing
Diazepam	Facilitates transmission at the GABA$_A$ receptors, one of the principal types of inhibitory synapses in the CNS	Sedation, decreased motor coordination, impaired attention and memory. Can cause overdose or withdrawal symptoms	0.12–0.8 mg/kg/d in divided doses or once daily at night
Baclofen	Binds to GABA$_B$ receptors in the spinal cord to inhibit reflexes that cause spasticity	Sedation, confusion, nausea, dizziness, hypotonia, muscle weakness, and ataxia. Can cause withdrawal symptoms	Start at 2.5–10 mg/d. Can taper up to a maximum of 40 mg/d divided tid or qid
Dantrolene	Acts at the site of skeletal muscle to inhibit calcium release from the sarcoplasmic reticulum	Sedation, diarrhea, and dizziness. Causes hepatotoxicity in 2%, so LFTs must be monitored	Start at 0.5 mg/kg/d. Can taper up to a maximum of 3 mg/kg administered qid
Tizanidine	α_2-Agonist that acts on the brain and spinal cord to decrease tone through hyperpolarization of motoneurons	Sedation, dizziness, dry mouth, elevated levels in LFTs, insomnia, muscle weakness	Start at 2 mg at bedtime. Can taper up to a maximum of 32 mg/d divided tid or qid

Abbreviations: CNS, central nervous system; LFT, liver function test.

proteins and prevents the release of acetylcholine, which causes muscle weakness.[34] The effects of botulinum toxin on the neuromuscular junction are reversible, so reinjection is required every 3 to 4 months. However, in some patients, the improvements outlast the direct effect on the nerve terminal.[35] Dosing is usually 10 to 12 U/kg, but it is not to exceed 400 U in any one procedure in most cases. Two serotypes, A and B, are available in the United States. Type A is marketed as BOTOX by Allergan, Inc (Irvine, CA, USA). Another preparation is marketed as Dysport by Ipsen Group (Brisbane, CA, USA) and Medicis Aesthetics (Scottsdale, AZ, USA). These preparations are approved for cervical dystonia, blepharospasm, hemifacial spasm, primary axillary hyperhidrosis, and strabismus. Type B is marketed as MYOBLOC by Solstice Neurosciences, Inc (South San Francisco, CA, USA) and is approved for cervical dystonia. Some other off-label uses include the treatment of spasticity in those with cerebral palsy, traumatic brain injury, spinal cord injury, and other diagnoses. MYOBLOC is also used to treat sialorrhea and myofascial pain. The most appropriate candidate for botulinum toxin injections is the patient in whom an appropriate diminution of spasticity of a limited number of muscles has the potential to provide meaningful benefit in care, comfort, or activity.[34] Patients with adequate selective motor control stand to have the best results, whereas those with longstanding contractures and deformities have poorer outcomes.[36] Botulinum toxin can also be used for focal and regional management of spasticity in conjunction with orthopedic surgery[37] or in combination with serial casting. Using serial casting in conjunction with botulinum toxin may decrease the time required to achieve the desired range-of-motion goals (**Table 2**).[38]

Neurosurgical Treatment of Spasticity

In cases in which spasticity cannot be managed with physical methods, oral medications, or injectable medications, surgical options such as selective dorsal rhizotomy and intrathecal baclofen therapy are used. Although these procedures are invasive, they are effective in those who have spasticity that is so severe that other methods of treatment have been ineffective or in cases in which the side effects of other various antispasticity treatments could not be tolerated.

Selective dorsal rhizotomy has been performed at several centers throughout the country since the late 1980s. The procedure was popularized in the United States by Warrick Peacock. The first rhizotomies for spasticity were performed by Foester in 1913. Fasano, in 1977, used electromyographic testing to identify populations of sensory nerve roots that were serving overactive lower motor nerves. In 1982, Peacock modified the procedure, identified appropriate candidates, and performed studies that examined long-term follow-up.[39–42] The procedure is usually performed by laminoplasty so that the dura can be opened. Dorsal rootlets from T12 through S1 are separated. Each rootlet is then stimulated, and the responses are recorded electromyographically. After targeting the rootlets that show an abnormal sustained

Table 2
Intramuscular medications for hypertonia

Medication	Mechanism	Site of Injection	Onset and Duration	Disadvantages/Risks	Cost
Phenol	Chemical neurolysis causes denervation via axonal degeneration	Injected into the motor points of the involved muscle	Takes effect immediately. Can last 3–12 mo	Can be painful and may require anesthesia. Can cause dysesthesias, numbness, or hematoma	Very low cost
Botulinum Type A	Presynaptic block of acetylcholine release	Intramuscular	Takes effect in 5–7 d. Can last 3–6 mo	Lasts only 3–4 mo and cannot be repeated in shorter intervals. Can cause swallowing and respiratory difficulties when used in large quantities in the neck muscles	Up to $600 per 100-U vial

or generalized response, the rootlets are severed. About 40% to 60% of nerve roots are cut during the procedure.[35,43] By severing overactive dorsal nerve rootlets, aberrant afferent activity from muscle spindles and spasticity are reduced.[34] The best candidates for selective dorsal rhizotomy are those children between the ages of 3 and 7 years who have spastic diplegia, good trunk control, and isolated leg movements.[44] After selective posterior rhizotomy, patients often have a significant amount of weakness, and extensive physical therapy is usually required. Many patients can require up to 6 months or more of therapy to reach their preoperative baseline. It is important to remember that in those who have significant underlying weakness before the procedure, functional improvement is unlikely once spasticity has been decreased.[35] This procedure should not be performed in patients who have dystonia.

Intrathecal baclofen pump placement is a surgical treatment that has also been used to treat severe spasticity. This method is best used to treat patients with multisegmental or extensive spasticity. The Food and Drug Administration has approved the use of baclofen intrathecally for spasticity of cerebral and spinal origin.[35] Intrathecal baclofen is delivered to the intrathecal space via a catheter attached to an implanted pump. Because of the direct delivery to the nervous system, the required dose is less than 1% of that delivered orally, thus limiting the side effects of lethargy that are sometimes seen with large amounts of oral baclofen administration.[33,45–47] Baclofen pumps are usually placed by a neurosurgeon, with the patient under general anesthesia. The pump is about the size of a hockey puck and is usually placed subcutaneously or submuscularly in the lower half of the abdomen. A catheter runs from the pump and is inserted into the intrathecal space in the low thoracic or lumbar spine. The catheter is usually inserted at the T11-T12 level of the spine but has been inserted at higher levels (even cervical) in some cases.[34] After the pump is placed, dosing adjustments are made with a remote via telemetry. Dosing is timed so that more or less medicine can be given at different times of the day as a patient's needs may dictate. Refills are delivered with the help of a needle that passes through the skin and enters the port of the pump. Refills are usually performed every 2 to 6 months depending on the patient's dosing needs. An alarm sounds when the pump reservoir is low, and patients should be informed that baclofen pump refills are not to be missed because of the dangerous side effects of baclofen withdrawal.

Withdrawal symptoms can include itching, paresthesias, rebound spasticity, priapism in men, tachycardia, hypotension or labile blood pressures, dysphoria, changes in mental status, and seizures.[33] Patients should also be educated about withdrawal symptoms because other complications such as catheter malfunction or kinking and pump malfunction can also cause baclofen to stop flowing into the intrathecal space and trigger symptoms of withdrawal. Good candidates for intrathecal baclofen therapy usually have spasticity in the lower extremities and are usually older than 3 years because the pump has to be safely and securely placed in the abdomen. Although not an absolute requirement, many surgeons will not implant the pump in children weighing less than 20 kg. Any patient who may benefit from intrathecal baclofen therapy should be sent for a baclofen trial, although there is controversy as to whether this step is absolutely necessary. During the screening test, baclofen is injected via lumbar puncture. If spasticity improves, there is a good chance that intrathecal baclofen placement will be of benefit to the patient.

TREATMENTS THAT TARGET DYSTONIA

Dystonia can be treated with oral medications, intramuscular injections, or in severe cases with surgical procedures such as intrathecal baclofen pump placement or deep brain stimulation. The method of treatment can sometimes depend on the severity and the location of the dystonia. For those with dystonia as a result of cerebral palsy, oral medications may be of benefit. In cases in which the dystonia is focal, intramuscular injections with botulinum toxin may be helpful. In patients with severe generalized spasticity and dystonia, intrathecal baclofen pump placement may be of benefit. In those with severe dystonia that cannot successfully be managed with oral medications, deep brain stimulation may be an option.

Oral Medications for the Treatment of Dystonia

All patients with childhood dystonia should receive a trial of carbidopa/levodopa because it is highly effective in dopa-responsive dystonias and other disorders affecting dopamine synthesis.[48] The drug is slowly titrated up to the maximum tolerated dose; central side effects such as memory impairment, confusion, and hallucinations usually limit dosing. Effects are usually seen with levodopa, less than 300 mg, when combined with carbidopa.[49]

If dopaminergic agents are ineffective, anticholinergics should be tried. In children who have a secondary dystonia caused by cerebral palsy,

Table 3
Comparison of carbidopa/levodopa and trihexyphenidyl for dystonia treatment

Drug	Mechanism of Action	Side Effects	Pediatric Dosing	Cost
Carbidopa/ Levodopa	Inhibits peripheral dopamine decarboxylation. Serves as a dopamine precursor	Dyskinesia, bradykinesia, hypotension, memory impairment, confusion, and hallucinations	Start at 10/100 mg bid and titrate up to 25/100 mg tid	$90–$115 for a 1-mo supply
Trihexyphenidyl	Antagonizes acetylcholine receptors	Dry mouth, blurry vision, dizziness, nausea, anxiety, glaucoma, anhidrosis, neuroleptic malignant syndrome, and tardive dyskinesia	Start at 2.5 mg/d and titrate up slowly as needed. Maximum dose is 15 mg/d	$25–$70 for a 1-mo supply

benefits have been seen with the use of trihexyphenidyl. Trihexyphenidyl is usually administered at 2.5 mg/d and then titrated up slowly to 60 to 80 mg/d.[50] This drug is usually tolerated well by children. The limiting factor for titrating trihexyphenidyl is usually its side effects. Side effects can include confusion, memory loss, nightmares, hallucinations, dry mouth, urinary retention, and blurred vision.[48]

When carbidopa/levodopa and anticholinergics are not effective, baclofen has been moderately effective in some cases, with fairly dramatic responses occurring in children.[49] Starting dose is 10 mg at bedtime followed by titration of 10 mg each week.[51]

Benzodiazepines such as clonazepam have also been used with starting doses of 0.25 mg at bedtime and gradually increasing the dosage to a maximum of 1 mg 4 times a day (**Table 3**).[51]

Intramuscular Medications for the Treatment of Dystonia

If oral medications fail, intramuscular injections of botulinum toxin are used to help manage dystonia. Botulinum toxin is most effective on focal dystonias but can also have good results in well-chosen muscles of patients with generalized dystonias.[48] Botulinum toxin injections should be placed in the most disabling or painful muscles and may be given in conjunction with the oral therapies mentioned earlier in this article.[49] Botulinum toxin may block involuntary movement but preserve

strength because the toxin is preferentially taken up by the most active muscle fibers.[52]

Neurosurgical Treatment of Dystonia

In patients who have been refractory to oral and intramuscular medications, surgical procedures such as intrathecal baclofen pump placement and deep brain stimulation may offer an effective treatment of dystonia. In those with spasticity and dystonia, baclofen pump placement may be a viable option despite this treatment being more effective for spasticity than dystonia.[53,54]

Pallidal stimulation, sometimes referred to as deep brain stimulation, has shown promising results in those with generalized dystonia. Pallidal stimulation offers the advantage of a bilateral intervention with an acceptable morbidity rate as well as the option for reversal or modification.[55,56] Deep brain stimulation is still new, and there are concerns about whether this method can continue to control dystonia for extended periods. For secondary generalized dystonia (cerebral palsy), results are highly variable, ranging from no benefit at all to significant improvement in some cases. This procedure is reserved for patients who have failed all other therapies.[57]

SUMMARY

The orthopedic surgeon is a constant participant in the care of children with cerebral palsy. Pediatric orthopedic surgeons are uniquely qualified to plan and orchestrate a program to decrease the risk of deformity and improve overall function. Treating both spasticity and dystonia during the growth years improves the orthopedic and functional outcomes of children with cerebral palsy. Being well acquainted with the hypertonic syndromes as well as being able to discriminate between them is important for the orthopedic surgeon.

Orthopedic surgeons are in an ideal position to begin treatment of hypertonia but may depend on other members of the team to monitor or expand on the treatment methods chosen. First-line medications are initiated by the orthopedic surgeon; however, children with cerebral palsy need close monitoring for dose adjustments, side effect monitoring, and evaluation of progress toward rehabilitation goals. A pediatric physiatrist, pediatric neurologist, or developmental pediatrician can typically provide expertise in tone management. The efforts of these professionals to control tone and manage the possible side effects of treatment will complement the work of the orthopedic surgeon.

Pediatric orthopedic surgeons pioneered the use of botulinum toxins in children with cerebral palsy.[58,59] The neurolytics can effectively control the focal tone that is found in both spasticity and dystonia. These procedures can be performed during office visits or concurrently during surgery.

Despite aggressive treatment of hypertonia, deformity can still occur. Decisions regarding the timing of treatments such as intrathecal baclofen therapy and selective posterior rhizotomy occur in the context of the overall functional and rehabilitation goals of the patient. These neurosurgical procedures are complementary and do not obviate careful orthopedic assessment.

REFERENCES

1. Little WJ. On the influence of abnormal parturition, difficult labours, premature birth, and asphyxia neonatorum, on the mental and physical condition of the child, especially in relation to deformities. Clin Orthop Relat Res 1966;46:7–22.

2. Tervo RC, Azuma S, Stout J, et al. Correlation between physical functioning and gait measures in children with cerebral palsy. Dev Med Child Neurol 2002;44(3):185–90.

3. Sanger TD, Delgado MR, Gaebler-Spira D, et al. Classification and definition of disorders causing hypertonia in childhood. Pediatrics 2003;111(1): e89–97.

4. Sanger TD. Toward a definition of childhood dystonia. Curr Opin Pediatr 2004;16(6):623–7.

5. Ito J, Araki A, Tanaka H, et al. Muscle histopathology in spastic cerebral palsy. Brain Dev 1996;18(4): 299–303.

6. Hoon AH Jr, Stashinko EE, Nagae LM, et al. Sensory and motor deficits in children with cerebral palsy born preterm correlate with diffusion tensor imaging abnormalities in thalamocortical pathways. Dev Med Child Neurol 2009;51(9):697–704.

7. Fahn S. Concept and classification of dystonia. Adv Neurol 1988;50:1–8.

8. Albanese A. The clinical expression of primary dystonia. J Neurol 2003;250(10):1145–51.

9. Marsden CD. The pathophysiology of movement disorders. Neurol Clin 1984;2(3):435–59.

10. Sanger TD. Childhood onset generalised dystonia can be modelled by increased gain in the indirect basal ganglia pathway. J Neurol Neurosurg Psychiatr 2003;74(11):1509–15.

11. Fenichel GM. Clinical pediatric neurology: a signs and symptoms approach. 6th edition. Philadelphia: Saunders/Elsevier; 2009. p. ix, 415.

12. Scholtes VA, Becher JG, Beelen A, et al. Clinical assessment of spasticity in children with cerebral palsy: a critical review of available instruments. Dev Med Child Neurol 2006;48(1):64–73.

13. Ashworth B. Preliminary trial of carisoprodol in multiple sclerosis. Practitioner 1964;192:540–2.

14. Bohannon RW, Smith MB. Interrater reliability of a Modified Ashworth Scale of muscle spasticity. Phys Ther 1987;67(2):206–7.

15. Peacock WJ, Staudt LA. Functional outcomes following selective posterior rhizotomy in children with cerebral palsy. J Neurosurg 1991;74(3):380–5.

16. Tardieu G, Shentoub S, Delarue R. [Research on a technic for measurement of spasticity]. Rev Neurol (Paris) 1954;91(2):143–4 [in French].

17. Boyd R. Objective measurement of clinical findings in the use of botulinum toxin type A for the management of children with cerebral palsy. Eur J Neurol 1999;6(Suppl 4):S23–35.

18. Barry MJ, VanSwearingen JM, Albright AL. Reliability and responsiveness of the Barry-Albright Dystonia Scale. Dev Med Child Neurol 1999;41(6):404–11.

19. Wiart L, Darrah J, Kembhavi G. Stretching with children with cerebral palsy: what do we know and where are we going? Pediatr Phys Ther 2008;20(2):173–8.

20. Pin T, Dyke P, Chan M. The effectiveness of passive stretching in children with cerebral palsy. Dev Med Child Neurol 2006;48(10):855–62.

21. Gracies JM, Elovic E, McGuire J, et al. Traditional pharmacological treatments for spasticity. Part II: general and regional treatments. Muscle Nerve Suppl 1997;6:S92–120.

22. Mathew A, Mathew MC. Bedtime diazepam enhances well-being in children with spastic cerebral palsy. Pediatr Rehabil 2005;8(1):63–6.

23. Mathew A, Mathew MC, Thomas M, et al. The efficacy of diazepam in enhancing motor function in children with spastic cerebral palsy. J Trop Pediatr 2005;51(2):109–13.

24. Patel DR, Soyode O. Pharmacologic interventions for reducing spasticity in cerebral palsy. Indian J Pediatr 2005;72(10):869–72.

25. Verrotti A, Greco R, Spalice A, et al. Pharmacotherapy of spasticity in children with cerebral palsy. Pediatr Neurol 2006;34(1):1–6.

26. Krach LE. Pharmacotherapy of spasticity: oral medications and intrathecal baclofen. J Child Neurol 2001;16(1):31–6.

27. Sanger TD. Pathophysiology of pediatric movement disorders. J Child Neurol 2003;18(Suppl 1):S9–24.

28. Terrence CF, Fromm GH. Complications of baclofen withdrawal. Arch Neurol 1981;38(9):588–9.

29. Saulino M, Jacobs BW. The pharmacological management of spasticity. J Neurosci Nurs 2006; 38(6):456–9.

30. Glenn MB, Whyte J. The practical management of spasticity in children and adults. Philadelphia: Lea & Febiger; 1990. p. xii, 325.

31. Utili R, Boitnott JK, Zimmerman HJ. Dantrolene-associated hepatic injury. Incidence and character. Gastroenterology 1977;72(4 Pt 1):610–6.

32. Young RR. Spasticity: a review. Neurology 1994;44 (11 Suppl 9):S12–20.

33. Tilton A. Management of spasticity in children with cerebral palsy. Semin Pediatr Neurol 2009;16(2):82–9.

34. Tilton AH. Therapeutic interventions for tone abnormalities in cerebral palsy. NeuroRx 2006;3(2):217–24.

35. Tilton AH. Approach to the rehabilitation of spasticity and neuromuscular disorders in children. Neurol Clin 2003;21(4):853–81, vii.

36. Graham HK, Aoki KR, Autti-Rämö I, et al. Recommendations for the use of botulinum toxin type A in the management of cerebral palsy. Gait Posture 2000;11(1):67–79.

37. Graham HK. Botulinum toxin type A management of spasticity in the context of orthopaedic surgery for children with spastic cerebral palsy. Eur J Neurol 2001;8(Suppl 5):30–9.

38. Booth MY, Yates CC, Edgar TS, et al. Serial casting vs combined intervention with botulinum toxin A and serial casting in the treatment of spastic equinus in children. Pediatr Phys Ther 2003;15(4):216–20.

39. Arens LJ, Peacock WJ, Peter J. Selective posterior rhizotomy: a long-term follow-up study. Childs Nerv Syst 1989;5(3):148–52.

40. Fasano VA, Broggi G, Barolat-Romana G, et al. Surgical treatment of spasticity in cerebral palsy. Childs Brain 1978;4(5):289–305.

41. Peacock W, Staudt L. Selective posterior rhizotomy: history and results. Neurosurgery 1989;4(2):403–8.

42. Lynn AK, Turner M, Chambers HG. Surgical management of spasticity in persons with cerebral palsy. PM R 2009;1(9):834–8.

43. Lazareff JA, Garcia-Mendez MA, De Rosa R, et al. Limited (L4-S1, L5-S1) selective dorsal rhizotomy for reducing spasticity in cerebral palsy. Acta Neurochir (Wien) 1999;141(7):743–51 [discussion: 751–2].

44. Engsberg JR, Ross SA, Park TS. Changes in ankle spasticity and strength following selective dorsal rhizotomy and physical therapy for spastic cerebral palsy. J Neurosurg 1999;91(5):727–32.

45. Albright AL, Cervi A, Singletary J. Intrathecal baclofen for spasticity in cerebral palsy. JAMA 1991; 265(11):1418–22.

46. Gilmartin R, Bruce D, Storrs BB, et al. Intrathecal baclofen for management of spastic cerebral palsy: multicenter trial. J Child Neurol 2000;15(2):71–7.

47. Van Schaeybroeck P, Nuttin B, Lagae L, et al. Intrathecal baclofen for intractable cerebral spasticity: a prospective placebo-controlled, double-blind study. Neurosurgery 2000;46(3):603–9 [discussion: 609–12].

48. Langlois M, Richer F, Chouinard S. New perspectives on dystonia. Can J Neurol Sci 2003;30(Suppl 1): S34–44.

49. Bressman SB. Dystonia update. Clin Neuropharmacol 2000;23(5):239–51.

50. Pranzatelli MR. Movement disorders in childhood. Pediatr Rev 1996;17(11):388–94.

51. Adler CH. Strategies for controlling dystonia. Overview of therapies that may alleviate symptoms. Postgrad Med 2000;108(5):151–2, 155–6, 159–60.

52. Hallett M, Glocker FX, Deuschl G. Mechanism of action of botulinum toxin. Ann Neurol 1994;36(3): 449–50.

53. Ford B, Greene P, Louis ED, et al. Use of intrathecal baclofen in the treatment of patients with dystonia. Arch Neurol 1996;53(12):1241–6.

54. Ford B, Greene PE, Louis ED, et al. Intrathecal baclofen in the treatment of dystonia. Adv Neurol 1998;78:199–210.

55. Krack P, Vercueil L. Review of the functional surgical treatment of dystonia. Eur J Neurol 2001;8(5): 389–99.

56. Pollak P. Neurosurgical treatment of dyskinesias: pathophysiological consideration. Mov Disord 1999;14(Suppl 1):33–9.

57. Volkmann J, Benecke R. Deep brain stimulation for dystonia: patient selection and evaluation. Mov Disord 2002;17(Suppl 3):S112–5.

58. Cosgrove AP, Corry IS, Graham HK. Botulinum toxin in the management of the lower limb in cerebral palsy. Dev Med Child Neurol 1994;36(5):386–96.

59. Koman LA, Mooney JF 3rd, Smith B, et al. Management of cerebral palsy with botulinum-A toxin: preliminary investigation. J Pediatr Orthop 1993;13(4):489–95.

Surgery of the Upper Extremity in Cerebral Palsy

L. Andrew Koman, MD*, Thomas Sarlikiotis, MD,
Beth P. Smith, PhD

KEYWORDS

- Cerebral palsy • Contracture release • Tendon transfer
- Osteotomy • Fusion

Functional activities of the upper extremity are limited in most individuals with a diagnosis of cerebral palsy (CP). However, surgical interventions are applied in fewer than 20% of pediatric patients with an upper extremity affected by CP,[1–5] in marked contrast to the lower extremity in which surgery is more frequently indicated. Apart from improving function, surgical procedures may decrease pain, prevent or fix upper limb deformity, and have a positive impact on the patient's caregiving, self-esteem, and appearance. Several conservative treatment methods are also available (eg, therapy, casting, electrical stimulation, oral spasmolytic medications, and parenteral neuromuscular blocking agents). These methods are primarily used to preserve joint range of motion (ROM), to delay tendon and muscle contractures, and to prevent upper extremity osseous deformities. In patients without competently functional antagonist muscles, passive stretch for a minimum of 6 out of 24 hours is required to maintain muscle length and to avoid development of a fixed contracture.[6,7] Occupational therapy and splinting alone do not accomplish long-term reduction of the involuntary spasm. Moreover, pharmacologic agents designed to decrease spasticity have not been validated as a definitive means of providing lasting improvement. In selected cases, surgery following conservative treatment has been reported to give satisfactory results.[8]

This article covers the surgical interventions used for the reconstruction of the upper limb in patients with CP. The optimal surgical approach for each deformity type is described. In addition, the various evaluation techniques of the upper extremity, the general principles of an operative treatment plan, and the appropriate postoperative care of these patients is presented.

EVALUATION
History and Physical Examination

A team approach to the management of the patient with CP is important; medical history and physical examination is the basis for the successful assessment of each individual. Input from the patient and his or her caregiver, and any involved health care worker should be provided. Functional classification systems (eg, House scale) as well as standardized testing regimens, such as the Melbourne Assessment of Unilateral Upper Limb Function (Melbourne), are helpful evaluation tools.[9–11] The Melbourne scale allows objective measurement of the upper extremity function in patients with CP.[12] Both active and passive ROM of the upper extremity joints should be assessed in a reliable and reproducible manner. In the authors' institution, the Upper Extremity Rating Scale (UERS) is used for this purpose. The UERS provides a composite score of the active and

The authors have nothing to disclose.
Department of Orthopedic Surgery, Wake Forest University School of Medicine, Medical Center Boulevard, Winston-Salem, NC 27157, USA
* Corresponding author.
E-mail address: lakoman@wfubmc.edu

orthopedic.theclinics.com

passive ROM of the shoulder, elbow, forearm, and wrist.[13] Degree of spasticity, and absence or presence and magnitude of involuntary movement disorders should also be evaluated and recorded. For patients with mild to moderate involvement, the use of the Melbourne scale and the Jebsen-Taylor Hand Function Test is suggested. A global instrument such as the WeeFIM (Uniform Data System for Medical Rehabilitation, University at Buffalo Foundation Activities, Inc, New York) is also available to measure self-care and functional skills. If possible, the patient is observed during ambulation, standing, and sitting to evaluate certain posturing and motion patterns. Several factors including fatigue level, anxiety, and even time of the day may affect the clinical findings; therefore, serial evaluations are necessary. Preoperatively, sensibility testing including evaluation of proprioception, stereognosis, and 2-point discrimination should also be performed.

Imaging Studies and Ancillary Testing

Evaluation of patients with CP is complex. Several examinations are necessary as part of the surgical planning process. Plain radiographs, computed tomography scans, and magnetic resonance imaging studies are helpful in assessing preoperative joint congruity. An individualized and detailed functional evaluation is also a critical component for developing the appropriate surgical plan. Dynamic electromyography (EMG) provides a qualitative and quantitative assessment of voluntary motor control and the type of motor activity of muscles being considered for transfer.[14–16] A videotaped evaluation of the upper extremity in children with CP provides an objective assessment of a patient's motor performance and functional capacity. Carlson and colleagues[17] reported changes to the initial preoperative plan following the study of videotaped evaluations, especially for procedures addressing the wrist, digit, and thumb. Motor blockade produced by injections of botulinum toxin A (BTX-A) or a topical anesthetic agent (eg, bupivacaine) into the muscles identified for surgery may serve as a diagnostic tool to select the proper operative interventions.[18]

General Principles of an Operative Treatment Plan

Diagnostic evaluation is helpful in identifying the suitable candidates for complex reconstructive procedures of the upper extremity. Selection of the appropriate intervention is required to achieve both specific and global outcomes individualized for each patient. However, it must be recognized that although some improvement in function and

appearance may be a realistic goal for properly selected patients, normality can rarely, if ever, be achieved. The type of joint deformity, the underlying neuromuscular disorder, the preoperative sensibility and functional capacity of the limb, the patient's intellectual status and goals, and the surgeon's preferences are the factors used to devise a treatment plan.[19]

Global surgical goals for best outcomes include (1) improved function, (2) facilitation of care, (3) pain reduction, and (4) enhancement of self-esteem. Specific surgical interventions may be performed at one or more levels (ie, shoulder, elbow, wrist, hand) to release overactive muscle groups, stabilize joints, and augment selective motor control of weak muscles by tendon transfer to achieve each patient's specific goals. Surgical interventions may be reduced to a checklist of options (**Table 1**). Proactive planning with multiple team members, including the development of an immediate postoperative regimen (eg, period and type of immobilization) and rehabilitation program, is the key to the success of the operative procedure.

Operative Procedures

Shoulder

Adduction and internal rotation shoulder deformity is common in patients with CP; the deformity is due to unbalanced spasticity of the internal rotators of the arm at the glenohumeral joint (pectoralis major, latissimus dorsi, subscapularis, and teres major).[20] A fixed contracture of the muscles (mentioned earlier) and the joint capsule may contribute to the deformity posture. Surgical interventions may need to address (1) the muscle/tendon and/or capsule contractures, and (2) the subluxation or dislocation of the humeral head in one or more planes of the shoulder joint. Inferior subluxation is the most common form in the hemiplegic shoulder.[21] Moreover, dysplasia of the glenoid or humeral head and/or arthritis of the glenohumeral joint should be encountered in the treatment plan. In dynamic deformities, the glenohumeral articulation is typically stable with congruous articular surface contact. Treatment options include muscle lengthening, tendon transfer, humeral osteotomy, and shoulder joint fusion.

Although surgical treatment is rare, the pectoralis major and subscapularis muscles should be lengthened to correct shoulder adduction and internal rotation deformity; capsular release may also be performed. Transfer of the latissimus dorsi and teres major may augment active external rotation of the arm (**Fig. 1**). In severe cases, release of the latissimus dorsi and teres major muscles in conjunction with the procedures described above

Table 1
Operative interventions of the upper extremity in CP

Joint	Aim	Options
Shoulder	Joint stabilization	Fusion, capsular reconstructions
	Improve external rotation	Lengthen pectoralis major/subscapularis; transfer LD and/or teres major; humeral osteotomy
	Improve internal rotation	Lengthen/release infraspinatus/teres minor
Elbow	Joint stabilization	Fusion
	Improve extension	Lengthen biceps brachii/brachialis; BR release; flexor-pronator mass release (slide); capsulotomy
Forearm	Improve supination	Reroute, lengthen, or release PT; radius/ulna osteotomy; flexor-pronator release (slide)
Wrist	Stabilization	Fusion
	Improve extension	Flexor tendon release; proximal row carpectomy; ECU transfer; FCU transfer to ECRB/ECRL/EDC
Thumb	Stabilization	Volar plate arthroplasty; MCP fusion
	Improve extension	Release/lengthen FPL; reinforce EPL
	Improve abduction	Release adductor pollicis; reinforce APL; EPL rerouting
Fingers	Flexion deformity	FDS to EDC transferflexor/pronator release (slide); FDS/FDP lengthening;FDS to FDP transfer
	Swan-neck deformity	PIP joint tenodesis; central slip tenotomy; intrinsic origin release

Abbreviations: APL, abductor pollicis longus; BR, brachioradialis; ECRB, extensor carpi radialis brevis; ECRL, extensor carpi radialis longus; ECU, extensor carpi ulnaris; EDC, extensor digitorum communis; EPB, extensor pollicis brevis; EPL, extensor pollicis longus; FCU, flexor carpi ulnaris; FDP, flexor digitorum profundus; FDS, flexor digitorum superficialis; FPL, flexor pollicis longus; LD, latissimus dorsi; MCP, metacarpophalangeal; PIP, proximal interphalangeal; PT, pronator teres.

may be required. If tendon/muscle release and/or transfer fail, a proximal or distal osteotomy of the humerus may be used to improve rotation of the arm. Osteotomy is also indicated for patients with dysplastic/subluxed or arthritic shoulder joints. Refractory arthritic pain may be addressed by shoulder fusion in individuals with CP; however, there is no experience with this procedure in the authors' institution.

Elbow

Flexion contracture of the elbow may interfere with the use of the limb by limiting reach activities of the hand. The associated abnormal attitude of the extremity, appearing during gait, is also a cosmetic disability and may impair self-image unless addressed. Increased muscle tone of the biceps brachii, brachialis, and brachioradialis muscles results in dynamic motor imbalance around the elbow joint. Secondary fixed contractures of the capsule and the adjacent flexor-pronator muscle/tendon units may contribute to elbow flexion deformity.[22] Subluxation/dislocation of the radial head due to associated hyperpronation of the forearm, accompanied with secondary dysplasia of the head may be an additional feature of elbow flexion deformity in children with CP. Pletcher and colleagues[23] identified a radial head dislocation in

approximately one-fourth of the children, with a combination of a flexion deformity of the elbow and a pronation contracture of the forearm. Most dislocations were posterior. The investigators proposed that preoperative elbow radiographs are required for all children with this combined deformity type.

Anterior elbow release is indicated for spastic elbow flexion deformity in patients with a diagnosis of CP. Operative treatment is seldom indicated unless extension loss exceeds 30°. For elbow deformities between 30° and 60°, soft tissue procedures (including excision of the lacertus fibrosus, Z-lengthening of the biceps, and fractional lengthening of the brachialis aponeurosis) are usually sufficient, and reliably decrease the degree of deformity (**Fig. 2**). For deformities exceeding 60°, a flexor-pronator origin slide accompanied with anterior elbow capsulotomy may also be required.

Anterior elbow release can improve active extension of the elbow, as well as both the functional use and aesthetic appearance of the involved upper extremity. Mital[22] reported the only large series of patients in whom elbow flexion deformity was addressed by weakening of both the brachialis (fractional lengthening) and the biceps muscles (release of lacertus

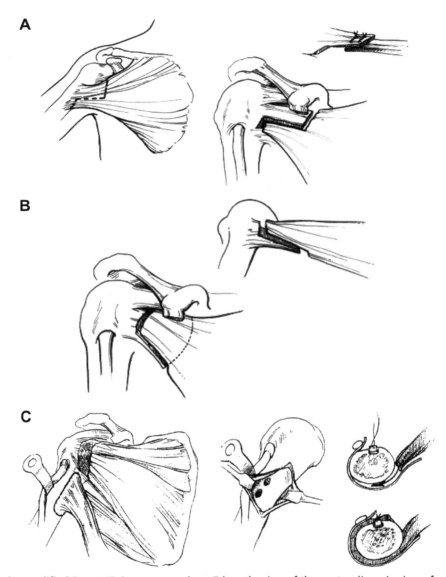

Fig. 1. For the modified Sever-L'Episcopo procedure, Z-lengthening of the pectoralis major is performed (*A*), the subscapularis is lengthened on the "flat" (*B*), and the latissimus dorsi and teres major are transferred to the posterolateral humerus using 1 incision (*C*) or 2 incisions (not shown). (*Reproduced from* Koman LA, editor. Wake Forest University School of Medicine orthopedic manual 2001. Winston-Salem (NC): Orthopaedic Press; 2001. © Wake Forest University Orthopaedic Press; with permission.)

aponeurosis, tendon Z-lengthening). Following this procedure the flexion posture angle was decreased, and the patient's ability to flex the elbow or supinate the forearm was retained. However, the risk of increasing pronation deformity following a biceps-lengthening procedure should be noted; rerouting or lengthening of the pronator teres (PT) muscle may prevent

increased pronation deformity after anterior elbow release.

Elbow fusion is considered as the last option for operative treatment of the elbow flexion deformity. It is reserved for patients who experience intractable elbow pain. However, this procedure is seldom used and has never been performed at the authors' institution.

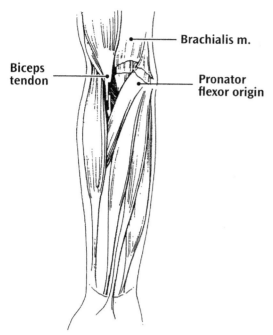

Biceps tendon

Brachialis m.

Pronator flexor origin

Fig. 2. Z-lengthening of the biceps tendon and fractional lengthening of the musculotendinous portion of the brachialis with or without flexor pronator release is appropriate for elbow flexion contractures. (*Reproduced from* Koman LA, editor. Wake Forest University School of Medicine orthopedic manual 2001. Winston-Salem (NC): Orthopaedic Press; 2001. © Wake Forest University Orthopaedic Press; with permission.)

Forearm

Pronation of the forearm is part of the typical pattern of the upper limb in patients with CP. The deformity may be fixed, dynamic, or a combination of both; hypertonicity of the PT and pronator quadratus muscles is the primary cause.[24] Inability to supinate the forearm in the absence of shoulder compensation interferes with hand function and compromises activities such as turning a doorknob or using a key. Multiple nonsurgical measures (muscle stretching, plaster casts, splints, braces, and BTX-A) have been advocated. Following extensive conservative treatment, operative procedures in properly selected patients are appropriate to improve forearm position and function. Allowing active supination to neutral should be considered a successful outcome.

Operations can be classified into 2 groups. In group I, procedures primarily designed to improve functions such as wrist dorsiflexion, elbow motion, and hand grasp and release are included. The release of the pronation contracture is incidental to these procedures.[25] The flexor-pronator release, primarily advocated to decrease flexion deformity of the wrist and fingers, has been reported to improve supination of the forearm.[26] However, the risk of supination deformity following excessive flexor-pronator release is increased.[27] Green[28] described a method to correct dynamic flexion deformity of the wrist; the flexor carpi ulnaris (FCU) tendon is transferred to augment either the extensor carpi radialis brevis (ECRB) or the extensor carpi radialis longus (ECRL) muscles. By transferring the FCU tendon from ulnar to radial, a supination moment is created and pronation deformity is potentially decreased.

In group II, procedures are designed exclusively for pronation deformity of the forearm. PT release tenotomy, fractional lengthening, Z-lengthening, and rerouting are described. In addition, rerouting of the brachioradialis has been reported to improve supination.[25,29,30] In none of the techniques mentioned here is the pronator quadratus released at the same time; thus, the risk of loss of active pronation is minimized. Dynamic EMG as well as clinical examination of the forearm helps decide the treatment plan. In the presence of passive supination, PT release, Z-lengthening, or fractional lengthening is appropriate for patients with a continuously firing PT by EMG. However, for patients with a phase-dependent PT muscle activity, PT rerouting is the preferred surgical option at the authors' institution (**Fig. 3**). If soft tissue procedures fail, radial osteotomy may be performed to improve forearm position. In severe cases, inferior radioulnar joint fusion may also be an option.[31]

Wrist

Flexion deformity of the wrist impairs grasp-and-release function of the hand. Common causes include hypertonic wrist flexors and/or weak wrist extensors with subsequent capsular contracture. Wrist joint deformities may be dynamic or static in nature. Management options include soft tissue and/or osseous procedures, depending on the severity and nature of the deformity.

Passively correctible deformities may benefit from transfer of a wrist flexor to the weak radial wrist extensors. Preoperative dynamic EMG and clinical testing of the muscles involved in active motion of the wrist determine the appropriate surgical intervention.[32] Functional sufficiency of the flexor carpi radialis muscle is crucial for a successful FCU tendon transfer.[33] Dynamic flexion deformities of the wrist can be managed by transferring the FCU to either the ECRB or the ECRL or the extensor digitorum communis (EDC) tendon (**Fig. 4**). Preferably, in patients with continuous FCU activity throughout the wrist motion arc, the FCU is transferred to the EDC; with this procedure, wrist and finger

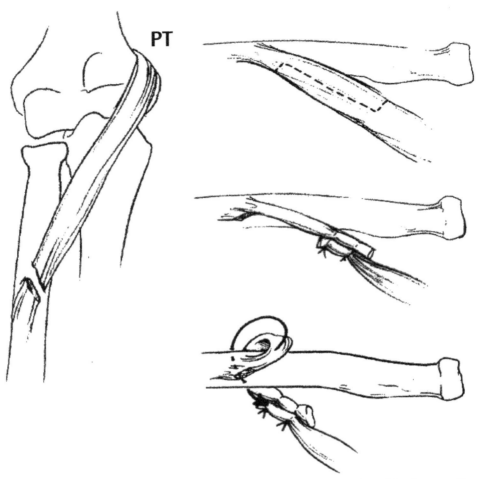

Fig. 3. The PT may be detached from the radius and rerouted to improve supination of the forearm. (*Reproduced from* Koman LA, editor. Wake Forest University School of Medicine orthopedic manual 2001. Winston-Salem (NC): Orthopaedic Press; 2001. © Wake Forest University Orthopaedic Press; with permission.)

extension is improved, finger flexion is permitted, and wrist extension deformity by FCU overpull is avoided.[14] If the combination of EMG and clinical testing demonstrates a phase-dependent FCU activity, improved voluntary wrist extension is achieved by transferring the FCU to the ECRB; when ulnar deviation of the wrist is an issue, the FCU to ECRL transfer is preferred. The latter procedure may be enhanced by transferring the extensor carpi ulnaris (ECU) tendon radially to the fourth metacarpal (**Fig. 5**).

Static wrist deformities are commonly associated with more than 45° of palmar flexion and may not respond to soft tissue release procedures in isolation. Static wrist deformities may require flexor tendon release combined with procedures such as wrist fusion (with or without carpal incisional resection)[34] and/or proximal row carpectomy (PRC).[35] Tendon transfers combined with PRC and flexor

tendon releases are reported to allow active extension of the wrist.[36] Wrist fusion maintains the wrist in a fixed neutral position and is indicated for patients that require pain relief and an improved cosmetic result.[37] Before considering a wrist stabilization procedure, finger flexion and extension capability should be evaluated in the desired corrected position. Wrist flexion is crucial for effective release in many patients, and wrist extension is often needed to achieve effective grasp. Therefore, procedures that limit motion should be reserved for patients with effective grasp-and-release in a position of the wrist close to neutral.[5,38]

Thumb and Finger Deformities

Finger flexion deformity
Finger flexion deformity typically is synchronous to other upper limb deformity types. Flexor digitorum

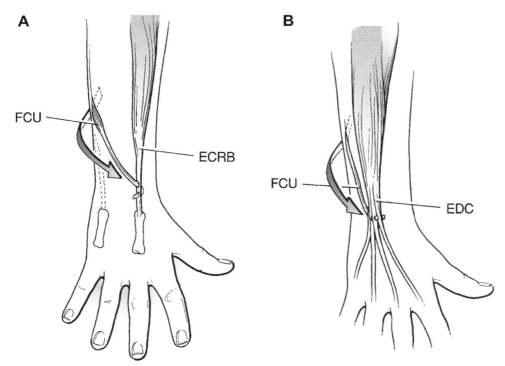

Fig. 4. Transfer of the FCU to the ECRB (*A*) or transfer of FCU to the EDC (*B*) improves wrist extension. The tendon may be transferred subcutaneously to provide a supination moment or through the interosseous membrane to provide more dorsiflexion without supination. (*Reproduced from* Koman LA, editor. Wake Forest University School of Medicine orthopedic manual 2001. Winston-Salem (NC): Orthopaedic Press; 2001. © Wake Forest University Orthopaedic Press; with permission.)

superficialis (FDS) and/or flexor digitorum profundus (FDP) spasticity is present; the digital extensors may also be weak. Lengthening of the shortened flexors is the appropriate treatment method for this deformity; power reinforcement of the finger extensors may also be performed. Preferably, the FCU or the FDS tendon of the ring finger is transferred to the EDC. One or two FDS tendons may be used; most frequently, the long and ring finger tendons are selected.

Depending on the severity of the deformity, flexor lengthening may be achieved by various interventions. Intramuscular BTX-A injections followed by serial muscle stretching is a nonoperative option. In mild to moderate cases, fractional lengthening of the individual FDS tendons combined with BTX-A injections into both the lengthened FDS and the nonlengthened FDP musculotendinous units is preferred in the authors' institution; stretching, casting, and therapy should be applied after the initial procedure. More involved deformities may require an additional fractional or Z-lengthening of the FDP tendons. The FDS to FDP transfer may also be performed.[33]

In severe cases, a flexor-pronator origin release (slide) is recommended. Caution should be

exercised when performing this procedure; the risk of overlengthening of the flexor-pronator mass is increased. This risk may be minimized by suturing the muscle mass in the optimal position to prevent overlengthening by injecting BTX-A or by a combination of both modalities.

Swan-neck deformity
The abnormal posture of the digits may adversely affect grasp function of the hand because of the inability to flex the fingers from the hyperextended position at the proximal interphalangeal (PIP) joint. Although effective treatment is difficult, the deformity can be managed by central slip tenotomy,[39] PIP tenodesis,[40] and lateral band translocation procedures.[41] Intrinsic origin release may also be beneficial.

Thumb-in-palm deformity
Thumb-in-palm deformity limits the grasp-and-release function of the hand in patients with CP. The deformity consists of static (due to contracture) and/or dynamic (due to spasticity) shortening of the adductor pollicis, first dorsal interosseous, and flexor pollicis longus (FPL) muscles; the adductors and flexors of the thumb may be

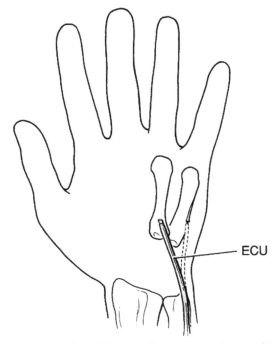

Fig. 5. Transfer of the ECU from its insertion on the fifth metacarpal to the fourth metacarpal decreases ulnar deviation and assist extension of the wrist. The extensor retinaculum should be released to allow dorsal translation of the ECU tendon. (*Reproduced from* Koman LA, editor. Wake Forest University School of Medicine orthopedic manual 2001. Winston-Salem (NC): Orthopaedic Press; 2001. © Wake Forest University Orthopaedic Press; with permission.)

affected in various combinations. In addition, muscles involved in active extension and abduction of the thumb may be weak; extensor pollicis brevis (EPB), extensor pollicis longus (EPL), and abductor pollicis longus (APL) are overstretched due to prolonged abnormal thumb and wrist position. The wide spectrum of contributing factors is completed by instability of the metacarpophalangeal (MCP) joint and the fixed contracture of the skin and soft tissue covering the first web space.

Surgical treatment of this complex deformity usually includes various combinations of muscle releases, tendon transfers, and joint stabilization procedures. Preoperative voluntary muscle control quality has been reported to be one of the most important factors in predicting the success of the operation. Limited sensory capability is a relative contraindication for the use of complex surgical procedures. Therefore, a careful assessment of the patient's thumb function must serve as the basis for all treatment decisions.[9]

Thumb adduction deformity can be managed with careful release of the adductor pollicis and/or first dorsal interosseous muscles. Z-lengthening of the adductor pollicis is another choice (**Fig. 6**). Adductor pollicis release is obtained by sectioning its origin from the third metacarpal through a palmar incision, along the thenar eminence crease.[42] In addition, a 4-flap Z-plasty rearranges the skin and soft tissues of the first web space (**Fig. 7**).

Surgery is indicated to hold the thumb out of the palm during grasp and to permit lateral pinch.

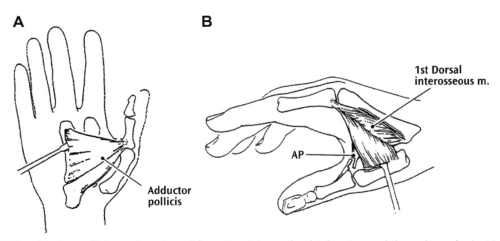

Fig. 6. The adductor pollicis may be released from its origin on the third metacarpal through a volar incision (*A*); alternatively, the adductor tendon may be Z-lengthened or transferred proximally to the first metacarpal to increase the first web space, (*B*) the first dorsal interosseous may be released from the first metacarpal. (*Reproduced from* Koman LA, editor. Wake Forest University School of Medicine orthopedic manual 2001. Winston-Salem (NC): Orthopaedic Press; 2001. © Wake Forest University Orthopaedic Press; with permission.)

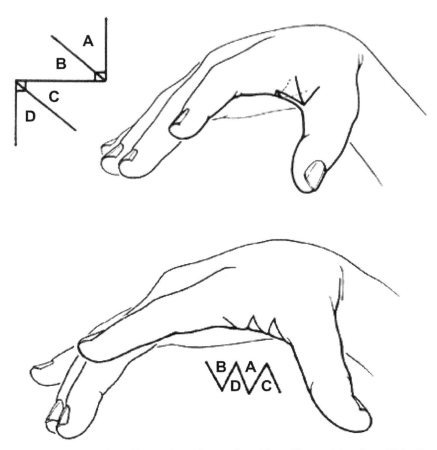

Fig. 7. Schematic presentation of a 4-flap Z-plasty. (*Reproduced from* Koman LA, editor. Wake Forest University School of Medicine orthopedic manual 2001. Winston-Salem (NC): Orthopaedic Press; 2001. © Wake Forest University Orthopaedic Press; with permission.)

Adduction deformity is not fully corrected unless the APL is reinforced. This reinforcement can be accomplished by transfer of the brachioradialis to the APL.[43] Rerouting of the EPL tendon radial to Lister's tubercle has also been described to augment thumb abduction.

Flexion deformity of the thumb may be an additional feature of the thumb-in-palm posture. Therefore, procedures designed to reinforce the thumb extensors should be included in the therapeutic protocol. The EPL tendon may be sectioned, rerouted through the first dorsal compartment, plicated, and reattached to the EPB at the MCP joint.[44] The brachioradialis or FDS tendon of the ring finger may be used to augment the thumb extensor. Before improving extensor power, fractional or Z-lengthening procedures are used to address FPL fixed contractures (**Fig. 8**). The contracted and spastic FPL is usually weak; either the brachioradialis or another tendon may be transferred to improve its overall strength.[5]

Pure MCP joint hyperextension instability may be improved by volar plate capsulodesis[45]; however, if this procedure fails, MCP fusion can be used to control thumb hyperextension.[46] Arthrodesis of the MCP joint has also proved to be a successful method for global instability of the thumb. In children, damage to the epiphyseal line can be minimized by the use of transitory thin fixation pins.[4] If tendon transfers fail to overcome an MCP flexion deformity, MCP fusion may be performed to improve the position of the thumb.[47]

POSTOPERATIVE CARE

Appropriate postoperative care is necessary to achieve the optimal surgical result. Preferably, input from therapists regarding the postoperative therapy and splinting regimen should be included in the preoperative planning. The initial 3 to 4 weeks of postoperative care are crucial for

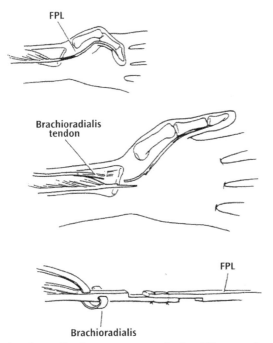

FPL

Brachioradialis tendon

FPL

Brachioradialis

Fig. 8. A fixed contracture of the FPL may be managed by Z-lengthening as demonstrated or more proximally by fractional lengthening (not shown). Reinforcement may be achieved as demonstrated by transfer of the brachioradialis proximal to the Z-lengthening. (*Reproduced from* Koman LA, editor. Wake Forest University School of Medicine orthopedic manual 2001. Winston-Salem (NC): Orthopaedic Press; 2001. © Wake Forest University Orthopaedic Press; with permission.)

a successful outcome; active and passive ROM of the contiguous joints (the operative site is protected by pins and rigid splinting or casting during this period) should be maintained or improved, and tendon transfers should be protected. Intramuscular injections of BTX-A may be used to protect tendon repairs associated with lengthening and/or transfer procedures; with this intervention, the postoperative pain is decreased, earlier active motion is permitted, and overlengthening following fractional procedures is prevented.[48] Following the initial healing phase, active and passive ROM protocols are implemented, and static splinting is used as indicated. At 6 to 10 weeks following surgery, a strengthening exercise program is initiated; the inclusion of a home program is an important component of the rehabilitation process.

SUMMARY

Although only a small percentage of children and adults with CP are candidates for upper extremity

surgery, the judicious use of the surgical procedures discussed in this article can result in positive outcomes and improve the health-related quality of life of patients. However, proper selection of patients is crucial to ensure reasonable postoperative results, and postoperative care must be coordinated with appropriately trained hand therapists for optimal results.

REFERENCES

1. Carroll RE. The surgical treatment of cerebral palsy. I. The upper extremity. Surg Clin North Am 1950;31:385–90.
2. Green WT, Banks HH. Flexor carpi ulnaris transplant and its use in cerebral palsy. J Bone Joint Surg Am 1962;44:1343–430.
3. Goldner JL. Upper extremity tendon transfers in cerebral palsy. Orthop Clin North Am 1974;5:389–414.
4. Goldner JL, Koman LA, Gelberman R, et al. Arthrodesis of the metacarpophalangeal joint of the thumb in children and adults. Adjunctive treatment of thumb-in-palm deformity in cerebral palsy. Clin Orthop Relat Res 1990;253:75–89.
5. Koman LA, Gelberman RH, Toby EB, et al. Cerebral palsy. Management of the upper extremity. Clin Orthop Relat Res 1990;253:62–74.
6. Eames NW, Baker R, Hill N, et al. The effect of botulinum toxin A on gastrocnemius length: magnitude and duration of response. Dev Med Child Neurol 1999;41:226–32.
7. Tardieu C, Lespargot A, Tabary C, et al. For how long must the soleus muscle be stretched each day to prevent contracture? Dev Med Child Neurol 1988;30:3–10.
8. Goldner JL. Reconstructive surgery of the hand in cerebral palsy and spastic paralysis resulting from injury to the spinal cord. J Bone Joint Surg Am 1955;37:1141–53.
9. House JH, Gwathmey FW, Fidler MO. A dynamic approach to the thumb-in palm deformity in cerebral palsy. J Bone Joint Surg Am 1981;63:216–25.
10. Johnson LM, Randall MJ, Reddihough DS, et al. Development of a clinical assessment of quality of movement for unilateral upper-limb function. Dev Med Child Neurol 1994;36:965–73.
11. Randall M, Carlin JB, Chondros P, et al. Reliability of the Melbourne assessment of unilateral upper limb function. Dev Med Child Neurol 2001;43:761–7.
12. Bourke-Taylor H. Melbourne Assessment of Unilateral Upper Limb Function: construct validity and correlation with the Pediatric Evaluation of Disability Inventory. Dev Med Child Neurol 2003;45:92–6.
13. Koman LA, Williams RM, Evans PJ, et al. Quantification of upper extremity function and range of motion

in children with cerebral palsy. Dev Med Child Neurol 2008;50:910—7.

14. Hoffer MM, Perry J, Melkonian GJ. Dynamic electromyography and decision-making for surgery in the upper extremity of patients with cerebral palsy. J Hand Surg Am 1979;4:424—31.

15. Hoffer MM, Lehman M, Mitani M. Long-term follow-up on tendon transfers to the extensors of the wrist and fingers in patients with cerebral palsy. J Hand Surg Am 1986;11:836—40.

16. Mowery CA, Gelberman RH, Rhoades CE. Upper extremity tendon transfers in cerebral palsy: electromyographic and functional analysis. J Pediatr Orthop 1985;5:69—72.

17. Carlson MG, Spincola LJ, Lewin J, et al. Impact of video review on surgical procedure determination for patients with cerebral palsy. J Hand Surg Am 2009;34:1225—31.

18. Autti-Ramo I, Larsen A, Peltonen J, et al. Botulinum toxin injection as an adjunct when planning hand surgery in children with spastic hemiplegia. Neuropediatrics 2000;31:4—8.

19. Zancolli EA, Zancolli E Jr. Surgical rehabilitation of the spastic upper limb in cerebral palsy. In: Lamb DW, editor. The paralysed hand. Edinburgh (UK): Churchill Livingstone; 1987. p. 153—68.

20. Landi A, Cavazza S, Caserta G, et al. The upper limb in cerebral palsy: surgical management of shoulder and elbow deformities. Hand Clin 2003;19:631—48, vii.

21. Braun RM, Botte MJ. Treatment of shoulder deformity in acquired spasticity. Clin Orthop Relat Res 1999;368:54—65.

22. Mital MA. Lengthening of the elbow flexors in cerebral palsy. J Bone Joint Surg Am 1979;61:515—22.

23. Pletcher DF, Hoffer MM, Koffman DM. Non-traumatic dislocation of the radial head in cerebral palsy. J Bone Joint Surg Am 1976;58:104—5.

24. Gschwind CR. Surgical management of forearm pronation. Hand Clin 2003;19:649—55.

25. Sakellarides HT, Mital MA, Lenzi WD. Treatment of pronation contractures of the forearm in cerebral palsy by changing the insertion of the pronator radii teres. J Bone Joint Surg Am 1981;63:645—52.

26. Page CM. Four cases of flexion contracture of the forearm treated by a muscle-sliding operation. Proc R Soc Med 1923;16:43—5.

27. Braun RM, Mooney V, Nickel VL. Flexor-origin release for pronation-flexion deformity of the forearm and hand in the stroke patient. An evaluation of the early results in eighteen patients. J Bone Joint Surg Am 1970;52:907—20.

28. Green WT. Tendon transplantation of the flexor carpi ulnaris for pronation-flexion deformity of the wrist. Surg Gynecol Obstet 1942;75:337—42.

29. Ozkan T, Tuncer S, Aydin A, et al. Brachioradialis rerouting for the restoration of active supination and correction of forearm pronation deformity in cerebral palsy. J Hand Surg Br 2004;29:265—70.

30. Pollock GA. Surgical treatment of cerebral palsy. J Bone Joint Surg Br 1962;44-B:68—81.

31. Tonkin MA. The upper limb in cerebral palsy. Curr Orthop 1995;9:149—55.

32. Perry J, Hoffer MM. Preoperative and postoperative dynamic electromyography as an aid in planning tendon transfers in children with cerebral palsy. J Bone Joint Surg Am 1977;59:531—7.

33. Carlson MG, Athwal GS, Bueno RA. Treatment of the wrist and hand in cerebral palsy. J Hand Surg Am 2006;31:483—90.

34. Van Heest AE. Surgical management of wrist and finger deformity. Hand Clin 2003;19:657—65.

35. Omer GE, Capen DA. Proximal row carpectomy with muscle transfers for spastic paralysis. J Hand Surg Am 1976;1:197—204.

36. Tonkin M, Gschwind C. Surgery for cerebral palsy: Part 2. Flexion deformity of the wrist and fingers. J Hand Surg Br 1992;17:396—400.

37. Hoffer MM, Zeitzew S. Wrist fusion in cerebral palsy. J Hand Surg Am 1988;13:667—70.

38. Szabo RM, Gelberman RH. Operative treatment of cerebral palsy. Hand Clin 1985;1:525—43.

39. Carlson MG, Gallagher K, Spirtos M. Surgical treatment of swan-neck deformity in hemiplegic cerebral palsy. J Hand Surg Am 2007;32:1418—22.

40. Swanson AB. Treatment of the swan-neck deformity in the cerebral palsied hand. Clin Orthop Relat Res 1966;48:167—71.

41. Tonkin MA, Hughes J, Smith KL. Lateral band translocation for swan-neck deformity. J Hand Surg Am 1992;17:260—7.

42. Matev I. Surgical treatment of spastic "thumb-in-palm" deformity. J Bone Joint Surg Br 1963;45:703—8.

43. McCue FC, Honner R, Chapman WC. Transfer of the brachioradialis for hands deformed by cerebral palsy. J Bone Joint Surg Am 1970;52:1171—80.

44. Manske PR. Redirection of extensor pollicis longus in the treatment of spastic thumb-in-palm deformity. J Hand Surg Am 1985;10:553—60.

45. Tonkin MA, Beard AJ, Kemp SJ, et al. Sesamoid arthrodesis for hyperextension of the thumb metacarpophalangeal joint. J Hand Surg Am 1995;20:334—8.

46. Tonkin M, Freitas A, Koman A, et al. The surgical management of thumb deformity in cerebral palsy. J Hand Surg Eur Vol 2008;33:77—80.

47. Tonkin MA, Hatrick NC, Eckersley JR, et al. Surgery for cerebral palsy part 3: classification and operative procedures for thumb deformity. J Hand Surg Br 2001;26:465—70.

48. Ma J, Shen J, Smith BP, et al. Bioprotection of tendon repair: adjunctive use of botulinum toxin A in Achilles tendon repair in the rat. J Bone Joint Surg Am 2007;89:2241—9.

Management of Spinal Deformity in Cerebral Palsy

Meghan N. Imrie, MD[a,b,c], Burt Yaszay, MD[d,e],*

KEYWORDS
- Cerebral palsy • Scoliosis • Neuromuscular scoliosis
- Surgical management

An understanding of the three-dimensional components of spinal deformity in children with cerebral palsy (CP) is necessary to recommend treatments that will positively affect these patients' quality of life. Management of these deformities can be challenging and orthopedic surgeons should be familiar with the different treatments available for this patient population.

INCIDENCE

The incidence of scoliosis in CP varies greatly, from 6% to almost 100%; but the generally accepted incidence in the overall CP population is 20% to 25%.[1–5] The rate varies depending on the particular study, the type of CP, the severity of neurologic involvement, and ambulatory status. The incidence is highest in patients with spastic CP (about 70%) and lowest in those with athetoid type (from 6%–50%).[2,6] Madigan and Wallace,[2] in their survey of institutionalized CP patients published in 1981, found that 64% of the 272 patients studied had scoliosis greater than 10 degrees on screening radiographs and that the incidence of scoliosis was related to severity of neurologic involvement. In support of this conclusion, they pointed to the inverse relationship of ambulatory status and scoliosis (44% of independent ambulators, 54% of dependent ambulators, 61% of independent sitters, and 75% of dependent sitters or bedridden residents). Patients with subluxated or dislocated hips (an indicator of disease severity) were also found to have a 75% to 77% incidence of scoliosis. Interestingly, there was no difference between patients with unilateral or bilaterally dislocated hips, underscoring the importance of severity of involvement rather than the balance of the pelvis. Kalen and colleagues[7] found that none of their patients with curves greater than 45 degrees were ambulators, whereas 34% of those with curves less than 45 degrees were. The incidence of scoliosis is directly related to their gross motor function classification system (GMFCS) level.

CAUSE

The cause of scoliosis in CP is not entirely clear, but is thought to be due to some combination of muscle weakness, truncal imbalance, and asymmetric tone in paraspinous and intercostal muscles. Whether the development of scoliosis is due to the primary cerebral insult or due to its secondary consequences is also unclear. In addition, there is some data to suggest that certain spasticity treatments, namely selective dorsal rhizotomy (SDR) and intrathecal baclofen, may result in progressive scoliosis. SDR is done with the intention of decreasing the spasticity. It has been implicated by some investigators in increasing spinal deformities with the incidence of scoliosis ranging from 16% to 57%.[8–15] Other

[a] Department of Orthopaedic Surgery, Stanford University, Stanford, CA, USA
[b] Lucile Packard Children's Hospital, Palo Alto, CA, USA
[c] 300 Pasteur Drive, Edwards Building, R 105, Stanford, CA 94305-5341, USA
[d] Department of Orthopaedic Surgery, Rady Children's Hospital and Health Center, 3030 Children's Way, Ste 410, San Diego, CA 92123, USA
[e] University of California, San Diego, CA, USA
* Corresponding author.
E-mail address: byaszay@rchsd.org

Orthop Clin N Am 41 (2010) 531–547
doi:10.1016/j.ocl.2010.06.008
0030-5898/10/$ – see front matter © 2010 Elsevier Inc. All rights reserved.

investigators, however, have demonstrated no significant spinal deformity following SDR. Spiegel and colleagues[12] reported scoliosis in only 17% of their ambulatory CP patients. Recently, Langerak and colleagues[8] evaluated the long-term follow-up of their patients who underwent SDR 17 to 26 years prior and compared this to the short-term results of those same patients. They found 57% of patients at long-term follow-up had scoliosis while none of the patients at short-term follow-up demonstrated scoliosis. The majority of curves were less than 30 degrees. Whereas this was statistically significant, it was not felt to be clinically important. The relationship between SDR and long-term, clinically significant spinal deformity is still unclear, but it is generally felt to be safe when done with great attention to maintaining the integrity of the laminae. The ideal candidates for a SDR are patients with pure spasticity and good trunk control (usually GMFCS I and II). These patients rarely develop scoliosis. SDR should probably not be performed in the GMFCS IV and V patients as they often have a mixed type CP with dystonia predominating.

In the case of intrathecal baclofen, there have been a few retrospective reviews and case reports suggesting more rapid progression of a scoliotic curve following baclofen pump insertion,[16–18] with the most recent of these studies reporting a sixfold increase.[16] In contrast, Shilt and colleagues[19] compared 50 patients with CP who had intrathecal baclofen pump insertion with matched controls and found no difference. Once again, the patients who receive a baclofen pump are usually the more severely involved patients and, therefore, their natural history is to have progressive scoliosis. As in the case of SDR, a causal relationship between intrathecal baclofen and progressive scoliosis has not been clearly established and further long-term, randomized, prospective study is needed.

DIFFERENCES WITH ADOLESCENT IDIOPATHIC SCOLIOSIS

There are several key differences between patients with CP and scoliosis and those with adolescent idiopathic scoliosis (AIS). The curves in patients with CP, especially those more profoundly affected, tend to occur at an earlier age than in AIS.[3] They, therefore, have a propensity to develop into larger, and stiffer, curves. As in AIS, larger curves are likely to progress after maturity. Thometz and Simon[4] found that curves greater than 50 degrees at skeletal maturity in patients with severe CP progressed at a rate of 1.4 degrees per year. Unlike AIS, severity of neural

involvement, ambulatory status, and curve location also impact the rate of curve progression following skeletal maturity.[3] In addition, skeletal maturity may be delayed in patients with CP; some maintain open growth plates early in the third decade.[20] The shape of the curve in CP may be different than that in AIS. In more severely affected patients with CP, long C-shaped curves and left-sided curves are not uncommon. Madigan and Wallace[2] found an equal distribution between single "C" curves and multiple or "S" curves in their institutionalized patients with scoliosis, although 67% of their bed-ridden group had "C" curves versus only 22% of the independent sitters. In that same study, 14 of the 42 thoracic "C" curves were convex to the left and 12 of the 28 double major curves had a thoracic component convex to the left. The CP curves also typically have greater deformity in the sagittal plane, either being kyphotic or lordotic. Finally, the associated pelvic obliquity seen in the CP patient separates their curve type from the typical AIS patient. As discussed later, these distinctions result in different approaches for the management of CP scoliosis and AIS. For example, bracing is less effective in halting curve progression in CP patients and is less tolerated due to patient comorbidities and movement disorders.[21–23] The planning and execution of spinal fusion is more difficult as these patients often require longer fusions to the pelvis. More important, many CP patients are more medically fragile than a typical idiopathic patient and often require multidisciplinary management.

NATURAL HISTORY

There have been several studies on the natural history of untreated scoliosis in patients with CP, looking at factors related to progression and at the impact untreated scoliosis may have on the patients' overall function and health. Factors implicated in progression include type of involvement (quadriplegia), poor functional status (nonambulatory), and curve location (thoracolumbar). Thometz and Simon[4] found that progression was most rapid for thoracolumbar curves, followed by lumbar curves, with thoracic curves having the slowest rate. Saito and colleagues[3] evaluated 37 institutionalized patients with severe spastic CP who were followed for an average of 17.3 years, from childhood to adulthood, and identified the following risk factors for progression: a spinal curve greater than 40 degrees before age 15 years, total body involvement, being bedridden, and a thoracolumbar curve. Untreated severe scoliosis is generally thought to have detrimental effects on patients' overall health and function specifically the cardiopulmonary system and sitting balance. Majd and colleagues,[6] in their survey of institutionalized adults with CP, found that those patients who experienced a decline in function had the greatest Cobb angle and rate of progression (80 vs 56 degrees and 4.4 vs 3.0 degrees per year respectively). Saito and colleagues[3] found that 20 of their 37 patients required increased amounts of nursing time to complete various activities of daily living. The average Cobb angle for those 20 patients was 73 degrees versus 34 degrees in those patients who did not require increased assistance. Conversely, Kalen and colleagues[7] did not demonstrate any difference in the incidence of decubiti, highest functional level achieved, functional loss, oxygen saturation, or pulse in CP patients with untreated scoliosis greater than 45 degrees as compared with those with mild or no curves. Finally, the importance of sitting balance in significantly affected patients cannot be underestimated. As curve severity increases beyond wheelchair modification capabilities, a patient may need to rely on his or her upper extremities to help maintain an upright position, thereby becoming a "functional quadriplegic."[24]

TREATMENT
Nonsurgical

The role of nonsurgical treatment in CP patients with scoliosis is very different than in the AIS population. Nonoperative treatment options still consist of observation and bracing, but also include seating modifications and medical management. The goals of any intervention are to maintain comfortable upright sitting and to allow the functional use of the upper extremities, thereby maximizing a patient's ability to interact with his or her environment. Observation is indicated for small curves that do not cause any functional deficit. Bracing is used in CP patients but, unlike in AIS, it is not used with the intention of stopping curve progression. There is some evidence that brace use may slow curve progression in CP patients.[21,25] Unfortunately, this is inconclusive with other investigators demonstrating no clinically significant effect of bracing on curve progression.[22,26,27] This may be caused by the great differences in achievement of skeletal maturity in CP. In general, soft braces are tolerated in spastic patients better than rigid orthoses, both in maintaining skin integrity[28] and minimizing respiratory compromise.[23] Bracing should remain an option for physicians treating scoliosis in CP patients, but for different intended purposes than in AIS. They can assist in sitting balance, as well as potentially slow curve progression—especially in young

patients or in hypotonic ambulatory patients with short thoracolumbar curves less than 40 degrees.[21]

Another option for patients that are wheelchair-dependent and cannot tolerate a brace is to provide seating modifications. This usually involves adapting a patient's wheelchair with various supports. It does not alter the natural history of the scoliosis. There are a variety of seating modifications that can be used—from custom-molded seatbacks for patients with severe spinal deformity to 2- and 3-point body support systems. The 3-point force configuration has been shown to achieve the best static correction of the scoliotic spine based on external measurements,[29] but modifications should be individually determined and tailored. Numerous alternative modalities have also been investigated, including physical therapy, electrical stimulation, and botulinum toxin A. Physical therapy and electrical stimulation have not been shown to be effective. Although botulinum toxin A is increasingly being used to treat limb spasticity in CP patients, there is scant evidence for its use in treating scoliosis. Nuzzo and colleagues[30] retrospectively reviewed patients with paralytic scoliosis who had a delay in surgical intervention that were treated with botulinum toxin as a supplement to other treatment modalities. No patient had any worsening of their scoliosis and some had a reduction in their Cobb angle.

Surgical

The definitive treatment for progressive, debilitating scoliosis in patients with CP is surgical intervention, with the goals being to halt progression, level the pelvis, and achieve good frontal and sagittal balance. There is no strict guideline for when surgery is absolutely indicated. Most investigators consider fusion for curves that progress beyond 50 degrees or for those that lead to a deterioration in functional sitting.[3,27,31-33] However, each patient, their families and caretakers, their deformity, and their specific comorbidities must be taken into consideration before embarking on treatment. The physician who treats neuromuscular scoliosis must be prepared to address the inherent complications routinely encountered in this patient population. Thorough preoperative evaluation, coherent multidisciplinary management, careful preoperative surgical planning, and safe intraoperative execution are all required for a successful outcome.

Preoperative evaluation
A comprehensive preoperative evaluation, including history, physical, laboratory, and

radiographic studies, is imperative and a multidisciplinary approach is helpful (**Table 1**).

Musculoskeletal The history should focus on ambulatory ability and GMFCS level, as well as the details of the patient's sitting or standing posture, upper extremity function, and any parent or caregiver concerns. In the physical examination, the clinician should note the patient's overall balance and ability to interact with his or her environment, as well as the level of voluntary muscle control. Depending on functional level, the curvature of the spine should be evaluated in the coronal and sagittal plane when standing, sitting, or supine. A push-pull examination can give some sense of the overall flexibility of the curve. A detailed lower extremity examination should note any hip flexion contractures, which may lead to lumbar hyperlordosis and may make intraoperative prone positioning more difficult. Any significant hamstring tightness should also be noted as it can severely limit hip flexion, leading to "sacral sitting" and decreased lumbar lordosis or increased thoracic kyphosis.[34] Finally, any hip adduction contracture or windswept deformity should also be noted because these are thought to be infrapelvic causes of pelvic obliquity. It is not entirely clear whether the scoliosis or hip asymmetry develops first, or if prevention of hip subluxation or dislocation decreases the frequency or severity of scoliosis,[35–41] but it is likely that hip asymmetry, pelvic obliquity, and scoliosis are interrelated and may exacerbate each other. In some cases, correction of the spinal deformity may worsen the hip positioning, necessitating further surgical intervention in the hip. Caregivers should be counseled on this before the spinal surgery. Finally, overall skin integrity should be evaluated and any areas of skin maceration or decubiti noted and appropriately treated.

Neurology Patients with CP may have a concomitant seizure disorder, and it is important to note the presence or absence of any seizure activity, medications used to control the condition, and whether the seizures are well controlled. Certain antiseizure medications have side effects that should factor into perioperative evaluation. Phenytoin, phenobarbital, and valproic acid have all been shown to alter vitamin D metabolism and intestinal calcium absorption. Patients taking any one of these medications will typically have lower bone mineral density,[42,43] which may impact implant fixation. In addition, valproic acid has been implicated in prolonged bleeding times, excessive blood loss, and increased need for blood products in those patients taking the medication and

undergoing spine surgery.[44,45] Chambers and colleagues[44] found a threefold increased risk of losing greater than 30 mL/kg of blood in patients taking valproic acid who had a single abnormal clotting test. Based on the concern for increased blood loss perioperatively, consideration should be given to replacing valproic acid with another antiepileptic medication, preferably at least 1 month before surgery. Finally, it should be noted whether the patient has had an intrathecal baclofen pump placed. In most cases, the pump must be turned off if intra-operative neuromonitoring is to be used. Proper supplies to repair the tubing should be available if an inadvertent break occurs during the course of the surgery. In some cases, an elective ligation can be done to minimize the risk of pulling it out of the thecal sac with a repair done before incision closure.

Pulmonary Patients with CP are already prone to poor pulmonary function due to many causes such as abnormal oropharyngeal tone and anatomic abnormalities. This diminished respiratory status may be further exacerbated by a large scoliotic curve. Formal pulmonary function tests are difficult and unreliable in significantly affected patients. Indirect signs of vital capacity include crying, laughing, and vocalizations.[46–48] Impaired vital capacity and forced expiratory volume in the first second increases the risk for prolonged mechanical ventilation.[49] The frequency of pneumonia over the preceding year is one of the predictors of postoperative pulmonary complications, and frequent coughing, choking, and sputtering during feedings may be a sign of aspiration risk. Patients at increased risk for aspiration may benefit from a gastrostomy tube (G-tube) and possible Nissen fundoplication before spine surgery.[46]

Gastrointestinal or nutritional Gastroesophageal reflux (GERD) and malnutrition play important roles in the perioperative evaluation. Many CP patients have significant GERD, which places them at increased risk of aspiration, reactive airway disease, and diminished nutritional status. Borkhuu and colleagues[50] recently demonstrated that preoperative GERD with feeding difficulties resulted in a 52% increased chance in developing postoperative pancreatitis, resulting in a longer hospital stay. Malnourishment has been shown to increase the risk of postoperative complications in this patient population; weight for chronologic age below the fifth percentile is associated with an increased postoperative complication score.[51] In addition, it has been shown that CP patients with a preoperative serum albumin less than

Table 1
Preoperative checklist when considering treatment of scoliosis in patients with CP

	Musculoskeletal	Neurologic	Pulmonary	Gastrointestinal or Nutritional	Hematologic
History	• GMFCS level • Caretaker concerns	• Seizure disorder controlled? Medications • Baclofen pump?	• Number of pneumonias in last year? • Respiratory hospital admissions? • Use of bipap or cpap?	• Assess aspiration risk • Intake: oral vs G-tube	• Bleeding with previous operation? • Any family history of bleeding disorders?
Physical Examination	• Coronal or sagittal balance • Hip examination • Skin integrity	• Any voluntary muscle control?	• Is child vocal • Assess airway obstruction	• Weight • Consider instrumentation prominence • Wound closure issues	—
Laboratory Tests	—	—		• Albumin/Prealbumin • Total blood lymphocyte count	• Blood count • Coagulation • Type and cross
Radiographs	• Sitting anteroposterior or lateral scoliosis films • Traction vs bend films	—	• Chest radiograph	—	—
Preoperative intervention	• Consider addressing hip contractures	• Consider changing to different seizure medicine if on valproic acid	• Consider G-tube if aspiration risk • Pulmonary evaluation	• Consider G-tube if aspiration risk • Increase nutritional support	• Correct coagulopathy
Perioperative considerations	• Intraoperative traction • Possible anterior release or fusion	• Neuromonitoring	• Postoperative mechanical ventilation	—	• Consider antifibrinolytic

35 g/L and total blood lymphocyte count less than 1.5 g/L have an increased infection rate, longer length of intubation, and longer hospital stay.[52] Preoperative labs should include measures of nutrition (albumin, prealbumin, total blood lymphocyte count) and, if low, procedures to optimize feeding orally or via G-tube should be taken to improve nutritional status before surgery.

Hematologic Patients with neuromuscular scoliosis are at risk for significant perioperative blood loss with some cases exceeding 200% of a patient's blood volume.[47] This may be due to many factors, including need for longer fusion, poor nutritional status, use of medications such as valproic acid, and a decrease in clotting factors.[53,54] Attention should be paid to any history of excessive bleeding in prior surgeries. Standard labs include hemoglobin level, prothrombin time, partial thromboplastin time, platelet count, and bleeding time. A more thorough coagulation work-up should be undertaken if there is a history of excessive bleeding during previous surgeries. Preoperative recombinant human erythropoietin, which has been shown to decrease perioperative transfusion rates in idiopathic and adult patients, has not been shown to have a significant clinical benefit in neuromuscular patients.[55]

Imaging studies Standard radiographs include anteroposterior and lateral of the entire spine, standing or seated if possible. The anteroposterior should be evaluated for curve type, curve magnitude, spinal balance, spinal rotation, and amount and direction of pelvic obliquity. Pelvic obliquity can be measured several ways, but is most reliable when measured from the horizontal; that is, the angle subtended by a line drawn across the top of the iliac crests and the perpendicular to a line drawn from T1 and S1.[56] The hips should be evaluated for subluxation or dislocation. The lateral is important for assessing overall sagittal balance, as well as evaluating for spondylolisthesis, because the incidence in patients with spastic diplegia has been reported as high as 21%.[57] A variety of special films can be taken to assess the flexibility of the spinal deformity, including bending, fulcrum bending, push-pull, and traction. In general, for this patient population, voluntary side-bending radiographs cannot be reliably obtained and traction radiographs are therefore preferred.

Surgical planning and perioperative considerations

There are several considerations to address when planning surgical correction of scoliosis in CP patients. These include the extent of the fusion, what type of instrumentation to use, and whether an anterior approach is indicated.

Extent of fusion For most CP scoliotic curves, the proximal instrumentation should end fairly high in the thoracic spine, generally around T2, to decrease the risk of proximal junctional kyphosis and pullout of proximal instrumentation.[58,59] This should also prevent any development of scoliosis above the instrumented level. The caudal extent of the fusion, most notably when to include the sacrum and pelvis, is a topic still under some debate, especially in an ambulatory patient. Several investigators report success fusing only to L5 when the pelvic obliquity is less than 15 degrees and there is some potential for ambulation.[60–62] Both Whitaker and colleagues[61] and McCall and Hayes[62] used pedicle screws at the most caudal level, and felt that this contributed to the stability of the construct. Even for nonambulatory patients, McCall and Hayes[62] have suggested that sparing the pelvis and maintaining a mobile L5/S1 segment may better absorb trunk movements during wheelchair activities. However, most investigators recommend fusing to the pelvis for curves that have significant pelvic obliquity.[31–33,59,63–66] Modi and colleagues[66] evaluated postoperative changes in pelvic obliquity in 55 neuromuscular patients with scoliosis with a minimum follow-up of 2 years. Those patients with pelvic obliquity greater than 15 degrees that had fixation to the pelvis had good correction of this obliquity and maintained it at follow-up. However, those with obliquity greater than 15 degrees that did not have pelvic fixation had good initial correction, but progressively lost this correction over time. Tsirikos and colleagues[67] found no alteration in ambulatory status in 24 ambulatory CP patients who underwent fusion to the pelvis, except in one patient who developed severe bilateral hip heterotopic ossification. In general, any patient with significant pelvic obliquity, ambulatory or not, should be fused to the pelvis.

Type of instrumentation Spinal instrumentation for neuromuscular scoliosis has evolved over the years since the introduction of the Harrington rod in 1962. Due to high pseudoarthrosis rates (11%–40%), modest initial correction (30%–55%), loss of correction over time (8%–28%), and need for prolonged bed rest or casting with Harrington rod instrumentation,[1,32,68,69] segmental spinal instrumentation as developed by Luque in 1976 was quickly adopted as a preferred method to treat scoliosis in neuromuscular patients. Numerous investigators demonstrated improved correction (40%–64%) with lower rates of pseudoarthrosis and decreased need for postoperative immobilization.[60,68,70–72] This was followed with a modification of the Luque-segmental spinal fixation in 1982 by Allen and Ferguson[63,73] to achieve pelvic fixation. This Galveston method was developed to extend the fusion to the pelvis to better correct pelvic obliquity and overall spinal balance (**Fig. 1**). Originally requiring intraoperative contouring of two separate Luque rods, the Galveston technique was later modified by Bell and colleagues[74] by developing the unit rod: a single, continuous stainless steel rod with a "U" bend at the rostral end and Galveston-type contouring at the caudal end. Numerous investigators have shown good correction with the unit rod. Bulman and colleagues[75] compared unit rod fixation to Luque rod instrumentation and found improved correction with the unit rod of both scoliosis (62% vs 49%) and pelvic obliquity (79% vs 50%). In one of the largest series, Tsirikos and colleagues[76] retrospectively evaluated 287 children treated with a unit rod; they reported an average Cobb correction rate of 68% and pelvic obliquity correction of 71%, with 96% caregiver satisfaction rate. The U-rod is similar to the unit rod, but it does not extend to the pelvis; instead, it ends in L5 pedicle screws.[62] Extending from its development and use in idiopathic scoliosis, multi-hook segmental systems such as the Cotrel-Dubousset and Isola instrumentation have also been used in neuromuscular patients, alone or as part of hybrid constructs.[65,77–79] Yazici and colleagues[79] evaluated 31 patients and reported scoliotic and pelvic obliquity correction rates of

64% and 82% respectively using Isola instrumentation with Galveston pelvic fixation. They suggested that this construct was the most effective in deformity correction as compared with Luque-Galveston, unit rod, or Cotrel-Dubousset instrumentation.

Recently, pedicle instrumentation has been successfully used for neuromuscular scoliosis. One of the first reports of its use in neuromuscular scoliosis is by Rodgers and colleagues[80] in patients with myelomeningocele. Since that time, there have numerous articles describing its successful use in CP patients.[81–85] The safety of pedicle screw placement in neuromuscular scoliosis patients using the free-hand technique has been evaluated; Modi and colleagues[82] evaluated 1,009 pedicle screws in 37 consecutive neuromuscular scoliosis patients by CT scan, and found that 93.3% were in the safe zone. In addition, Modi and colleagues[84] published the three-year follow-up data of 52 CP patients who underwent posterior spinal fusion with pedicle screw construct, reporting a 63% scoliosis correction and 56% pelvic obliquity correction. There were 17 major and minor complications in 15 patients; one of these was canal impingement by a screw causing leg weakness and urinary retention, which resolved following screw removal. Watanabe and colleagues[85] compared the radiographic outcomes of curves greater than 100 degrees, of which the majority were neuromuscular, treated at the apical level with either Luque wires, hooks, or pedicle screws. They found that the greatest Cobb correction rate, smallest loss of correction,

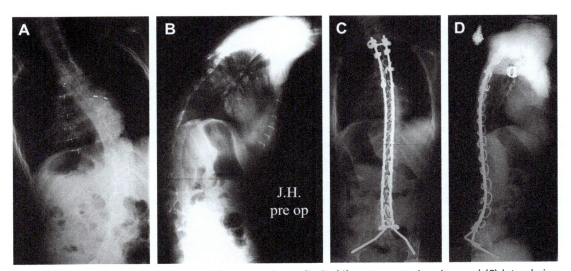

Fig. 1. Twelve-year-old GMFCS V male with progressive scoliosis: (*A*) anteroposterior view and (*B*) lateral view. Patient underwent a T2-pelvis posterior spinal fusion using Luque-Galveston instrumentation: (*C*) anteroposterior view and (*D*) lateral view. (*Courtesy of* Peter Newton, MD.)

and greatest amount of apical vertebral translation was in the pedicle screw group.

Similar to the many constructs used to instrument the spine, there are also many methods of addressing pelvic obliquity. The Galveston technique is the most popular and most tested, but iliac and sacral screws, spinopelvic transiliac fixation,[86] and an S-contoured rod that wraps over the sacral ala[87] have also been used. There are advantages and disadvantages to each method but, biomechanically, it appears to be important that the construct crosses a point anterior to the caudal projection of the middle column.[88] Peelle and colleagues[89] compared 20 neuromuscular patients treated with the Galveston method to 20 neuromuscular patients treated with iliac screws and found that there was no difference in Cobb correction, but better pelvic obliquity correction in the iliac screw group. In addition, there were four broken rods and two reoperations in the Galveston group versus one broken screw and no reoperations in the iliac screw group. Sponseller and colleagues,[90] on the other hand, recently compared unit rods with custom bent rods that commonly used iliac screws in 157 CP patients treated for scoliosis. They found improved pelvic obliquity correction with the unit rods, but with higher transfusion requirements and infection rates. In summary, Luque segmental spinal fixation with Galveston pelvic fixation has been successfully used since the 1980s and provides predictable and inexpensive correction, but not without complications. Increased use of pedicle screws has resulted in some improvement in deformity correction. It may also even further decrease the risk of pseudoarthrosis and a loss in correction. There is some controversy, however, whether this justifies the greater financial cost associated with pedicle screws. Currently, a prospective multicenter study is being conducted to evaluate the operative treatment of scoliosis in CP patients. Since various instrument types are included, some of these controversies may be answered.

Role of anterior approach Traditionally, the inclusion of anterior release and fusion has been to improve flexibility in large, stiff curves and to prevent crankshaft in young patients. To improve curve flexibility and, therefore, correction, anterior release and fusion is usually considered for curves greater than 70 to 100 degrees,[70,90,91] or those that do not bend down to 50 to 70 degrees on flexibility radiographs.[33,91,92] Significant sagittal deformity[92] and persistent pelvic obliquity on flexibility radiographs are also indications for anterior release.[31,93–95] However, the use of pedicle screws with more aggressive posterior-based releases or osteotomies have challenged these indications for an anterior procedure. There have been a few studies suggesting anterior release may not be necessary even in large, stiff curves. Suk and colleagues[96] reviewed 35 patients with curves over 70 degrees treated with posterior pedicle screw instrumentation and fusion only. Thoracic curve correction averaged 66% and lumbar curve correction averaged 59%. They concluded that severe curves of 70 to 105 degrees and greater than 25% flexibility can be successfully treated by posterior spinal fusion without anterior release. They did comment that an anterior release was performed for curves greater than 110 degrees and flexibility less than 20%. Watanabe and colleagues[85] reviewed 68 patients, 44 neuromuscular, with curves greater than 100 degrees treated (at the apical level) with wires, hooks, or pedicle screws. The pedicle screw group had the lowest rate of an anterior procedure with the best rate of correction. The investigators concluded that curves of 100 to 159 degrees can be acceptably and safely treated by posterior-only instrumentation and fusion using pedicle screw constructs. In the only study of exclusively neuromuscular patients, Suh and colleagues[97] reviewed 13 patients with curves greater than 100 degrees treated by posterior-only approach using pedicle screws and posterior multilevel vertebral osteotomies at the apex. The average preoperative Cobb was 118 degrees with only 20% flexibility. The average Cobb correction was 59.4% with 46.1% pelvic obliquity correction. There no neurologic or vascular injuries.

With regard to crankshaft, there is some evidence to suggest that an anterior approach is not always needed in younger patients. Smucker and Miller[98] looked at 50 CP patients with open triradiate cartilages treated with posterior-only spinal fusion with the unit rod. Twenty-nine had a closed triradiate on their most recent films and the mean absolute curve change postoperatively was 0.6 degrees (−9 to14 degrees). They concluded that posterior spinal fusion alone is adequate to control crankshaft in this skeletally immature population. Westerlund and colleagues[99] also found that acceptable curve correction and maintenance of correction can be achieved with posterior-only unit rod instrumentation, even in very skeletally immature patients.

For certain neuromuscular patients (deficient posterior elements, very young patients, ambulatory, nonprogressive curve), some surgeons recommend a selective anterior-only fusion.[100,101] Although this has not been widely studied in CP patients, the authors routinely perform an anterior instrumentation and fusion to control progressive scoliosis and pelvic obliquity in patients who are too young to undergo a typical T2 to pelvis fusion. This obviates the need for repeated surgeries with methods such as growing rods (**Fig. 2**). Typically, these patients will require a posterior fusion once they are more skeletally mature.

Perioperative traction Some investigators have recommended perioperative traction for very stiff, severe curves. Traction can be used preoperatively, intraoperatively, or between staged anterior and posterior procedures. Preoperative traction can consist of halo-gravity, halo-pelvic, halo-femoral, or halo-tibial methods. Halo-gravity has the benefit of allowing continued mobility without constant high traction forces. Proponents site improved trunk balance with decreased risk of neurologic complications.[102,103] Intraoperative traction has also been shown to safely improve postoperative alignment. Vialle and colleagues[95] compared the use of intraoperative asymmetric halo-lower extremity traction with standard intraoperative distraction and compression techniques in nonambulatory CP patients. They found better Cobb correction (63% vs 44%), better pelvic obliquity correction (81% vs 56%), and shorter operative times (282 minutes vs 334 minutes) in the traction group. The complication rate was comparable. Huang and Lenke[104] described their technique of intraoperative halo-femoral traction in a patient with CP and severe pelvic obliquity and scoliosis. They reported on their technique as a way to "straighten the scoliotic spine, level the pelvis, and thereby facilitate the posterior instrumentation." Takeshita and colleagues[105] followed this case report up with a retrospective review of 20 nonambulatory patients treated with intraoperative halo-femoral traction versus a control cohort of nonambulatory patients treated without traction. Their intraoperative traction set-up used a 4-pin halo and a 0.32-mm distal femoral Kirschner wire on the elevated pelvis side. Initially, 15 lbs of traction was placed on the halo side while an increasing amount of weight (average of 25 lbs) was placed on the femoral side until the pelvis was level. The investigators reported better pelvic obliquity correction in the traction group than in the control group, 78% versus 52%, with no traction-related complications. Halo-gravity traction can also be used safely between staged procedures to maximize the effect of the release and decrease the need for more aggressive intraoperative techniques.[106]

Neuromonitoring Despite their underlying neurologic disorder, intraoperative multimodality spinal cord monitoring generally has been recommended for CP patients.[107–109] As in idiopathic scoliosis, use of both transcranial electric motor evoked potentials (TceMEPs) and somatosensory evoked potentials (SSEPs) can be used. There is some concern about the use of TceMEPs in those patients with a seizure disorder, which can be common in many patients with CP. TceMEPs have been shown to reliably detect an impending injury to the corticospinal tract to allow for prompt corrective action before a neurologic deficit develops. SSEPs have been used for many years

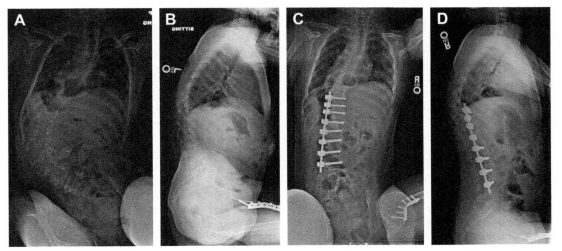

Fig. 2. Eight-year-old GMFCS V with 110 degrees scoliosis and severe pelvic obliquity had difficulty with sitting and hygiene at concavity of curvature: (*A*) anteroposterior view and (*B*) lateral view. Patient underwent anterior spinal fusion and instrumentation T9 to L4 to allow for continued growth in the minimally deformed thoracic spine: (*C*) anteroposterior view and (*D*) lateral view. It is anticipated she will undergo a T2 to pelvis when she is more skeletally mature.

to assess the dorsal sensory columns.[110] DiCindio and colleagues[107] looked at the reliability and applicability of TceMEP and SSEP monitoring in neuromuscular patients and found that SSEPs were reliably detected in 82% of patients with CP. TceMEPs were not attempted in patients with a history of active seizure disorder, but were measurable in 100% of the mild and moderate CP patients tested, and in 90% of the severe CP patients. Three of their CP patients had significant neurophysiologic changes detected: two during passage of sublaminar wires and one with evidence of an impending brachial plexopathy. Corrective measures were taken and there were no resulting permanent neurologic deficits. More recently, Vitale and colleagues[108] looked at a large heterogeneous group of scoliosis patients with intraoperative spinal monitoring during corrective surgery, and reported 77% success of SSEP monitoring in CP patients with either scoliosis or kyphosis and 47% success of TceMEP monitoring, with an overall neuromonitoring success rate of 88%. They were able to detect three true electrophysical effects, which, after appropriate intervention, lead to no detectable neurologic change postoperatively. Therefore, despite being technically more difficult and slightly less reliable than in idiopathic patients, intraoperative monitoring is recommended for CP scoliosis surgery.

Antifibrinolytic agent use Perioperative blood loss can be quite significant in this patient population, so there has been interest in the use and effectiveness of antifibrinolytics, including tranexamic acid (TXA), aprotinin, and epsilon-aminocaproic acid.[111–116] Tzortzopoulou and colleagues[113] reviewed the existing literature for the Cochrane Database on antifibrinolytic use in pediatric scoliosis surgery and found that its use reduced blood loss and the amount of blood transfused, but did not necessarily decrease the number of children requiring transfusion. Thompson and colleagues[112] investigated the use of Amicar (aminocaproic acid) in neuromuscular patients and reported significantly less estimated intraoperative blood loss (1125 mL vs 2194 mL), total perioperative blood loss (1805 mL vs 3055 mL), and transfusion requirements (660 mL vs 1548 mL) in the Amicar group versus control. Aprotinin, known for its use in cardiac surgery, has also been used in pediatric spine surgery. Kasimian and colleagues[111] compared neuromuscular patients undergoing scoliosis surgery with perioperative aprotinin use against a control group that did not. The aprotinin group had significantly less total blood loss, as well as less blood loss per kilogram, and fewer intraoperative

transfusions. The investigators, using the cost of drug therapy, operating room time, and blood product use, calculated that aprotinin saved an average $8,577 per patient. It is important to note, however, that the manufacturers of aprotinin halted its production in 2007 over concern for a higher mortality rate following cardiac surgery.[114] Finally, TXA has been shown to safely decrease the total amount of blood transfused in the perioperative period following pediatric spine surgery[115,116]; however, it has not been specifically studied in the CP population.

Bone graft choices To maximize the opportunity for fusion in these generally osteopenic, often malnourished, patients, both autograft and allograft are used routinely.[117,118] Autograft is usually obtained locally and may be supplemented with iliac crest bone graft. The benefit of adding antibiotics to allograft bone has been investigated. Borkhuu and colleagues[119] compared the infection rate after posterior spinal fusion with unit rod instrumentation with or without gentamicin-impregnated allograft bone in 220 CP patients. All patients received a mixture of morcellized freeze-dried corticocancellous allograft and morcellized autograft from the spinous processes. Those patients who were in the antibiotic group also received a second allograft mixture consisting of freeze-dried corticocancellous allograft bone soaked with liquid gentamicin. The deep wound infection rate in the antibiotic allograft group was 3.9% versus 15.2% in the nonantibiotic impregnated allograft group.

Author's preferred method

We attempt to brace young patients with small, flexible curves. In very young patients, with progressive curves that are not controlled with bracing or wheelchair modifications, we consider the following temporizing measures to allow for chest wall development in these already respiratory-compromised patients: growing rods or limited anterior thoracolumbar fusion at the apex of the curve (see **Fig. 2**). For patients with limited growth remaining, we consider spinal fusion for curves greater than 50 degrees that are progressive and functionally limiting. This decision, however, is based on the patient's overall health and comorbidities and only after extensive discussion with the patient, family, or caregivers so that the decision reached is a mutual one. For the typical C-shaped curve with associated pelvic obliquity that is less than 100 degrees and bends down at least 50% on traction films, we proceed with posterior-only fusion with pedicle screw instrumentation. The extent of fusion is usually from T2 or T3 to the pelvis; we favor iliac screws over the Galveston technique for better pelvic fixation. We routinely use multimodality neuromonitoring. To assist with leveling the pelvis and manage large curve, we commonly use intraoperative traction. The tension used is dependent both on the deformity correction as well as reliability of the baseline neuromonitoring. At any point during the operation if there is a change from baseline, the traction is released. A standard posterior approach to the spine and facetectomies are completed, and two large iliac screws are placed from the posterior superior iliac spine between the inner and outer table of the pelvis toward the anterior inferior iliac spine. Pedicle screws are then placed at either every or every other level depending on curve size, bone quality, and skeletal maturity. Transverse process hooks are placed at the most rostral level to minimize proximal dissection in an effort to decrease the risk of proximal junctional kyphosis. If the curve is stiffer, Ponte-type releases are performed at the apex of the curves and the density of screws is increased to help distribute the corrective forces applied to the spine. The rods are then contoured and connected to each other with a temporary crosslink before placement in the patient, thereby creating a unit rod-equivalent construct. The spine is then reduced to the rods and secured; final decortication is performed and a mixture of autograft from the spinous processes and facets

and corticocancellous allograft mixed with antibiotics and demineralized bone matrix is placed (**Fig. 3**). A postoperative brace may be prescribed to facilitate transfers, in patients with active seizures or those with severely osteopenic bone. Whereas our indications for an anterior release continue to evolve, we generally perform one if the curve is greater than 120 degrees, has poor flexibility, or is associated with severe pelvic obliquity or sagittal deformity. If doing both anterior and posterior procedures, we prefer to do this in a single stage. The anterior procedure is done first, either thoracoscopically if localized to the thoracic spine or open if for a thoracolumbar deformity. In many cases an open thoracolumbar release will also be instrumented to maximize correction and to decrease the difficulty of the posterior procedure (**Fig. 4**). This also allows for a delay in the second stage (up to several weeks to months) if it is not safe to proceed that same day. The patient may be allowed to recover physiologically, at home if necessary, before proceeding with the posterior procedure. If the correction achieved with anterior release is not ideal and further posterior release is needed, then the spine is not instrumented anteriorly, but left "loose" so that further correction can be obtained from the second stage.

COMPLICATIONS

Complications in CP scoliosis surgery should be considered the rule, rather than the exception.

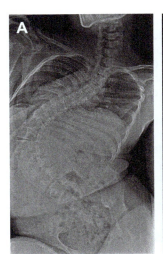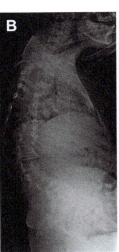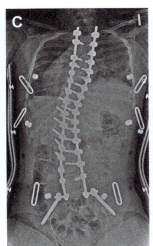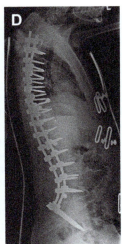

Fig. 3. Twelve-year-old GMFCS V with 120 degrees of scoliosis had difficulty with sitting and hygiene: (*A*) anteroposterior view and (*B*) lateral view. Patient had multilevel posterior Ponte-type osteotomies followed by posterior spinal instrumentation and fusion from T1 to pelvis with iliac screw fixation: (*C*) anteroposterior view and (*D*) lateral view. Intraoperative traction as well as 3 months postoperative bracing (for transfers) was used.

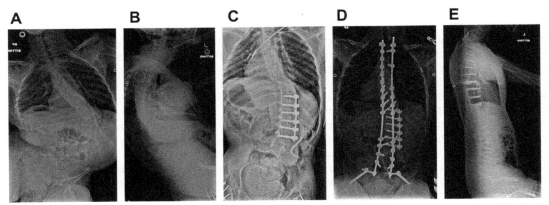

Fig. 4. (*A, B*) Eighteen-year-old GMFCS V CP patient had 117 degrees of scoliosis and severe pelvic obliquity. (*C*) Patient underwent staged anterior instrumentation and fusion from T11 to L4 with significant correction of spinal deformity. (*D, E*) Same-day second stage was then performed with a posterior fusion and instrumentation from T2 to pelvis.

The complication rate varies, depending on the study, from 40% to 80%[120] with a 0% to 7% mortality rate.[5] Tsirikos and colleagues,[76] in their extensive review of 287 consecutive CP patients, reported a 1% mortality rate, 6% deep infection rate, and 16% instrumentation problems.

Respiratory

Pulmonary complications are common in this compromised patient population, and range from prolonged intubation to atelectasis. The rate ranges from 8% to 35%,[59] and postoperative intensive care unit management should be anticipated. Preoperative coordination with a pulmonologist may be beneficial.

Wound Infections

The rate of postoperative wound infection is greater in CP patients than in idiopathic patients and ranges from 5% to 15%. The infection often is polymicrobial with gram-negative bacteria.[59] Although the risk of correction loss and pseudoarthrosis increase after infection,[121,122] it can usually be successfully treated with irrigation and debridement and closure over drains along with antibiotic administration. Occasionally, implant removal is required. With the increasing popularity of the vacuum-assisted device (VAC) in other areas of orthopedics, this technique is being applied to postoperative wound management in neuromuscular patients as well. Van Rhee and colleagues[123] reported on six consecutive neuromuscular patients with deep wound infection treated with irrigation and debridement, antibiotic administration, and VAC placement. Wound closure averaged 3 months, infection parameters

normalized by 6 weeks, and no patient required removal of instrumentation. Canavese and colleagues[124] had a slightly larger series of 14 patients with deep infection after spinal instrumentation, 12 of which were neuromuscular patients, and again found that none required implant removal to successfully treat the infection. The VAC system should be considered in the armamentarium for successful treatment of postoperative spinal wound infections.

Pseudoarthrosis

Pseudarthrosis has traditionally been thought to occur more frequently in CP patients than in idiopathic patients and is thought to be related to postoperative infection,[122] curve magnitude, and instrumentation technique. Pseudoarthrosis rates of as high as 11% to 40% with Harrington rod instrumentation improved following the use of Luque instrumentation (0%–13%).[59] In their large series of 287 CP patients using unit rod instrumentation, Tsirikos and colleagues[76] had only one pseudoarthrosis. In their three-year follow-up series of 52 CP patients treated with pedicle screws, Modi and colleagues[84] reported no pseudoarthroses. Implant failure, such as rod-breakage or screw pull-out, may herald an established or impending pseudoarthrosis. Revision surgery for this implant failure should only be undertaken for pain or clinically significant loss of correction.

PATIENT OUTCOMES

As with any surgical intervention, especially one with risk of complications, it is important to objectively evaluate outcomes in scoliosis surgery for patients with CP. In a review of the literature on quality-of-life outcomes in neuromuscular patients undergoing spinal fusion, Mercado and colleagues[125] found low-level evidence that surgery improves the quality of life in CP patients. Comstock and colleagues[126] looked at patient and caregiver satisfaction following surgery for scoliosis in total-body-involvement CP; despite 68% of patients experiencing complications, 85% of parents or caregivers were very satisfied with results of the surgery. They noted a beneficial impact on patients' sitting ability, physical appearance, ease of care, and comfort. The only major criticism from parents and caregivers was the lack of preparation for the difficulty of the postoperative course, including time in the ICU, amount of pain, and appearance of the child with multiple lines and tubes during their hospital stay. Most recently, Watanabe and colleagues[127] developed a questionnaire specifically devised for the patient or parent in the assessment of patients with neuromuscular deformity. They reviewed the questionnaire results of 84 spastic CP patients and families of patients who underwent spinal fusion. The overall satisfaction rate was 92% with an overall complication rate of 27%. Improvements in sitting balance, cosmesis, and quality life were reported in 93%, 94%, and 71% respectively. The investigators analyzed a subgroup of patients with less satisfaction and found that this group had a higher late complication rate, less correction of the major curve, and hyperlordosis of the lumbar spine after surgery. Scoliosis in CP patients is relatively complicated and nonsurgical treatment is not effective in preventing curve progression. Although surgical treatment of CP scoliosis is challenging and associated with frequent complications, the overall satisfaction of patients and caregivers and the improvement in patients' quality of life justify an operative approach, albeit a thoughtful and careful one.

REFERENCES

1. Balmer GA, MacEwen GD. The incidence and treatment of scoliosis in cerebral palsy. J Bone Joint Surg Br 1970;52(1):134–7.

2. Madigan RR, Wallace SL. Scoliosis in the institutionalized cerebral palsy population. Spine 1981; 6(6):583–90.

3. Saito N, Ebara S, Ohotsuka K. Natural history of scoliosis in spastic cerebral palsy. Lancet 1998; 351(9117):1687–92.

4. Thometz JG, Simon SR. Progression of scoliosis after skeletal maturity in institutionalized adults who have cerebral palsy. J Bone Joint Surg Am 1988;70(9):1290–6.

5. McCarthy JJ, D'Andrea LP, Betz RR, et al. Scoliosis in the child with cerebral palsy. J Am Acad Orthop Surg 2006;14(6):367–75.

6. Majd M, Muldowny D, Holt R. Natural history of scoliosis in the institutionalized adult cerebral palsy population. Spine 1997;22(13):1461–6.

7. Kalen V, Conkin MM, Sherman FC. Untreated scoliosis in severe cerebral palsy. J Pediatr Orthop 1992;12(3):337–40.

8. Langerak NG, Vaughan CL, Hoffman EB, et al. Incidence of spinal abnormalities in patients with spastic diplegia 17 to 26 years after selective dorsal rhizotomy. Childs Nerv Syst 2009;25(12):1593–603.

9. Golan JD, Hall JA, O'Gorman G, et al. Spinal deformities following selective dorsal rhizotomy. J Neurosurg 2007;106(Suppl 6):441–9.

10. Steinbok P, Hicdonmez T, Sawatzky B, et al. Spinal deformities after selective dorsal rhizotomy for spastic cerebral palsy. J Neurosurg 2005;102 (Suppl 4):363–73.

11. Johnson MB, Goldstein L, Thomas SS, et al. Spinal deformity after selective dorsal rhizotomy in ambulatory patients with cerebral palsy. J Pediatr Orthop 2004;24(5):529–36.

12. Spiegel DA, Loder RT, Alley KA, et al. Spinal deformity following selective dorsal rhizotomy. J Pediatr Orthop 2004;24(1):30–6.

13. Turi M, Kalen V. The risk of spinal deformity after selective dorsal rhizotomy. J Pediatr Orthop 2000; 20(1):104–7.

14. Peter JC, Hoffman EB, Arens LJ. Spondylolysis and spondylolisthesis after five-level lumbosacral laminectomy for selective posterior rhizotomy in cerebral-palsy. Childs Nerv Syst 1993;9(5):285–7.

15. Peter JC, Hoffman EB, Arens LJ, et al. Incidence of spinal deformity in children after multiple level laminectomy for selective posterior rhizotomy. Childs Nerv Syst 1990;6(1):30–2.

16. Ginsburg GM, Lauder AJ. Progression of scoliosis in patients with spastic quadriplegia after the insertion of an intrathecal baclofen pump. Spine 2007; 32(24):2745–50.

17. Sansone JM, Mann D, Noonan K, et al. Rapid progression of scoliosis following insertion of intrathecal baclofen pump. J Pediatr Orthop 2006;26(1):125–8.

18. Segal LS, Wallach DM, Kanev PM. Potential complications of posterior spine fusion and instrumentation in patients with cerebral palsy treated with intrathecal baclofen infusion. Spine 2005; 30(8):E219–24.

19. Shilt JS, Lai LP, Cabrera MN, et al. The impact of intrathecal baclofen on the natural history of scoliosis in cerebral palsy. J Pediatr Orthop 2008; 28(6):684–7.

20. Gilbert SR, Gilbert AC, Henderson RC. Skeletal maturation in children with quadriplegic cerebral palsy. J Pediatr Orthop 2004;24(3):292–7.

21. Terjesen T, Lange JE, Steen H. Treatment of scoliosis with spinal bracing in quadriplegic cerebral palsy. Dev Med Child Neurol 2000;42(7):448–54.

22. Olafsson Y, Saraste H, Al-Dabbagh Z. Brace treatment in neuromuscular spine deformity. J Pediatr Orthop 1999;19(3):376–9.

23. Leopando MT, Moussavi Z, Holbrow J, et al. Effect of a Soft Boston Orthosis on pulmonary mechanics in severe cerebral palsy. Pediatr Pulmonol 1999; 28(1):53–8.

24. Shook JE, Lubicky J. Paralytic spinal deformity. Scoliosis. In: Bridwell KH, DeWald RL, editors. The textbook of spinal surgery. 1st edition. Philadelphia: Lippincott-Raven; 1991. p. 279–322.

25. Kotwicki T, Drumala J, Czubak J. Bracing for neuromuscular scoliosis: orthosis construction to improve the patient's function. Disabil Rehabil Assist Technol 2008;3(3):161–9.

26. Miller A, Temple T, Miller F. Impact of orthoses on the rate of scoliosis progression in children with cerebral palsy. J Pediatr Orthop 1996;16(3):332–5.

27. Renshaw TS, Green NE, Griffin PP, et al. Cerebral palsy: orthopaedic management. Instr Course Lect 1996;45:475–90.

28. Letts M, Rathbone D, Yamashita T, et al. Soft Boston Orthosis management of neuromuscular scoliosis: a preliminary report. J Pediatr Orthop 1992;12(4):470–4.

29. Holmes KJ, Michael SM, Thorpe SL, et al. Management of scoliosis with special seating for the nonambulant spastic cerebral palsy population—a biomechanical study. Clin Biomech 2003;18(6): 480–7.

30. Nuzzo RM, Walsh S, Boucherit T, et al. Counterparalysis for treatment of paralytic scoliosis with botulinum toxin type A. Am J Orthop 1997;26(3):201–7.

31. Lonstein J. Spine deformities due to cerebral palsy. In: Weinstein S, editor. The pediatric spine: principles and practices. Philadelphia (PA): Lippincott, Wiliams, and Wilkins; 2001. p. 797–807.

32. Lonstein JE, Akbarnia A. Operative treatment of spinal deformities in patients with cerebral palsy or mental retardation. An analysis of one hundred and seven cases. J Bone Joint Surg Am 1983; 65(1):43–55.

33. Thomson JD, Banta JV. Scoliosis in cerebral palsy: an overview and recent results. J Pediatr Orthop B 2001;10(1):6–9.

34. Rang M, Douglas G, Bennet GC, et al. Seating for children with cerebral palsy. J Pediatr Orthop 1981; 1(3):279–87.

35. Persson-Bunke M, Hagglund G, Lauge-Pedersen H. Windswept hip deformity in children with cerebral palsy. J Pediatr Orthop B 2006; 15(5):335–8.

36. Senaran H, Shah SA, Glutting JJ, et al. The associated effects of untreated unilateral hip dislocation in cerebral palsy scoliosis. J Pediatr Orthop 2006; 26(6):769–72.

37. Cooperman DR, Bartucci E, Dietrick E, et al. Hip dislocation in spastic cerebral palsy: long-term consequences. J Pediatr Orthop 1987;7(3): 268–76.

38. Lonstein JE, Beck K. Hip dislocation and subluxation in cerebral palsy. J Pediatr Orthop 1986;6(5): 521–6.

39. Letts M, Shapiro L, Mulder K, et al. The windblown hip syndrome in total body cerebral palsy. J Pediatr Orthop 1984;4(1):55–62.

40. Pritchett JW. The untreated unstable hip in severe cerebral palsy. Clin Orthop 1983;173:169–72.

41. Samilson R. Orthopaedic aspects of cerebral palsy. Philadelphia: Lippincott; 1975.

42. Farhat G, Yamout B, Mikati MA. Effect of antiepileptic drugs on bone density in ambulatory patients. Neurology 2002;58(9):1348–53.

43. Sheth RD, Wesolowksi CA, Jacob JC. Effect of carbamazepine and valproate on bone mineral density. J Pediatr 1995;127(2):256–62.

44. Chambers HG, Weinstein CH, Mubarak SJ, et al. The effect of valproic acid on blood loss in patients with cerebral palsy. J Pediatr Orthop 1999;19(6): 792–5.

45. Winter SL, Kriel RL, Novacheck TF, et al. Perioperative blood loss: the effect of valproate. Pediatr Neurol 1996;15(1):19–22.

46. Winter SL. Preoperative assessment of the child with neuromuscular scoliosis. Orthop Clin North Am 1994;25(2):239–45.

47. Pruijs JE, van Tol MJ, van Kesteren RG, et al. Neuromuscular scoliosis: clinical evaluation pre- and postoperative. J Pediatr Orthop B 2000;9(4): 217–20.

48. Soudon P, Hody JL, Bellen P. Preoperative cardiopulmonary assessment in the child with neuromuscular scoliosis. J Pediatr Orthop B 2000;9(4): 229–33.

49. Udink ten Cate FE, van Royen BJ, van Heerde M, et al. Incidence and risk factors of prolonged mechanical ventilation in neuromuscular scoliosis surgery. J Pediatr Orthop B 2008;17(4):203–6.

50. Borkhuu B, Nagaraju D, Miller F, et al. Prevalence and risk factors in postoperative pancreatitis after spine fusion in patients with cerebral palsy. J Pediatr Orthop 2009;29(3):256–62.

51. Lipton GE, Miller F, Dabney KW, et al. Factors predicting postoperative complications following spinal fusions in children with cerebral palsy. J Spinal Disord 1999;12(3):197–205.

52. Jevsevar DS, Karlin LI. The relationship between preoperative nutritional status and complications after an operation for scoliosis in patients who have cerebral palsy. J Bone Joint Surg Am 1993;75(6):880–4 [Erratum in: J Bone Joint Surg Am 1993;75(8):1256].

53. Brenn BR, Theroux MC, Dabney KW. Clotting parameters and thromboelastography in children with neuromuscular and idiopathic scoliosis undergoing posterior spinal fusion. Spine 2004;29(15): E310–4.

54. Kannan S, Meert KL, Mooney JF. Bleeding and coagulation changes during spinal fusion surgery: a comparison of neuromuscular and idiopathic scoliosis patients. Pediatr Crit Care Med 2002; 27(19):2137–42.

55. Vitale MG, Privitera DM, Matsumoto H, et al. Efficacy of preoperative erythropoietin administration in pediatric neuromuscular scoliosis patients. Spine 2007;32(24):2662–7.

56. Gupta MC, Wijesekera S, Sossan A, et al. Reliability of radiographic parameters in neuromuscular scoliosis. Spine 2007;32(6):691–5.

57. Hennrikus WL, Rosenthal RK, Kasser JR. Incidence of spondylolisthesis in ambulatory cerebral palsy patients. J Pediatr Orthop 1993;13(1):37–40.

58. Sanders JO, Evert M, Stanley EA, et al. Mechanisms of curve progression following sublaminar (Luque) spinal instrumentation. Spine 1992;17(7): 781–9.

59. Newton PO, Capelo RM. Spinal deformity in cerebral palsy. In: Kim DH, Betz RR, Huhn SL, et al, editors. Surgery of the pediatric spine. New York: Thieme; 2008. p. 441–56.

60. Sussman MD, Little D, Alley RM. Posterior instrumentation and fusion of the thoracolumbar spine for treatment of neuromuscular scoliosis. J Pediatr Orthop 1996;16(3):304–13.

61. Whitaker C, Burton DC, Asher M. Treatment of selected neuromuscular patient with posterior instrumentation and arthrodesis ending with lumbar pedicle screw anchorage. Spine 2000;25 (18):2312–8.

62. McCall RE, Hayes B. Long-term outcome in neuromuscular scoliosis fused only to lumbar 5. Spine 2005;30(18):2056–60.

63. Allen BL Jr, Ferguson RL. L-rod instrumentation for scoliosis in cerebral palsy. J Pediatr Orthop 1982; 2(1):87–96.

64. Maloney WJ, Rinsky LA, Gamble JG. Simultaneous correction of pelvic obliquity, frontal plane, and sagittal plane deformities in neuromuscular scoliosis using a unit rod with segmental sublaminar wires: a preliminary report. J Pediatr Orthop 1990;10(6):742–9.

65. Neustadt JB, Shufflebarger HL, Cammisa FP. Spinal fusions to the pelvis augmented by Cotrel-Dubousset instrumentation for neuromuscular scoliosis. J Pediatr Orthop 1992;12(4):465–9.

66. Modi HN, Suh SW, Song HR, et al. Evaluation of pelvic fixation in neuromuscular scoliosis: a retrospective study in 55 patients. Int Orthop 2010;34 (1):89–96.

67. Tsirikos AI, Chang WN, Shah SA, et al. Preserving ambulatory potential in pediatric patients with cerebral palsy who undergo spinal fusion using unit rod instrumentation. Spine 2003;28(5):480–3.

68. Sullivan JA, Conner SB. Comparison of Harrington instrumentation and segmental spinal instrumentation in the management of neuromuscular spinal deformity. Spine 1982;7(3):299–304.

69. Bonnett C, Brown JC, Grow T. Thoracolumbar scoliosis in cerebral palsy. Results of surgical treatment. J Bone Joint Surg Am 1976;58(3):328–36.

70. Herring JA, Wenger DR. Segmental spinal instrumentation: a preliminary report of 40 consecutive cases. Spine 1982;7(3):285–98.

71. Gersoff WK, Renshaw TS. The treatment of scoliosis in cerebral palsy by posterior spinal fusion with Luque-rod segmental instrumentation. J Bone Joint Surg Am 1988;70(1):41–4.

72. Gau YL, Lonstein JE, Winter RB, et al. Luque-Galveston procedure for correction and stabilization of neuromuscular scoliosis and pelvic obliquity: a review of 68 patients. J Spinal Disord 1991;4(4): 399–410.

73. Allen BL Jr, Ferguson RL. The Galveston technique for L rod instrumentation of the scoliotic spine. Spine 1982;7(3):276–84.

74. Bell DF, Moseley C, Koreska J. Unit rod segmental spinal instrumentation in the management of patients with progressive neuromuscular spinal deformity. Spine 1989;14(12):1301–7.

75. Bulman WA, Dormans JP, Ecker ML, et al. Posterior spinal fusion for scoliosis in patients with cerebral palsy: a comparison of Luque rod and Unit Rid instrumentation. J Pediatr Orthop 1996;16(3):314–23.

76. Tsirikos AI, Lipton G, Chang WN, et al. Surgical correction of scoliosis in pediatric patients with cerebral palsy using the unit rod instrumentation. Spine 2008;33(10):1133–40.

77. Guidera KJ, Hooten J, Weatherly W, et al. Cotrel-Dubousset instrumentation. Results in 52 patients. Spine 1993;18(4):427–31.

78. Wimmer C, Wallnofer P, Walochnik N, et al. Comparative evaluation of luque and isola instrumentation for treatment of neuromuscular scoliosis. Clin Orthop Relat Res 2005;439:181–92.

79. Yazici M, Asher MA, Hardacker JW. The safety and efficacy of Isola-Galveston instrumentation and arthrodesis in the treatment of neuromuscular spinal deformities. J Bone Joint Surg Am 2000;82 (4):524–43.

80. Rodgers WB, Williams MS, Schwend RM, et al. Spinal deformity in myelodysplasia. Correction with posterior pedicle screw instrumentation. Spine 1997;22(20):2435–43.

81. Modi HN, Suh SW, Song HR, et al. Treatment of neuromuscular scoliosis with posterior-only pedicle screw fixation. J Orthop Surg Res 2008;3:23.

82. Modi HN, Suh SW, Fernandez H, et al. Accuracy and safety of pedicle screw placement in neuromuscular scoliosis with free-hand technique. Eur Spine J 2008;17(12):1686–96.

83. Modi HN, Suh SW, Yang JH, et al. Surgical complications in neuromuscular scoliosis operated with posterior-only approach using pedicle screw fixation. Scoliosis 2009;4:11.

84. Modi HN, Hong JY, Mehta SS, et al. Surgical correction and fusion using posterior-only pedicle screw construct for neuropathic scoliosis in patients with cerebral palsy: a three-year follow-up study. Spine 2009;34(11):1167–75.

85. Watanabe K, Lenke LG, Bridwell KH, et al. Comparison of radiographic outcomes for the treatment of scoliotic curves greater than 100 degrees: wires versus hooks versus screws. Spine 2008;33(10):1084–92.

86. King AG, Thomas KA, Eiserloh HL III, et al. Analysis of the STIF technique for spino-pelvic fixation: clinical results in 19 patients with neuromuscular scoliosis. J Pediatr Orthop 2000;20(5):667–76.

87. McCarthy RE, Bruffett WL, McCullough FL. S rod fixation to the sacrum in patients with neuromuscular spinal deformities. Clin Orthop Relat Res 1999;364:26–31.

88. McCord DH, Cunningham BW, Shono Y, et al. Biomechanical analysis of lumbosacral fixation. Spine 1992;17(Suppl 8):S235–43.

89. Peelle MW, Lenke LG, Bridwell KH, et al. Comparison of pelvic fixation techniques in neuromuscular spinal deformity correction: Galveston rod versus iliac and lumbosacral screws. Spine 2006;31(20):2392–8.

90. Sponseller PD, Shah SA, Abel MF, et al. Scoliosis surgery in cerebral palsy: differences between unit rod and custom rods. Spine 2009;34(8):840–4.

91. Swank SM, Cohen DS, Brown JC. Spine fusion in cerebral palsy with L-rod segmental spinal instrumentation. A comparison of single and two-stage combined approach with Zielke instrumentation. Spine 1989;14(7):750–9.

92. Bridwell KH. Surgical treatment of idiopathic adolescent scoliosis. Spine 1999;24(24):2607–16.

93. Auerbach JD, Spiegel DA, Zgonis MH, et al. The correction of pelvic obliquity in patients with cerebral palsy and neuromuscular scoliosis: is there a benefit of anterior release prior to posterior spinal arthrodesis? Spine 2009;34(21):E766–74.

94. McCarthy RE. Management of neuromuscular scoliosis. Orthop Clin North Am 1999;30(3):435–49.

95. Vialle R, Delecourt C, Morin C. Surgical treatment of scoliosis with pelvic obliquity in cerebral palsy: the influence of intraoperative traction. Spine 2006;31(13):1461–6.

96. Suk SI, Kim JH, Cho KJ, et al. Is anterior release necessary in severe scoliosis treated by posterior segmental pedicle screw fixation? Eur Spine J 2007;16(9):1359–65.

97. Suh SW, Modi HN, Yang JH, et al. Posterior multilevel vertebral osteotomy for correction of severe and rigid neuromuscular scoliosis: a preliminary study. Spine 2009;34(12):1315–20.

98. Smucker JD, Miller F. Crankshaft effect after posterior spinal fusion and unit rod instrumentation in children with cerebral palsy. J Pediatr Orthop 2001;21(1):108–12.

99. Westerlund LE, Gill SS, Jarosz TS, et al. Posterior-only unit rod instrumentation and fusion for neuromuscular scoliosis. Spine 2001;26(18):1984–9.

100. Tokala DP, Lam KS, Freeman BJ, et al. Is there a role for selective anterior instrumentation in neuromuscular scoliosis? Eur Spine J 2007;16(1):91–6.

101. Basobas L, Mardjetko S, Hammerberg K, et al. Selective anterior fusion and instrumentation for the treatment of neuromuscular scoliosis. Spine 2003;28(20):S245–8.

102. Rinella AR, Lenke L, Whitaker C, et al. Perioperative halo-gravity traction in the treatment of severe scoliosis and kyphosis. Spine 2005;30(4):475–82.

103. Sink EL, Karol LA, Sangers J, et al. Efficacy of perioperative halo-gravity traction in the treatment of severe scoliosis in children. J Pediatr Orthop 2001;21(4):519–24.

104. Huang MJ, Lenke LG. Scoliosis and severe pelvic obliquity in a patient with cerebral palsy: surgical treatment utilizing halo-femoral traction. Spine 2001;26(19):2168–70.

105. Takeshita K, Lenke LG, Bridwell KH, et al. Analysis of patients with nonambulatory neuromuscular scoliosis surgically treated to the pelvis with intraoperative halo-femoral traction. Spine 2006;31(20):2381–5.

106. Sponseller PD, Takenaga RK, Newton PO, et al. The use of traction in the treatment of severe spinal deformity. Spine 2008;33(21):2305–9.

107. DiCindio S, Theroux M, Shah S, et al. Multimodality monitoring of transcranial electric motor and somatosensory-evoked potentials during surgical correction of spinal deformity in patients with cerebral palsy and other neuromuscular disorders. Spine 2003;28(16):1851–5.

108. Vitale MG, Moore DW, Matsumoto H, et al. Risk factors for spinal cord injury during surgery for spinal deformity. J Bone Joint Surg Am 2010;92(1):64–71.

109. Langeloo DD, Journee HL, Polak B, et al. A new application of TCE-MEP: spinal cord monitoring in patients with severe neuromuscular weakness undergoing corrective spine surgery. J Spinal Disord 2001;14(5):445–8.

110. Deletis V, Sala F. Neurophysiological monitoring during pediatric spine surgery. In: Kim DH, Betz RR, Huhn SL, et-al, editors. Surgery of the pediatric spine. New York: Thieme; 2008. p. 441–56.

111. Kasimian S, Skaggs DL, Sankar WN, et al. Aprotinin in pediatric neuromuscular scoliosis surgery. Eur Spine J 2008;17(12):1671–5.

112. Thompson GH, Florentino-Pineda I, Poe-Kochert C, et al. Role of Amicar in surgery for neuromuscular scoliosis. Spine 2008;33(24):2623–9.

113. Tzortzopoulou A, Cepeda MS, Schumann R, et al. Antifibrinolytic agents for reducing blood loss in scoliosis in children. Cochrane Database Syst Rev 2008;3:CD006883.

114. Gill JB, Chin Y, Levin A, et al. The use of antifibrinolytic agents in spine surgery: a meta-analysis. J Bone Joint Surg Am 2008;90(11): 2399–407.

115. Neilipovitz DT, Murto K, Hall L, et al. A randomized trial of tranexamic acid to reduce blood transfusion for scoliosis surgery. Anesth Analg 2001;93(1):82–7.

116. Grant JA, Howard J, Luntley J, et al. Perioperative blood transfusion requirements in pediatric scoliosis surgery: the efficacy of tranexamic acid. J Pediatr Orthop 2009;29(3):300–4.

117. McCarthy RE, Peek RD, Morrissey RT, et al. Allograft bone in spinal fusion for paralytic scoliosis. J Bone Joint Surg Am 1986;68(3):370–5.

118. Yazici M, Asher MA. Freeze-dried allograft for posterior spinal fusion in patients with neuromuscular spinal deformities. Spine 1997;22(13): 1467–71.

119. Borkhuu B, Borowski A, Shah SA, et al. Antibiotic-loaded allograft decreases the rate of acute deep wound infection after spinal fusion in cerebral palsy. Spine 2008;33(21):2300–4.

120. Koop SE. Scoliosis in cerebral palsy. Dev Med Child Neurol 2009;51(Suppl 4):92–8.

121. Sponseller PD, Shah SA, Abel MF, et al. Infection rate after spine surgery in cerebral palsy is high and impairs results: multicenter analysis of risk factors and treatment. Clin Orthop Relat Res 2010;468:711–6.

122. Sponseller PD, LaPorte DM, Hungerford MW, et al. Deep wound infections after neuromuscular scoliosis surgery: a multicenter study of risk factors and treatment outcomes. Spine 2000;25 (19):2461–6.

123. Van Rhee MA, de Klerk LW, Verhaar JA. Vacuum-assisted wound closure of deep infections after instrumented spinal fusion in six children with neuromuscular scoliosis. Spine J 2007;7(5): 596–600.

124. Canavese F, Gupta S, Krajbich JI, et al. Vacuum-assisted closure for deep infection after spinal instrumentation for scoliosis. J Bone Joint Surg Br 2008;90(3):377–81.

125. Mercado E, Alman B, Wright JG. Does spinal fusion influence quality of life in neuromuscular scoliosis? Spine 2007;32(19S):S120–5.

126. Comstock CP, Leach J, Wenger DR. Scoliosis in total-body-involvement cerebral palsy: analysis of surgical treatment and patient and caregiver satisfaction. Spine 1998;23(12):1412–24.

127. Watanabe K, Lenke LG, Daubs MD, et al. Is spine deformity surgery in patients with spastic cerebral palsy truly beneficial? A patient/parent evaluation. Spine 2009;34(20):2222–32.

Management of Hip Deformities in Cerebral Palsy

Francisco G. Valencia, MD

KEYWORDS

- Hip • Deformities • Cerebral palsy

The incidence and spectrum of hip abnormalities in children with cerebral palsy vary greatly. The reported incidence ranges from 2% to 75%.[1] These reports include children who have significantly different degrees of neurologic involvement. The severity and pathology ranges from an alteration of gait or muscle contracture to painful neuromuscular dislocation. This wide spectrum raises several challenges for how best to identify the risk of hip deformities and how best to address their needs.

One of the major obstacles is having a reproducible system to allow comparison of different patient populations and different treatments. Currently, most common clinical descriptions of patients with cerebral palsy incorporate the movement abnormality (spastic vs athetoid) and a geographic description of the areas involved (diplegia or quadriplegia). However, children with the same diagnosis, such as spastic diplegia, do not necessarily have the same functional impairment or clinical course. Stratifying patients by functional capacity helps identify the risk relative to their level of independent function.[2] Lonstein and Beck[2] reported the incidence of hip abnormalities to be 7% in independent ambulators and up to 60% in nonindependent sitters. More recently, the Gross Motor Function Classification Score (GMFCS) categorizes youths and children with cerebral palsy.[3–5] This system classifies patients into 5 levels based on self-initiated motor function. It is not intended to classify children's best performance or potential for improvement; emphasis is paid to sitting, walking, and wheeled mobility in the community (ie, daily function). The classification has been updated to incorporate individuals in late adolescence.[4] The full classification is available online at www.canchild.ca

Level I: walks without limitation
Level II: walks with limitations
Level III: walks using a hand-held mobility device
Level IV: self-mobility with limitations; may use power device
Level V: transported in manual wheelchair.

The GMFCS classification has gained clinical acceptance as a means of simplifying communication amongst researchers and as a means to guide treatment plans. Using the GMFCS, Soo[6] identified the incidence of hip displacement as 0% for children with GMFCS level I and 90% for those with GMFCS level V. Compared with children with GMFCS level II, those with levels III, IV, and V had significantly higher relative risks of hip displacement (2.7, 4.6, and 5.9, respectively).

NATURAL HISTORY

In the normal hip, balanced muscle use promotes the symbiotic development of the acetabulum and femoral head. Upright posture and ambulation promotes remodeling of neonatal femoral anteversion. Children with cerebral palsy are born with normal hips. However, these hips are soon subjected to abnormal muscle forces that lead to hip abnormalities.

The ability to ambulate determines the fate of the hips. Children who become independent ambulators by age 5 years develop enough muscle balance to stabilize the hips; they may develop acetabular dysplasia or femoral head deformities

Financial Disclosure: The author has nothing to disclose.
University Orthopedic Specialist, 1555 East River Road, Tucson, AZ 85718, USA
E-mail address: fvalencia@uorthospec.com

Orthop Clin N Am 41 (2010) 549–559
doi:10.1016/j.ocl.2010.07.002
0030-5898/10/$ — see front matter © 2010 Published by Elsevier Inc.

but do not dislocate. Children who ambulate with crutches, walkers, or canes may develop silent and painless subluxation of hips that may not be a clinical issue for years. Nonambulators may begin to dislocate before the age of 7 years.[7]

In a mathematical model of the spastic hip, the increased tone to the spastic muscles creates a hip-force magnitude 3^3 times that of the normal hip.[8] It is thought that the main muscle deformers of the hip joint are the adductors, hip flexors, and hamstrings. The hip joint has a ball-and-socket configuration that presumably maximizes contact between the femoral head and the acetabulum throughout a wide range of different positions including flexion and extension. However, a computer model has demonstrated "very little 'containment' of the posterior and lateral surfaces of the femoral head"[9(p354)] in the sitting position. The persistent femoral anteversion redirects the head away from the depth of the socket toward the rim.

The combination of spastic muscle activity and altered sitting posture redirects the femoral head to the superolateral and posterior aspects of the acetabulum. If the weak abductors and extensors are unable to offset the adductor spasticity, a contracture of the adductors and the inferomedial joint capsule develops in time. The femoral head is directed and restricted to the lateral rim of the socket. The abnormal forces on the chondroepiphysis of the acetabulum presumably lead to suppression of normal growth. Based on computed tomography (CT) scans, the deficiency is usually in the superolateral or posterior aspect of the acetabulum.[10,11] It is unclear whether the acetabulum is dysplastic or is enlarging. Recent three-dimensional (3D) reconstruction study has shown that, once the hip dislocates, the acetabular deformity becomes global and the volume of the acetabulum decreases in much the same way that a saucer holds less volume than a cup.[10] The greatest deformation of the acetabulum and femoral head occurs when the migration index is 52% to 68%.[12] In cases in which the spasticity of the legs is asymmetric, a windblown deformity develops with the infrapelvic obliquity. The high side usually dislocates, although exceptions do occur. Subluxation and dislocation of the hip correlate with muscle imbalance and not pelvic obliquity.[2,9]

With progressive subluxation, the femoral head presses up to the lateral edge of the acetabulum. The lack of mobility and increased pressure on the medial aspect of the femoral head leads to flattening and a loss of sphericity. The superior portion of the femoral head remodels, resulting in the characteristic triangular-shaped femoral head, and the articular cartilage of the femoral head is denuded **Fig. 1**. It is debatable whether the loss of articular cartilage is caused by degeneration caused by immobility and lack of contact with the opposing articular surface, pressure from the superior rim of the acetabulum, or from compression from the overlying soft tissues.[9] There are no reports of mirror image articular cartilage lesions on the acetabular side. Regardless of the cause, the combination of remodeling and articular cartilage degeneration produces a femoral head that is not considered to be reconstructable.

CLINICAL EVALUATION

A clinical evaluation of the child with cerebral palsy should be part of an ongoing comprehensive surveillance program that incorporates a history of the child's functional capabilities, clinical examination, and radiographic evaluation. In patients who are ambulatory, the inquiry should detail age-appropriate activities such as standing, walking with assistance, or independent walking. The ability to walk, and the age at which this is achieved, is one of the strongest prognostic indicators of hip problems. Scrutton[13] found that no child who could walk by 30 months developed a hip problem. In children who walked between 30 months and 5 years, the incidence was 15%. Changes in standing or walking should raise the suspicion of possible hip abnormalities. However, this is not the universal finding, because children, especially with severe hemiplegia, can develop hip problems later in life.

In patients who are nonambulatory, changes in mobility, comfort and pain, sitting, contractures, and hygiene difficulties are indicators of hip problems. The input of family, therapists, and other

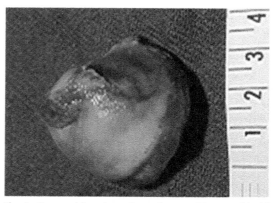

Fig. 1. Femoral head specimen from a 17-year-old girl with painful dislocation of the hip. Note the triangular shape of the femoral head and extensive loss of articular cartilage.

caregivers can be helpful in identifying problems and critical in developing reasonable treatment plans and expectations.

The physical examination of patients with cerebral palsy has been outlined by Horstmann and Bleck.[9] The different tests were developed to assess the different contributions of the hip adductors, flexors, and hamstrings to the development of hip displacement. Passive abduction of less than 40 degrees with the hips in flexion should raise a suspicion of hip instability. Dislocation can be suspected by leg-length discrepancy, but early subluxation is difficult to assess by physical examination.[13,14] The presence of severe dystonia can make it difficult to differentiate between tone and contracture. In these instances, serial examinations or even examination under anesthesia (in comparison with the awake examination) can help guide surgical decisions.

Stance and gait help identify functional impairments, such as crouch gait, scissor posture, and rotational abnormalities. Spinal deformities, pelvic obliquity, and other joint abnormalities should be assessed.

The radiologic evaluation complements the clinical examination. The mainstay is the anteroposterior (AP) and frog lateral images. Obtaining standardized radiographs can be challenging. Pelvic obliquity, lumbar lordosis, and contractures interfere with proper positioning and measurements. The hips should be flexed to overcome the lumbar lordosis. Several radiographic measurements have been reported,[15–18] but the most widely used are the acetabular index and Reimers migration index.

The acetabular index is a helpful predictor of instability. Cooke and colleagues[14] identified an acetabular index of greater than 30 degrees as a predictor of future instability in children more than the 4 years old.[15] The acetabular index varies with pelvic orientation. It decreases with lordosis and increases with flexion, and also varies with rotational malposition.

The Reimers migration index measures the degree of subluxation on the AP view.[18] It is a simple, reliable, and reproducible measurement. In a healthy child, the 90th percentile for migration percentile is 10%.[18] The upper limit of normal is 25% in a 4 year old. A migration index of 30 % is considered abnormal. In a normal child, the spontaneous progression is less than 1%. In children with cerebral palsy, an annual increase of 7.7 % was observed in those unlikely to walk, and 4% in those with walking potential.[16] Spontaneous stabilization and correction without treatment were observed in some children with a migration index of 33 %.[15] Although the migration index is the more valuable, both the acetabular index and migration index are useful (**Fig. 2**).[16] The use of these indices combined with changes over time seem to be the most valuable criteria for determining surgical intervention.

Children with cerebral palsy have altered proximal femoral anatomy.[19] This includes increased neck shaft angles along with persistent femoral anteversion when compared with individuals without cerebral palsy. The valgus deformity appreciated on plain films tends to be overstated because of the presence of femoral anteversion. True neck shaft measurements require maximum profile views.

CT scans and 3D reconstructions are helpful in identifying the location and degree of acetabular deformity and assist in preoperative planning. The most common deformity is in the superolateral portion of the acetabulum, but exceptions do occur.[11] 3D CT is recommended to help preoperative planning. Volumetric analysis has shown the volume of the acetabulum to increase after acetabuloplasty.[10]

The most important aspect of the clinical evaluation is developing a systematic surveillance program. Several reports have documented the benefits of surveillance for prevention of dislocation.[15,16,20,21] Dobson and colleagues[20] reported a significant drop in the incidence of dislocation and palliative surgical procedures, with a concomitant increase in preventative surgical procedures.

When should surveillance be initiated? There is no consensus. The range is 12 to 30 months.[9,13,16,20] Using the GMFCS as a guide,[22] children categorized as GMFCS I and II should have an initial radiograph at 12 to 24 months and

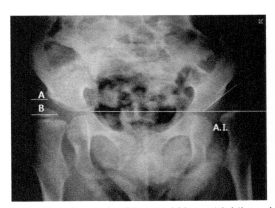

Fig. 2. AP radiograph of 5-year-old boy with bilateral hip subluxation. Migration index is calculated by A/B×100. A.I., acetabular index.

a follow-up at 4 years, if clinically stable. For patients who are GMFCS III to V, the surveillance should be conducted every 6 months.[22] If the migration index is stable, Wynter and colleagues[22] recommended follow-up every 12 months, if the migration percentage is stable, until skeletal maturity.

NONSURGICAL TREATMENT

Nonsurgical treatments have been directed at either reducing the amount of spasticity or stretching a tight or contracted tendon. Tone-reducing agents include baclofen and diazepam. Baclofen is a γ-aminobutyric acid (GABA) analogue and blocks GABA receptors.[23] It crosses the blood-brain barrier and can lead to sedation or weakness in other muscle groups, which limits the clinical usefulness of the oral form. Intrathecal baclofen bypasses the blood-brain barrier and has been used to control lower-extremity tone while minimizing the sedation side effects. It is recommended in patients who are nonambulatory with moderate to severe spasticity. Patients with intrathecal pumps require close monitoring of the pumps and periodic fillings.

Botulinum toxin is also an effective tone-reduction adjunct. It blocks the release of acetylcholine at the neuromuscular junction. The denervation effect can last up to 6 months but tends to diminish with repeated injections. It has been most commonly used in the lower extremity in conjunction with serial casting to manage gastrosoleus contractures.[24] Spasticity of the hip is more difficult to address.[25,26] Dose/weight limitations and the number of spastic muscles limit the effectiveness of botulinum injections. Technically, the muscles in and around the hip are more difficult injection sites, especially the iliopsoas muscle.[26] In a randomized trial of Botox and bracing, Graham and colleagues[26] found that there may be a small treatment benefit for the combined intervention of intramuscular injection of botulinum toxin A and abduction hip bracing in the management of spastic hip displacement in children with cerebral palsy. However, progressive hip displacement continued to occur in the treatment group, and the data did not support recommending this treatment.

Phenol has also been used as a chemical denervator and a lower-cost alternative to botulinum toxin. The effects can last up to twice as long as botulinum toxin. Phenol injections carry significant injection-site side effects, so it has limited widespread use.[9]

Physical therapy is a widely used modem of maximizing the neurodevelopment of the child with cerebral palsy. However, no studies have identified its effectiveness in preventing a neuromuscular subluxation or dislocation of the hip.[9]

Bracing regimens have been recommended for patients with subluxating hips, but there is no evidence to support that they halt the progression of the subluxation. Postoperative bracing has been reported to improve results in both mild and severe subluxation in children less than 6 years of age.[27] Abduction contractures have been reported with prolonged use of braces.

SURGICAL TREATMENT

The surgical management of hip abnormalities in children with cerebral palsy can be divided into 3 levels.[16,25,28] Level 1 consists of soft tissue releases intended to prevent or halt subluxation. Level 2 incorporates bony osteotomies and addresses advanced subluxation or dislocation of the hip associated with acetabular and/or femoral dysplasia. Palliative measures are indicated in the treatment of a painful, arthritic dislocated hip, and these are level 3 surgery. There is no agreement on the threshold for intervention.

Treatment Adductor Tenotomy

Adductor tenotomy is the indicated surgical treatment of adduction contraction and early subluxation of the hip. A range of motion of less than 30 degrees abduction with the hips and knees flexed is an indication for soft tissue releases. Radiographically, a migration index of 30% to 40%, or progression of more than 10% in 1 year, is an indication for soft tissue release.[28–30] If a contracture of the iliopsoas or the hamstrings is also identified by clinical examination, it is important to address all of these in a comprehensive manner.

Open release of the adductor muscles is accomplished through a medial adductor approach. The adductor longus is released in the tendinous portion, which reduces the amount of bleeding. The adductor brevis lies deep to the longus and is usually spastic. The brevis has a small tendon and thus requires a myotomy, as does the gracilis muscle. It is common to have asymmetric releases to achieve symmetric range of motion. Most reports agree that soft tissue releases of the adductor longus, adductor brevis, gracilis, iliopsoas, and hamstrings is necessary to rebalance the hips.[8,9,29] Muscles are released until 50 degrees of symmetric abduction is obtained. Unilateral surgery should be avoided in cases in which spasticity is present in both lower extremities, even if only 1 hip is subluxed.[31,32]

The anterior branch of the obturator nerve lies on the anterior surface of the adductor brevis. Historically, division of the nerve had been used as an adjunct to reduce the recurrence of an adduction contracture, but has been associated with creation of an abduction contracture after surgery. It is difficult to delineate whether the neurectomy, overly aggressive tenotomies, or prolonged abduction splinting is the cause of this complication. Although a neurectomy is no longer advocated, the author has used temporary interruption of the signal with a crush neurectomy in nonambulatory settings without leading to an abduction-posture complication. Phenol can also be placed directly on the nerve at the time of surgery.

Hip Flexion Deformities

Hip flexion contractures usually present as part of the combined hip adduction, flexion, and rotation deformities. They are seen in nonambulatory, bilateral ambulatory, and type IV hemiplegic individuals. The clinical importance of the iliopsoas in the progression of hip subluxation is supported by the relatively high failure rates of adductor myotomies alone.[9]

In patients who are ambulatory, recession of the iliopsoas at the level of the pelvic brim has been advocated. The preservation of hip flexor power and the ability to climb stairs in individuals who are ambulatory has been used as the rationale for this recommendation.[33] Historically, the release of the iliopsoas at the lesser trochanter had been reserved for patients who are nonambulatory. Recent gait study information has challenged this surgical recommendation.[34] Bialik and colleagues[34] compared the results of patients treated either with iliopsoas tenotomy at the level of the lesser trochanter or recession at the pelvic brim. The improvement of hip extension parameters was more robust in patients who underwent release at the lesser trochanter. There was no adverse kinematic or kinetic change in hip function after surgery. The authors stated that, "Because there were no adverse effects of iliopsoas release from the lesser trochanter and improvement in hip extension is greater, this approach should be considered in ambulatory patients."[34] Postoperative hip flexion strength was found to be comparable.

Postoperative regimen after soft tissue releases varies. The benefits of long-term postoperative bracing are debated. Houkam and colleagues[27] reported improved results in both mildly and severely involved individuals, especially in children less than 6 years of age.

The use of combined adductor and iliopsoas release can lead to good clinical and radiographic results. Successful outcome is related to age of intervention, a low migration index, and ambulatory status. Horstmann and Bleck[9] reported the best results with soft tissue if performed before the age of 5 years. Miller reported 80% good or fair outcomes at 39-months follow-up in a population that included 69% nonambulators undergoing soft tissue releases at an age of 4.5 years. More than 50% of quadriplegics had satisfactory results.[33] Intervention, even at an age of 2 to 3 years, may be warranted.

A migration index of more than 30% is considered to be the threshold for intervention. There is also no absolute cutoff value for the migration index for a good result, but a migration index of 40% is a good guide in most cases.[35] Satisfactory results have been reported up to a migration index of 60%.[29] The success of soft tissue releases can be appreciated by 6 months, and migration index at 1 year is predictive of outcome.

The importance of long-term follow-up after soft tissue release is essential because tendons can reattach and subluxation recurs, especially for individuals who are nonambulatory. Although the primary goal of soft tissue releases is to halt the early progression of hip subluxation, they can also be considered as a way to slow the rate of progression. In severely involved children who are nonambulatory and who are not healthy enough to undergo a more extensive procedure, early soft tissue intervention can gain time and defer a complex reconstruction until the child is bigger, healthier, and has better bone stock.

RECONSTRUCTIVE PROCEDURES

In spite of soft tissue releases, or in late presenting children, the bony anatomy needs to be addressed. In children with limited or no ambulatory potential, the femur and acetabulum need to be evaluated and treated accordingly. Ambulatory children with cerebral palsy may not have significant subluxation but may benefit from bony procedures to address rotational deformities.

Rotational Deformities

Internal rotation deformities are considered to be caused by a combination of dynamic and structural elements. Electromyogram studies have identified the medial hamstrings as the main internal rotator of the hip and a weakness of the gluteus medius. The bony deformity is caused by persistent femoral anteversion. Internal rotation posture is a common deformity in individuals who have type IV hemiplegia and children with crouch gait and spastic diplegic.[29,36-38] The medial rotation posture of the foot and leg are offset by retraction of the ipsilateral pelvis. The medial rotation posture does not correct in time.

Soft tissue releases have not led to favorable long-term results.[39] A derotation osteotomy is the procedure of choice. The indications for treatment are a functional impairment of gait, such as tripping or catching the involved leg, internal rotation of greater than 60 degrees, external rotation of 25 degrees, and a femoral anteversion of 40 to 45 degrees. The functional impairment is usually exacerbated by a heelcord and/or hamstring contracture that should also be addressed. Good results have been described for both intertrochanteric- and supracondylar-level osteotomies.[38,40] Rigid internal fixation (plates and screws or intramedullary fixation in patients who are nearly or fully skeletally mature) is associated with decreased pain and allows for early mobilization. The goal should be to retain approximately 30 degrees of passive internal rotation; over-rotation; can lead to posterior instability. If hip subluxation or coxa valgus is present, a proximal varus derotation osteotomy (VDRO) is preferred. Derotation osteotomies improve the ease of ambulation. Postsurgical gait analysis shows improved sagittal and transverse plane parameters.[36,37,39] Younger children are at additional risk of recurrence of deformity.[41]

In individuals who have impaired mobility or are nonambulatory (GFMCS III, IV, V) are at highest risk for progression of subluxation and dislocation of the hip. In spite of dedicated surveillance strategies and protocols and aggressive soft tissue surgery, progression of subluxation can occur in up to half of the patients. Bony surgery is indicated in situations in which the migration index exceeds 40% and there is a deformity of the proximal femur. In the absence of significant acetabular dysplasia, proximal femoral VDROs have been recommended. Children with a migration index of greater than 60% or residual acetabular dysplasia have a higher incidence of recurrent subluxation with only VDRO and benefit from comprehensive treatment.[42]

The goal is to redirect the femoral head into the deepest part of the acetabulum, thereby mitigating the deforming forces on the superolateral acetabulum and femoral head. The femoral anteversion can be corrected and the extremity shortened. In a computer model of the spastic hip, correcting for anteversion and neck shaft angle did little to influence the direction or magnitude of forces. The shortening component of the VDRO relaxes the muscle tendon unit and helps to rebalance the forces about the hip.

Karol and colleagues[39] reported 84% of their patients to have a stable pain-free hip in a treatment group that included 2/3 patients who were nonambulatory spastic and quadriparetic at a mean age of 7.7 years. Reducing the migration index and improved *center-edge* angle were associated with good radiographic outcomes at final follow-up. Insufficient varus and the inability to achieve good lateral coverage after the osteotomy are associated with recurrent subluxation. Effective acetabular remodeling cannot be expected at more than 4 years of age in children with spastic quadriplegia.[9,30,41]

Age at the time of surgery is an important determinant of long-term results. Schmale and colleagues[30] cautioned that children who underwent proximal femoral osteotomies at a young age are at risk for reoperation. At the 5-year follow-up, 74% of the children had undergone reoperation for recurrent subluxation. Of 38 patients who underwent only VDROs, 35 were classified as spastic tetraplegics. In one of the longest follow-up studies of VDROs (15-year mean follow-up), Brunner and Baumann[43] found that 96% of the valgus had recurred and that there was a 40% loss of the femoral anteversion. The loss of correction was greater the younger the child at the time of surgery and the more severe the spastic symptoms. After age 8 years, the change in the neck shaft angle and the anteversion were found to be small, therefore they recommended delaying bony procedures until after age 8 years. This recommendation underscores the importance of long-term follow-up, especially for younger children with higher GMFCS scores.

POSTOPERATIVE TREATMENT

Successful surgical outcomes begin with appropriate preoperative planning. A comprehensive team approach is key to anticipating and addressing multiple underlying comorbidities such as seizures disorders, pulmonary status, and nutritional status before they become clinical issues. Timely pain and spasticity control is important. Manipulation of spastic muscles adds to the level of surgical pain. Pain control with narcotics and antispasmodics is effective but needs to be used with caution in this population. Drooling, poor gag reflex, and compromised swallowing make the risk of oversedation and aspiration a clinical concern. Regional anesthetics, such as nerve blocks, caudals and epidurals, offer attractive alternatives. The anesthetic can be single shot or continuous, and can consist of local anesthetics with or without the addition of narcotics. They limit spasms and control pain while curtailing the amount of systemic sedation and respiratory compromise.

Regional blocks carry the risk of urinary retention and infection, especially with indwelling catheters. The risk of masking a compartment syndrome is a significant concern in tibial osteotomies but has not been of concern for hip surgeries.

Traditionally, cast immobilization has been used after both soft tissue and bony surgeries. Well-padded casts allow control of postoperative pain and spasms, but at the expense of mobility. Prolonged immobilization can lead to pressure sores, weakness, and osteopenia. The osteopenia can lead to postoperative insufficiency fractures when physical therapy is initiated. Postoperative immobilization after bony surgery can lead to a prolonged recovery of presurgical functional levels. Schafer and colleagues[44] showed a 4-month difference in time to presurgical functional levels after VDROs in ambulatory children allowed weight bearing as tolerated versus a period of cast immobilization. The recent trend has been to decrease the length of immobilization and initiate early movement. In cases of soft tissue surgery, removable braces and splints versus long-leg abduction casts allow for early range of motion. In bony surgery, stronger internal fixation has reduced the period of cast mobilization. Certain investigators dispense with postoperative immobilization completely and follow a program of early mobilization.[21,29]

COMPREHENSIVE TREATMENT

Progressive subluxation leads to dysplasia of the acetabulum. Once the presence of dysplasia is established, the acetabulum shows poor remodeling potential, especially after the age of 4 years, whether treated with soft tissue release or VDROs.[9,42] Progressive deformity of the hip requires comprehensive treatment that addresses the soft tissue contractures, femoral head displacement, and dysplasia of the hip.

One-stage treatment of the high-grade subluxation or dislocation has become the predominant treatment in the last 20 years.[9,28,29,45–48] Single-stage surgical relocation has been shown to be an effective treatment in both short- and long-term follow-up studies. Even hips with relative incongruity and femoral head irregularity are candidates for surgical reconstruction.[47] If preoperative radiographs indicate remodeling of the femoral head, it should be inspected at the time of surgery for degenerative changes. Although the technical details differ between different institutions, the operation consists of relocation of the hip, soft tissue lengthening, femoral osteotomy with shortening, and pelvic osteotomy.

Several pelvic osteotomies have been described to address the acetabular dysplasia. The periacetabular osteotomy is a reliable, fairly safe, and effective osteotomy.

The osteotomy is performed through an anterior ilioinguinal approach.[28] The interval between the sartorius and tensor fascia is developed. The external oblique is reflected off the iliac crest. The crest is divided, allowing exposure of the outer table. The dissection is carried down to the sciatic notch. The inner table is similarly exposed. The anterior and posterior columns are divided to allow easier hinging of the osteotomy. The posterior column is divided with Kerrison rongeur. A flat 1.9 cm osteotome is used to make the initial cut on the outer cortex. A curved osteotome is used to make a curvilinear cut under fluoroscopic guidance down to the level of the triradiate cartilage or slightly cephalad to the triradiate cartilage. The osteotomy is gently levered with the osteotome or a small lamina spreader. Triangular wedges cut from the iliac crest or bone from the VDRO are recessed into the osteotomy. The size and placement of the wedges can be modified to give the desired correction (**Fig. 3**). Standard closure is performed.

The hinging effect of the periacetabular osteotomy relies on the presence of an open triradiate. The osteotomy allows effective treatment of the superolateral acetabular deficiency. The osteotomy can be tailored to provide more anterior or posterior coverage depending on the abnormality. The correction is held by a bone graft that is wedged into place. The osteotomy is stable and internal fixation is not required. The indication for addition of pericapsular acetabuloplasty includes open triradiate cartilage, acetabular dysplasia (acetabular index of >25 degrees), and subluxation or dislocation with a migration percentage of more than 40%.[28,47]

Complications of the combined single-stage reconstruction include infection, avascular necrosis, femoral fractures, and premature closure of the triradiate cartilage. The avascular necrosis can occur from injury to the femoral head circulation during the open reduction, injury to the medial circumflex artery with iliopsoas release, or increased pressure between femoral head and acetabulum.[47]

Older children who present with a neuromuscular dislocation and closed triradiate cartilage are usually not candidates for a periacetabular osteotomy. In these cases, nonanatomic coverage is created by a lateral bony buttress using a Chiari,

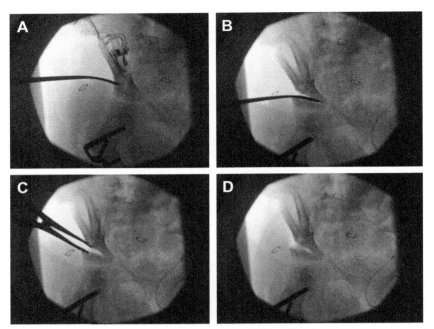

Fig. 3. Periacetabular pelvic osteotomy in a 5-year-old boy GMFCS IV.(*A*) Osteotomy starts above the hip capsule and a curved osteotome is directed toward the triradiate cartilage. (*B*) The osteotomy hinges on the triradiate cartilage or slightly cephalad to the triradiate cartilage. (*C*) Small laminar spreader holds the correction and facilitates placement of graft. (*D*) Bone graft from VDRO in place. No internal fixation is required.

or slotted augmented shelf osteotomy.[9,49] The hip capsule is used as the interposition material between the femoral head and the ilium. In time, the capsule undergoes metaplasia and fibrocartilage mimics the function of articular cartilage. The complication peculiar to the Chiari osteotomy is a sciatic neuropathy.

TREATMENT OF THE PAINFUL DISLOCATED HIP

Even with the institution of hip surveillance programs and aggressive preventative and reconstruction procedures, spastic hips can still dislocate. If aggressive treatment is recommended to prevent a dislocation, do dislocated hips merit aggressive treatment? If so, what is the best option?

Not all patients with dislocated hips are destined to lead a painful existence.[50,51] A review of 234 adult individuals with spastic hip dislocation reported an overall incidence of pain of 47%. Only a 25% incidence of painful hips required surgical intervention.[50] There is no single factor that identifies the painful from nonpainful dislocated hip. With the exceptions of hygiene or sitting issues, dislocated hips that are not painful should be left alone.

The painful dislocated hip poses a significant challenge. Several treatment options have been recommended over the years, and there is no preferred solution. The options available have been adapted from the treatment of monoarticular degenerative processes, such as untreated developmental dislocation of the hip or posttraumatic arthritis. The options available are valgus redirectional osteotomy, hip arthrodesis, femoral head resection, interposition arthroplasty, and total joint arthroplasty.

Valgus osteotomy points the dislocated head away from the acetabulum.[52] It was initially used in irreducible congenital hip dislocations. The Hass osteotomy redirected the femoral head from the acetabulum but allowed the indirect transfer of load through the subtrochanteric region. In cerebral palsy, the goal is to redirect the femoral head away from the acetabulum while abducting the leg to improve perineal care.

The surgical procedure consists of a subtrochanteric valgus osteotomy. The advent of specially designed locking plates has simplified the operation and eliminated the need for postoperative immobilization. Hogan and colleagues[52] reported that most patients were doing well. Caregivers reported increased ease of perineal care, and 14/15 caregivers would recommend the procedure.

Hip arthrodesis in a young, active laborer for isolated posttraumatic degenerative disease is well documented and has favorable results even in individuals who are nonambulatory[53,54] The long-term results are dependent on the viability of the contralateral hip and spine. Arthrodesis may be an option for individuals who are unilaterally ambulatory.

Resection arthroplasty has been used as a salvage procedure for failed total joints. In cerebral palsy, resection arthroplasty has been performed with good outcomes.[51,55,56] The surrounding tissues are used as an interpositional arthroplasty. Traction has been recommended during the healing phase to limit proximal migration, but it is of questionable benefit. Postoperative complications include persistent pain, infection, pressure sores, pneumonia, and heterotopic ossification (HO). Postoperative pain can last for up to a year. HO has been reported after resection. The risk factors for HO are repeat surgery and capsulotomy. However, the number of individuals who require resection is small.

There is a reluctance to use total joints in neuromuscular conditions. Patients with these conditions are prone to dislocation because of poor volitional muscle control. Infection, HO, loosening and longevity of the components, stiffness, and pain are other potential complications. The appeal is the ability to preserve movement and functional capacity while eliminating pain. Encouraging results have been reported by using arthroplasty to achieve pain relief and ease of care.[54,57] In a series by Root and colleagues,[54] 14 out of 15 patients reported pain relief. Ten patients had some walking ability, indicating some abductor muscle control. However, Root and colleagues[54] commented that "total body involvement in eight patients did not adversely influence the success of the procedure." Dislocation did not seem to preclude patients from being pain free and able to sit.[57]

SUMMARY

Hip abnormalities affect most children with cerebral palsy. Dedicated surveillance programs have been shown to be effective means of identifying hips at risk and preventing pathologic dislocation. Patients who are ambulatory and correlate with GMFCS I and II experience deformities that affect mobility and gait, but rarely dislocations. Marginal and nonambulatory patients parallel the GMFCS III, IV, and V and have an increasing risk of dislocation. Once subluxation has been identified, early surgical intervention is indicated. Surgical treatment can be grouped as soft tissue (preventative), bony procedures (reconstructive), and palliative (salvage). Soft tissue releases should address the spastic adductors, iliopsoas, and hamstrings. Long-term postoperative follow-up is needed to monitor for recurrence. Individuals who recur or who do not respond to initial soft tissue releases benefit from bony surgery. Comprehensive reconstruction of the hip has become the predominant treatment approach when acetabular and proximal femoral dysplasia is present. The painful arthritic dislocated hip has numerous treatment options. Hip arthroplasty procedures show promising results and may supplant other salvage options in the future.

REFERENCES

1. Bagg MR, Farber J, Miller F. Long term follow-up of hip subluxation in cerebral palsy patients. J Pediatr Orthop 1993;13:32–6.
2. Lonstein JE, Beck RPT. Hip dislocation and subluxation in cerebral palsy. J Pediatr Orthop 1986;6(5):521–6.
3. Palisano RJ, Cameron D, Rosenbaum PL, et al. Stability of the gross motor function classification system. Dev Med Child Neurol 2006;48:424–8.
4. Palisano RJ, Rosenbaum P, Bartlett D, et al. Content validity of the expanded and revised gross motor function classification system. Dev Med Child Neurol 2008;50:744–50.
5. Palisano R, Roesenbaum P, Walter S, et al. Development and reliability of a system to classify gross motor function in children with cerebral palsy. Dev Med Child Neurol 1997;39:214–23.
6. Soo B, Howard JJ, Boyd RN, et al. Hip displacement in cerebral palsy. J Bone Joint Surg Am Jan 2006;88:121–9.
7. Samilson RL, Tsou P, Aamoht G, et al. Dislocation and subluxation of the hip in cerebral palsy. J Bone Joint Surg Am 1972;54:863–73.
8. Miller F, Slomczykowski M, Cope R, et al. Computer modeling of the pathomechanics of spastic hip dislocation in children. J Pediatr Orthop 1999;19(4):486–94.
9. Horstmann HM, Bleck EE. Orthopedic management in cerebral palsy. 2nd edition. London: Mackieth Press; 2007.
10. Chung CY, Park MS, Cho IH, et al. Morphometric analysis of acetabular dysplasia in cerebral palsy. J Bone Joint Surg Br 2006;88:243–7.
11. Kim HT, Wenger DR. Location of acetabular deficiency and associated hip dislocation in neuromuscular hip dysplasia: three-dimensional computed tomographic analysis. J Pediatr Orthop 1997;17(2):143–51.
12. Heinrich SD, MacEwen GD, Zembo MM. Hip dysplasia, subluxation, and dislocation in cerebral

palsy: an arthrographic analysis. J Pediatr Orthop 1991;11(4):488–93.

13. Srcutton D, Baird G, Smeeton N. Hip dysplasia in bilateral cerebral palsy: incidence and natural history in children 18 months to 5 years. Dev Med Child Neurol 2001;43:586–600.

14. Cooke PH, Cole WG, Carey RP. Dislocation of the hip in cerebral palsy: natural history and predictability. J Bone Joint Surg Br 1989;71:441–6.

15. Hagglund G, Andersson S, Duppe H, et al. Prevention of dislocation of the hip in children with cerebral palsy: the first ten years of a population based prevention programme. J Bone Joint Surg Br 2005; 87:95–101.

16. Gordon GS, Simkiss DE. A systematic review of the evidence for surveillance in children with cerebral palsy. J Bone Joint Surg 2006;88:1492–6.

17. Miller F, Girardi H, Lipton G, et al. Reconstruction of dysplastic spastic hip with peri-ilial pelvic and femoral osteotomy followed by immediate mobilization. J Pediatr Orthop 1997;17:592–602.

18. Reimers J. Stability of the hip in children a radiographic study of muscle surgery in cerebral palsy. Acta Orthop Scand Suppl 1980;184:1–100.

19. Robin J, Graham HK, Selber P, et al. Proximal femoral geometry in cerebral palsy: a population-based cross-sectional study. J Bone Joint Surg Br 2008;90(10):1372–9.

20. Dobson F, Boyd RN, Parrott J, et al. Hip surveillance in children with cerebral palsy: impact of the surgical management of spastic hip disease. J Bone Joint Surg Br 2002;84:720–6.

21. Miller F, Dias RC, Dabney KW, et al. Soft-tissue release for spastic hip subluxation in cerebral palsy. J Pediatr Orthop 1997;17(5):571–84.

22. Wynter M, Gibson N, Kentish M, et al. Consensus statement on the hip - surveillance for children with cerebral palsy. Australian Standards of Care; 2008. Available at: www.cpaustralia.com.au/ausacpdm. Accessed July 20, 2010.

23. Dabney KW, Miller F. In: Abel MF, editor. Cerebral palsy in orthopedic knowledge update, pediatrics 3. Rosemont (IL): American Academy of Orthopedic Surgeons; 2006.

24. Preiss A, Condie DN, Rowley DI, et al. The effects of botulinum toxin (btx-a) on spasticity of the lower limb and on gait in cerebral palsy. J Bone Joint Surg Br 2003;85:943–8.

25. Graham HK, Selber P. Musculoskeletal aspects of cerebral palsy. J Bone Joint Surg Br 2003;85:157–66.

26. Graham HK, Boyd R, Dobson F, et al. Does botulinum toxin combined with bracing prevent hip displacement in children with cerebral palsy and "hips at risk". J Bone Joint Surg Am 2008;90:23–33.

27. Houkam JA, Roach JW, Wenger DR, et al. Treatment of acquired hip subluxation in cerebral palsy. J Pediatr Orthop 1986;6:285–90.

28. Mubarak SJ, Valencia FG, Wenger D. One stage correction of the spastic dislocated hip: use of pericapsular osteotomy to improve coverage. J Bone Joint Surg Am 1992;74:1347–57.

29. Flynn JM, Miller F. Management of hip disorders in patients with cerebral palsy. J Am Acad Orthop Surg May June 2002;10(3):198–209.

30. Schmale GA, Eilert RE, Chang F, et al. High reoperation rates after early treatment of subluxating hips in children with spastic cerebral palsy. J Pediatr Orthop 2006;26(5):617–23.

31. Carr C, Gage JR. The fate of the nonoperated hip in cerebral palsy. J Pediatr Orthop 1987;7(3): 262–7.

32. Noonan KJ, Walker TL, Kayes KJ, et al. Effect of surgery on the nontreated hip in severe cerebral palsy. J Pediatr Orthop 2000;20(6):771–5.

33. Sutherland DH, Zilberfarb JL, Kaufman KR, et al. Psoas release at the pelvic brim in ambulatory patients with cerebral palsy: operative technique and functional outcome. J Pediatr Orthop 1997; 17(5):563–70.

34. Bialik GM, Pierce R, Dorociak R, et al. Ilipsoas tenotomy at the lesser trochanter versus at the pelvic brim in ambulatory children with cerebral palsy. J Pediatr Orthop 2009;29:251–5.

35. Cornell MS, Hatrick NC, Boyd R, et al. The hip in children with cerebral palsy. Predicting the outcome of soft tissue surgery. Clin Orthop Relat Res 1997; 340:165–71.

36. Ounpuu S, Deluca P, Davis R, et al. Long term effects of derotation osteotomies: an evaluation using three dimensional gait analysis. J Pediatr Orthop 2002;22:139–45.

37. Murray-Weir M, Root L, Peterson M, et al. Proximal femoral varus rotation osteotomy in cerebral palsy: a perspective gait study. J Pediatr Orthop 2003;23: 321–9.

38. Kay RM, Rethlefsen SA, Hale JM, et al. Comparison of proximal and distal rotational femoral osteotomy in children with cerebral palsy. J Pediatr Orthop 2003; 23(2):150–4.

39. Karol LA. Surgical management of the lower extremity in ambulatory children with cerebral palsy. J Am Acad Orthop Surg May June 2004;12(3).

40. Pirpiris M, Trivett A, Baker A, et al. Femoral derotation osteotomy in spastic diplegia: proximal or distal? J Bone Joint Surg Br Mar 2003;85:265–72.

41. Kim H, Aiona M, Sussman M. Recurrence after femoral derotational osteotomy in cerebral palsy. J Pediatr Orthop 2005;25(6):739–43.

42. Song H-R, Carroll NC. Femoral varus derotation osteotomy with or without acetabuloplasty for unstable hips in cerebral palsy. J Pediatr Orthop 1998;18(1): 62–8.

43. Brunner R, Baumann JU. Long term effect of varus derotation osteotomy on femur and acetabulum in

spastic cerebral palsy: an 11 to 18 year follow-up study. J Pediatr Orthop 1997;17:585–91.

44. Schaefer MK, McCarthy JJ, Josephic K. Effects of early weight bearing on the functional recovery of ambulatory children with cerebral palsy after bilateral proximal femoral osteotomy. J Pediatr Orthop September 2007;27(6):668–70.

45. Al-Ghadir M, Masquijo JJ, Guerra LA, et al. Combined femoral and pelvic osteotomies versus femoral osteotomy alone in the treatment of hip dysplasia in children with cerebral palsy. J Pediatr Orthop 2009;29(7):779–83.

46. Debnath UK, Guha AR, Karlakki S, et al. Combined femoral and pelvic osteotomies for the reconstruction of the painful subluxation or dislocation of the hip in cerebral palsy. J Bone Joint Surg Br 2006; 88:1373–8.

47. McNerney NP, Mubarak SJ, Wenger DR. One stage correction of the dysplastic hip in cerebral palsy with the San Diego acetabuloplasty: results and complications in 104 hips. J Pediatr Orthop 2000;20(1):93.

48. Sankar WN, Spiegel DA, Gregg JR, et al. Long term follow-up after one-stage reconstruction of dislocated hips in patients with cerebral palsy. J Pediatr Orthop 2006;26(1):1–7.

49. Luegmair M, Vuillerot C, Cunin V, et al. Slotted acetabular augmentation alone or as part of a combined one-stage approach for treatment of hip dysplasia in adolescent with cerebral palsy: results and complications in 19 hips. J Pediatr Orthop 2009;29(7):784–91.

50. Hodgkinson I, Vadot JP, Metton G, et al. Hip pain in 234 nonambulatory adolescents and young adults with cerebral palsy; a cross-sectional multicenter study. Dev Med Child Neurol 2001;43: 806–8.

51. Knapp DR Jr, Cortes H. Untreated hip dislocation in cerebral palsy. J Pediatr Orthop 2002;22(5):668–71.

52. Hogan KA, Blake M, Gross RH. Subtrochanteric valgus osteotomy for the treatment of chronically dislocated spastic hips. J Bone Joint Surg Am 2007;89:226–31.

53. Fucs PM, Svartman C, deAsumpcao RMC, et al. Treatment of chronically dislocated and subluxated painful hip in with arthrodesis. J Pediatr Orthop 2003;23(4):529–34.

54. Root L, Goss JR, Mendes J. The treatment of painful hip in cerebral palsy by total hip replacement or hip arthrodesis. J Bone Joint Surg 1986;68(4):590–8.

55. Baxter MP, D'Astous JL. Proximal femoral resection-interposition arthroplasty: salvage hip surgery for the severely disabled child with cerebral palsy. J Pediatr Orthop 1986;6(6):681–5.

56. Widmann RF, Do TT, Doyle SM, et al. Resection arthroplasty of the hip for patients with cerebral palsy: an outcome study. J Pediatr Orthop 1999;19(6): 805–10.

57. Gabos PG, Miller F, Galban MA, et al. Prosthetic interposition for palliative treatment of end stage spastic hip disease in nonambulatory patients with cerebral palsy. J Pediatr Orthop 1999;19(6): 796–804.

Management of the Knee in Spastic Diplegia: What is the Dose?

Jeffrey L. Young, MD[a],*, Jill Rodda, PhD[b],
Paulo Selber, MD, FRACS[a,c], Erich Rutz, MD[a],
H. Kerr Graham, MD, FRCS (Ed), FRACS[a,b,d,e]

KEYWORDS

- Cerebral palsy • Spastic diplegia • Knee dysfunction
- Treatment

The principal topographic patterns of involvement in cerebral palsy (CP) are spastic hemiplegia, spastic diplegia, and spastic quadriplegia. From the orthopedic surgeon's point of view, it is convenient to think of the orthopedic priorities for each of these 3 main groups. In children with spastic hemiplegia, there is much more involvement of the foot and ankle than of the hip and knee. Orthopedic interventions usually address deformity of the foot and ankle, of which spastic equinus, equinovarus, and equinovalgus feet are the most common problems. On the opposite end of the severity spectrum, patients with spastic quadriplegia are more affected by deformities of the hip, pelvis, and spine. These deformities may preclude comfortable sitting. Deformities at the knee, foot, and ankle are often present and are sometimes significant, but spastic hip dislocation, pelvic obliquity, and scoliosis dominate orthopedic priorities.

In the lower limbs of children with spastic diplegia there is multilevel involvement, with the common pattern being equinovalgus at the foot/ankle, flexion with stiffness at the knee, and flexion with internal rotation at the hip. Contractures of the biarticular muscles, such as the hamstrings, rectus femoris, and gastrocnemius, create a challenge in selecting the most appropriate interventions to achieving sagittal plane balance. For example, hamstring lengthening may improve knee extension but at the expense of causing increased anterior pelvic tilt. A wide range of interventions has been described to manage knee dysfunction, but the indications and outcomes are not clearly established. Selber and colleagues[1] introduced the concept of surgical dose in CP, whereby the surgical intervention should match the severity of dysfunction. The authors apply this concept to the management of knee dysfunction in children with CP, with a special emphasis on spastic

---

[a] Orthopaedic Department, The Royal Children's Hospital, Melbourne, 50 Flemington Road, Parkville, Victoria, 3052, Australia
[b] Hugh Williamson Gait Laboratory, The Royal Children's Hospital, Melbourne, 50 Flemington Road, Parkville, Victoria, 3052, Australia
[c] Orthopaedic Department, The Children's Hospital at Westmead, Locked Bag 4001, Westmead, New South Wales, 2145, Australia
[d] The University of Melbourne and Murdoch Childrens Research Institute, 50 Flemington Road, Parkville, Victoria, 3052, Australia
[e] National Health and Medical Research Council (NHMRC) Centre of Research Excellence in Gait Rehabilitation, 50 Flemington Road, Parkville, Victoria, 3052, Australia
* Corresponding author.
E-mail address: jly829@hotmail.com

Orthop Clin N Am 41 (2010) 561–577
doi:10.1016/j.ocl.2010.06.006
0030-5898/10/$ — see front matter © 2010 Elsevier Inc. All rights reserved.

diplegia. Some of these principles may be applied in children with hemiplegia and quadriplegia.

EVALUATION

For a complete evaluation of the child with spastic diplegia, information from several sources needs to be gathered and synthesized. Formalized by Davids and colleagues[2] in the diagnostic matrix, information is gathered from the following 5 sources (**Fig. 1**):

1. Clinical history
2. Physical examination
3. Instrumented gait analysis
4. Special investigations including radiology
5. Examination under anesthesia.

An appropriate integration of information from these sources provides a comprehensive view of an individual patient's musculoskeletal pathology and gait pathology. This information provides the basis on which management can be planned and outcomes can be measured. For example, in crouch gait, the patient may present with fatigue and anterior knee pain (clinical history). Physical examination may indicate spastic hamstring contracture (increased popliteal angle, fixed flexion deformity at the knee). Radiographs may show patella alta and fragmentation at the inferior pole of the patella. Motion analysis may show a stiff flexed knee gait pattern. Examination under anesthesia gives an opportunity to accurately assess the degree of fixed flexion deformity without the effects of spasticity, which is valuable in selecting the most appropriate intervention.

PHYSICAL EXAMINATION

In spastic diplegia, knee flexion deformity predominates. Differentiating among joint contracture,

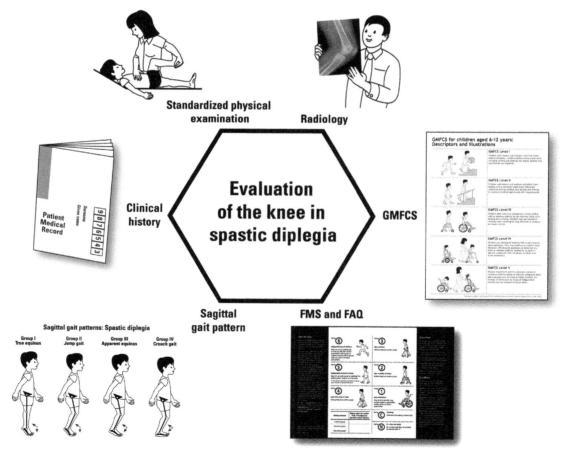

Fig. 1. The diagnostic matrix takes into consideration the clinical history, the physical examination, the gait analysis, the radiology results, and an examination under anesthesia when determining a patient's musculoskeletal pathology, formulating a treatment plan, and assessing outcomes. GMFCS, Gross Motor Function Classification System; FMS, Functional Mobility Scores; FAQ, Functional Assessment Questionnaire.

muscle contracture, and muscle spasticity helps guide appropriate interventions. Joint contractures are quantified by measurements of fixed flexion deformity at the knee. Maximum knee extension is measured with the hip in neutral extension.[3] Extending the hip relaxes the hamstrings at this level and eliminates their contribution to knee flexion. Contracture of the hamstrings, described by measuring the popliteal angle, is tested by measuring knee extension with the hip in the flexed position, placing the hamstrings at their maximal stretch across the hip and knee.[3] Muscle spasticity is assessed by performing the maneuver mentioned earlier at varying speeds to determine the velocity-dependent contribution to limited knee extension. The Duncan-Ely test, performed by placing the patient in the prone position with the hip extended and flexing the knee, assesses rectus femoris spasticity.[4]

GAIT ANALYSIS

Gait analysis is essential in evaluating and quantifying gait dysfunction. Understanding the gait pattern and the interrelationship of the hip, knee, and ankle helps guide treatment.[2]

Sagittal Knee Patterns

One of the earliest and most useful categorical descriptions of knee dysfunction was by Sutherland and Davids[5] in 1993. Using a combination of physical examination and sagittal kinematics, the investigators identified 4 sagittal patterns at the knee. These patterns were jump knee, crouch knee, stiff knee, and recurvatum knee. In jump knee, there is increased knee flexion in early stance, followed by near-normal knee extension in late stance. In crouch knee, there is both increased knee flexion and ankle dorsiflexion throughout stance. In stiff knee, there is decreased knee flexion and decreased knee range of motion (ROM) during swing phase, resulting in inefficient foot clearance. In recurvatum knee, there is a hyperextension deformity in mid to late stance. Recognizing these knee patterns helps target interventions.

Sagittal Gait Patterns

Sagittal gait patterns describe the knee and the entire sagittal plane of the lower extremity, which includes the pelvis, hip, knee, and ankle. The 4 gait patterns described are true equinus, jump gait, apparent equinus, and crouch gait (**Fig. 2**).[6] Each group has progressively less ankle equinus, increasing proximal contractures, a shift of the ground reaction force from in front of the knee to behind the knee, and decreasing plantar flexion/

knee extension coupling. In true equinus the ankle is in equinus, the knee is normal or with recurvatum, and the hip has normal extension. Jump gait is characterized by increased knee flexion and ankle equinus. The pelvis is usually normal or anteriorly tilted, and the hip is usually flexed. Apparent equinus is a transitional group between jump gait and crouch gait. In apparent equinus, the child may be seen to be "toe walking," with the heel never contacting the floor. However, the sagittal ankle kinematics is within the normal range and the toe walking is imposed by flexion contractures at the knee and hip. The importance of this pattern is that further intervention to the calf, such as injection of botulinum toxin A (BoNT-A) or lengthening of the gastrocsoleus, is contraindicated because it may produce rapidly progressive crouch gait.

Crouch gait is defined as excessive flexion at the knee and calcaneus at the ankle during stance. Calcaneus at the ankle distinguishes crouch gait from the other flexed knee gait patterns (jump gait, and apparent equinus). In crouch gait there is also excessive hip flexion, although the pelvis position is variable and can be posterior, neutral, or anterior. In patients with posterior pelvic tilt, the hamstrings are short and may well benefit from lengthening. In patients with a neutral pelvis, the hamstrings are typically normal in length. In patients with an anterior pelvic tilt and crouch gait, the hamstrings are already excessively long and should not be lengthened. This observation is counterintuitive because the consistent clinical examination findings in patients with crouch gait include a dramatically increased popliteal angle (typically 70°–90°) as well as a fixed flexion deformity at the knee. However, popliteal angle has a very poor correlation with knee flexion during walking.[7,8] It seems appropriate in such patients to assume that distal hamstring lengthening would be the primary way to correct this gait pattern. In a patient with crouch gait, distal hamstring lengthening may improve knee extension but at the expense of further increasing anterior pelvic tilt.[9] This occurrence is a classic example of the usefulness of the diagnostic matrix for better understanding the subject's gait pattern and for better planning of intervention.

KNEE INTERVENTIONS IN SPASTIC DIPLEGIA
Nonoperative Management

Musculoskeletal strengthening for knee dysfunction

Weakness is an important contributor to gait dysfunction in children with CP. Physical therapists are often the first to identify this problem

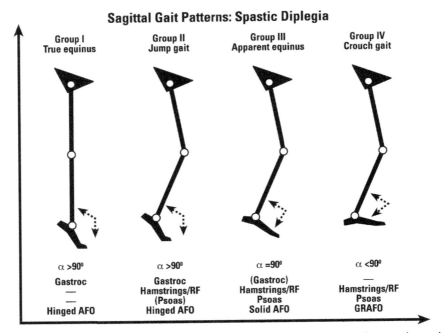

Sagittal Gait Patterns: Spastic Diplegia

Fig. 2. There are 4 main sagittal gait patterns: true equinus, jump gait, apparent equinus, and crouch gait. These patterns describe sagittal plane alignment of the entire lower extremity, which includes the pelvis, hip, knee, and ankle, during stance phase. AFO, ankle-foot orthosis; GRAFO, ground reaction ankle-foot orthosis; RF, rectus femoris. (*Reproduced and adapted with permission* and copyright © of the British Editorial Society of Bone and Joint Surgery [Rodda JM, Graham HK, Carson L, Galea MP, Wolfe R. Sagittal gait patterns in spastic diplegia. J Bone Joint Surg [Br] 2004;86-B:251–8. (Figure 1)].)

because they have the expertise to address this issue. Orthopedic surgeons, on the other hand, may focus more on contractures and deformities because they have the tools to correct these problems. In reality, gait dysfunction often results from a combination of weakness and contractures.

Strengthening, therefore, is an integral part in the management of children with diplegia, both before and after multilevel orthopedic surgery, as well as in children with mild gait deviations. Isometric strengthening exercises improved the strength of targeted muscle groups in short-term studies.[10,11] However, detraining occurred as early as 6 weeks after stopping the exercises.[11] In addition, the relationship between improved strength and gait improvements is not certain. Damiano and colleagues[12] showed a wide variability of gait kinematics after an 8-week progressive resistance exercise program.

Spasticity management for knee dysfunction

Spasticity management in the child with spastic diplegic CP is a complex issue. Recent publications discuss spasticity management in CP at length.[13,14] Options include oral medications, injections of BoNT-A, selective dorsal rhizotomy (SDR) in carefully selected cases, and occasionally

intrathecal baclofen (ITB) pump for severe generalized spasticity. Oral benzodiazepines, such as diazepam (Valium), are most useful for managing acute postoperative pain and spasm but are rarely used for chronic spasticity management.

Injections of BoNT-A are effective in the short term, particularly as a means of deferring multilevel orthopedic surgery until an appropriate age. Injecting the hamstrings with BoNT-A improved knee extension at initial contact by 6° and maximal knee extension in stance phase by 8° at 2 weeks after injection.[15] However, these improvements were no longer present at 12 weeks. The effects of BoNT-A are short lived and never definitive. As a temporizing measure before multilevel surgery, BoNT-A injections provide significant benefit. As shown by Molenaers and colleagues,[16] children receiving multilevel BoNT-A injections for spastic muscle contractures were less likely to have undergone surgery by 8 years of age, 10% versus 27% (*P*<.0025).

More generalized lower limb spasticity, including severe cocontraction at the knee, may be managed in carefully selected children by SDR. Finally, when hypertonia is mixed with a combination of spastic and dystonic features, severe and generalized throughout the lower limbs, the most appropriate intervention may be an ITB (**Fig. 3**A).[13]

Surgical Correction of Knee Gait Dysfunction in Spastic Diplegia

A wide range of surgical procedures has been described for the management of knee problems in children with spastic diplegia, and recently, several new procedures have been either reintroduced or described for the first time. These procedures include various combinations of lengthening of the distal hamstrings, transfer of the distal hamstrings, lengthening or transfer of the rectus femoris, extension osteotomy of the distal femur, and distal femoral growth plate surgery. Information on the outcomes of these various procedures is limited by study design and the lack of randomized trials.

The authors do not think that it is sufficient for orthopedic surgeons to have a single approach to a problem such as flexed knee gait. The

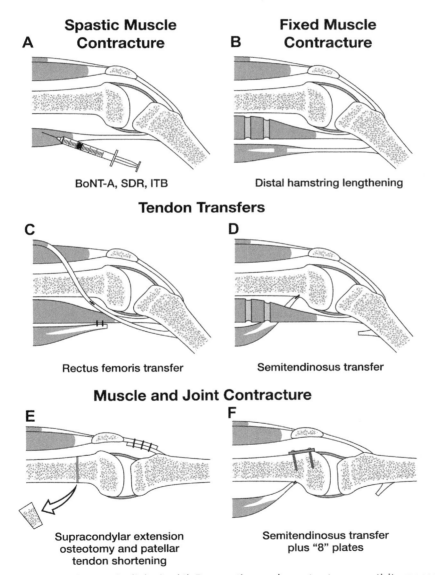

Fig. 3. Knee interventions in spastic diplegia. (*A*) For spastic muscle contracture, spasticity management may include BoNT-A, SDR, and occasionally ITB. (*B*) Fixed muscle contractures are addressed by medial distal hamstring lengthening. (*C, D*) Useful tendon transfers include a rectus femoris transfer or semitendinosus transfer. (*E*) Fixed knee flexion contracture may be addressed by supracondylar extension osteotomy and patellar tendon shortening. (*F*) When growth is remaining, guided growth can be used, applying eight-Plates across the anterior distal femoral physis.

variations in age and the severity of pathology are so extensive that a range of interventions is required. In this context, it is appropriate to consider the "surgical dose," as first described by Selber.[1] Intuitively, the use of BoNT-A in the management of spastic hamstrings is based on an understanding that a different dose of BoNT-A would be used for children of different ages, of different weights, and with different degrees of hamstring spasticity. In the same manner, orthopedic surgeons need to consider the patient's age, Gross Motor Function Classification System (GMFCS) level, sagittal gait pattern, and severity of the knee dysfunction when determining the appropriate surgical dose.

Distal hamstring lengthening

Hamstring contractures are common in CP, and its management often includes distal hamstring lengthening. The precise indications for distal hamstring lengthening are not clearly established. Muscle length modeling studies suggest that short contracted hamstrings are less prevalent than previously thought and distal hamstring lengthening has almost certainly been overused in children with spastic diplegia.[17]

The patient's level of activity and function may help guide management. In nonambulatory spastic quadriplegic patients, GMFCS IV or V, hamstring contractures may interfere with sitting. Therefore, lengthening of the proximal hamstrings[18,19] in combination with adductor lengthening may be appropriate. In contrast, distal hamstring lengthening has been the preferred technique in the management of ambulant children with spastic diplegia. For the independent ambulators, GMFCS I and II, carefully controlled lengthening of the hamstrings is mandatory.

Various techniques are described. The semimembranosus and biceps are usually lengthened by several circular stripes in the fascia over the distal muscle followed by gentle extension of the knee. With this technique, lengthening in continuity is observed, with preservation of the underlying muscle and presumably its long-term function. Lengthening of the gracilis and semitendinosus is more controversial because of the relevant distal anatomy. Described techniques include simple tenotomy, Z-lengthening, and intramuscular lengthening.

The role of lateral hamstring lengthening is more controversial and less well defined than medial hamstring lengthening. Kay and colleagues[20] compared medial and lateral hamstring lengthening and demonstrated similar clinical outcomes in both groups. No statistically significant differences were noted in postoperative popliteal angle,

postoperative knee extension during stance, or postoperative knee extension at terminal swing. There was no change in hip extension during stance. Recurvatum during stance occurred in 5 of 21 patients (8 limbs) undergoing both medial and lateral hamstring lengthening versus 1 of 6 patients (1 limb) undergoing isolated medial hamstring lengthening. This difference was not statistically significant, but highlights the risk of recurvatum with hamstring-lengthening surgery. Recurvatum was associated with increased knee extension ROM, decreased ankle dorsiflexion ROM, and increased calf spasticity.

Another risk of distal hamstring lengthening is increased anterior pelvic tilt. DeLuca and colleagues[21] reported an increase in pelvic tilt after combined medial and lateral distal hamstring lengthening for patients with normal preoperative pelvic tilt. Pelvic tilt increased from a mean of 6° to 15° when medial and lateral hamstring lengthening was performed. Medial hamstring lengthening alone did not result in significant increases in anterior pelvic tilt. In this study by DeLuca and colleagues,[21] psoas lengthening over the brim did not protect against increasing anterior pelvic tilt after medial and lateral hamstring lengthening.

The authors' preferred method The authors are less commonly performing isolated distal hamstring lengthening because they believe that the knee dysfunction is often too mild or too severe to benefit. When distal hamstring lengthening is performed, only the medial hamstrings are lengthened to minimize the risk of increased anterior pelvic tilt. To maintain the integrity of the muscle-tendon unit, the semimembranosus is fractionally lengthened with 1 or 2 circumferential stripes in the fascia and the semitendinosus and gracilis are lengthened by intramuscular technique, similar to that described for the lengthening of the tibialis posterior (see **Fig. 3**B).[22] In this technique, the tendons are divided well above the muscle-tendon junction and the knee is gently extended. For mild to moderate degrees of fixed flexion deformity at the knee, greater than 5°, distal hamstring lengthening is often inadequate and results in incomplete correction with increased anterior pelvic tilt.[9] Instead, the authors combine distal hamstring lengthening with other procedures such as a semitendinosus transfer, described later.

Rectus femoris transfer

Many published studies confirm the value of distal hamstring lengthening as part of multilevel surgery in children with spastic diplegia. However, those with instrumented gait analysis have often reported that hamstring lengthening alone improves knee extension during stance phase but results in decreased flexion during swing phase and increased stiffness,[23] which may result in clearance problems, toe scuffing, and increased energy expenditure.[24] A solution to this problem is to combine medial hamstring lengthening with transfer of the rectus femoris. The indications for this procedure and its outcomes have been described in several studies.[25–33] It is important to consider the GMFCS level because the best results of rectus femoris transfer are at GMFCS levels I and II.[34] Another important consideration is the spasticity of the rectus femoris, confirmed by the Duncan-Ely or prone rectus test.[24,25] Kinematic variables that are helpful in decision making regarding whether to transfer the rectus femoris include a decreased peak knee flexion in swing phase,[25] decreased knee ROM during swing phase,[24,26] decreased overall knee ROM during the gait cycle, and delay in the timing of peak knee flexion.[25] Dynamic electromyography showing prolonged rectus firing during swing phase is useful information too.[24,26]

At this time, there is persuasive evidence that transferring the distal rectus femoris yields better results than either proximal or distal rectus femoris lengthening.[26–28] There is no evidence that one site of transfer is superior to another.[29,30] Medially, the most commonly used recipient tendons for the rectus femoris transfer are the semitendinosus, gracilis, or sartorius. Laterally, the iliotibial band has been used as a recipient tendon. The current literature reports improvement in peak knee flexion to be between 10° and 26°.[24,26,31,32] The total knee ROM has shown an improvement of between 7° and 15°.[29,32,33,35]

The authors' preferred method The authors prefer to transfer the rectus femoris medially to the semitendinosus tendon. The rectus femoris tendon, when "tubed" into a round construct, is often a good match for the distal semitendinosus stump after the semitendinosus is divided (see **Fig. 3**C). A sound tendon-to-tendon transfer and secure repair allow early active and passive mobilization techniques postoperatively. The proximal segment of the semitendinosus is cross-sutured to the semimembranosus to preserve proximal hip extensor function.

The indications for rectus femoris transfer in the context of multilevel surgery are not always clear cut. The authors consider delaying rectus femoris transfer when the clinical and kinematic indications for rectus femoris transfer are borderline, the anticipated immediate postoperative rehabilitation may be too complex for the child or the family to be sure of achieving a good result, or there is concern of precipitating crouch gait in a child who already has an excessive knee flexion throughout stance phase. During the surgery to remove fixation plates, such as blade plates, after a femoral osteotomy, a second opportunity arises for a rectus femoris transfer. If knee extension has been successfully restored, the authors' preferred technique is then to transfer the rectus femoris laterally to the fascia lata.

Medial hamstring lengthening combined with semitendinosus transfer to the adductor tubercle

In the past, transfer of some or all of the hamstrings to the distal femur was described by Eggers.[36] However, the procedure was abandoned when it was found that intractable recurvatum developed quickly.[37] To improve knee extension without causing recurvatum, some centers transferred a single hamstring instead.

The indications for semitendinosus transfer in the authors' center include severe knee flexion throughout the stance phase of gait in combination with a knee flexion deformity, typically in the range of 5° to 20°, when examined under anesthesia. In patients without a fixed knee flexion contracture, semitendinosus transfer is contraindicated given the high risk of recurvatum. The typical patient functions at GMFCS level III or IV, although some young children categorized under GMFCS level II with early fixed flexion contractures may also qualify.

The authors' outcomes after semitendinosus transfers to the adductor tubercle combined with medial hamstring lengthening showed improvement of fixed knee flexion deformity by approximately 15°, from 18° preoperatively to 3° postoperatively.[38] Knee flexion at initial contact improved by 17° and minimum knee flexion during stance phase improved by 18°. Pelvic tilt did not deteriorate. Significant improvements were noted in the Functional Mobility Scores (FMS) at 5 and 50 m. The authors concluded that distal hamstring lengthening, combined with the transfer of the semitendinosus to the adductor tubercle, results in significant improvements in dynamic knee function, reduced knee flexion deformity, and improved gait and functioning in the context of multilevel surgery for selected children with bilateral spastic CP.

The authors' preferred method Semitendinosus transfers may be indicated for patients with a flexed knee gait and fixed knee flexion contractures in the range of 5° to 20°. Age and GMFCS level should also be considered. This procedure involves harvesting the semitendinosus distally from its attachment to the pes anserinus and transferring it to the adductor magnus tendon with a strong nonabsorbable suture. The procedure is performed in combination with the conventional lengthening of the semimembranosus by fascial striping and an intramuscular lengthening of the gracilis (see **Fig 3**D).

One negative aspect of the procedure is an exaggeration of the knee stiffness problems in swing. The authors' approach to this aspect is to accept knee stiffness in the short term. Once the correction of the sagittal plane is stable with no residual knee flexion deformity and good extension during stance phase, an isolated transfer of the rectus femoris to the fascia lata may be considered. The benefits of combined distal medial hamstring lengthening, combined with transfer of the semitendinosus to the adductor tubercle, can be further extended by the use of distal femoral growth plate surgery for residual knee flexion deformity, as described in a later section (**Fig. 4**).

Supracondylar extension osteotomy and patellar tendon shortening

Children with spastic diplegia who have optimal early management, including access to BoNT-A injections to the hamstrings, the provision of solid ankle-foot orthoses (AFOs), avoidance of Achilles tendon lengthening, and a good physical therapy program, do not usually develop severe knee flexion deformities. Some patients, however, have limited access to specialist care and present with a severe flexed knee gait.

Distal hamstring lengthening in the presence of knee flexion deformity of more than 5° to 10° is ineffective and may be dangerous. The procedure risks complications such as common peroneal nerve stretch injuries, and may worsen anterior pelvic tilt. Correction of knee flexion deformity by a supracondylar extension osteotomy (SEO) in combination with patellar tendon shortening (PTS) is more effective. Indications for SEO-PTS include severe crouch gait, knee flexion deformity of 10° to 30°, an extensor lag greater than 10° to 20°, and patella alta on radiographs. The combination of an SEO and a PTS addresses the static knee flexion contracture and the dynamic extensor lag. SEO is performed by excision of a trapezoid wedge from the distal femur and stable internal fixation with a blade plate. The patellar tendon may be advanced or shortened.

Stout and colleagues[39] retrospectively reviewed their outcomes after isolated distal femur

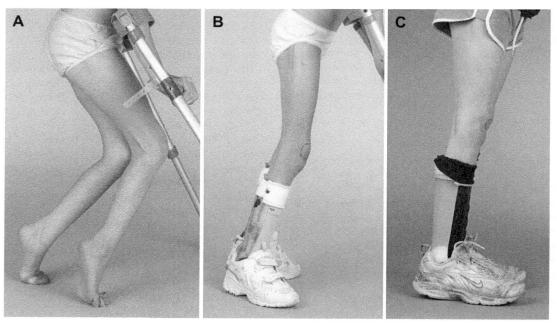

Fig. 4. Jump gait alignment. (*A*) An 8-year-old patient with spastic diplegia and GMFCS III, who demonstrates jump gait alignment, with flexed hips, flexed knees, and equinus ankles. (*B*) After multilevel surgery consisting of bilateral varus derotation osteotomies of the proximal femur, bilateral distal medial hamstring lengthening with semitendinosus transfer, and bilateral Strayer calf lengthening, the patient had improved alignment but had residual knee flexion and out-toed stance. The lever arm dysfunction and incomplete correction were likely to lead to relapse. (*C*) The lever arm deformities have been corrected with os calcis lengthening and supramalleolar osteotomies of the tibia. Eight-Plates applied to the distal femoral physis helped improve residual knee flexion. The combination of semitendinosus transfer (for spastic hamstring contracture) and eight-Plates (for residual flexion deformity) is a powerful tool for the correction of severe knee flexion during gait.

osteotomy versus isolated patellar tendon advancement and after each technique, versus a combination of both. The combined distal femoral osteotomy and patellar tendon advancement procedures showed the most favorable outcome: improvement of extensor lag (14°) and postoperative kinematic measurements (ie, 16° improvement of knee flexion at initial contact and 29° improvement in minimum knee flexion during stance phase). The data supported performing distal femoral extension osteotomy and patellar tendon advancement in combination.

The authors' preferred method SEO and PTS are performed in skeletally mature patients or skeletally immature patients with less than 2 years of growth remaining, who have a severe flexed knee gait and knee flexion between 10° and 30°. The procedure is safer, is easier, and results in less secondary deformity in individuals who have already reached skeletal maturity because the fixation and the osteotomy can be placed more distally. When the distal femoral growth plate is open, the blade plate must be inserted between 1 and 2 cm proximal to the growth plate, which results in more secondary translation deformity.

The authors' technique for PTS was adopted from the Association for Assistance of the Disabled Child in São Paulo, Brazil, as shown in **Fig. 3**E.[40] The first step is transecting the patellar tendon in its midsubstance. The distal segment is prepared with a nonabsorbable suture and passed proximally through 2 drill holes along the longitudinal axis of the patella. The proximal segment is repaired over the distal segment to reinforce the repair. Postoperatively, the lower extremity is immobilized in a long leg cast for 6 weeks. Afterwards, a solid AFO is combined with a 3-point splint or rigid knee splint for 6 more weeks. Immobilization of the knee in extension for periods of up to 3 months is inconvenient but has no bearing on long-term function. In spastic diplegia, the knee does not become stiff in extension, but it may do so in flexion. The Ferraretto and Selber technique is safe and effective. The technique can be safely used in skeletally immature children in whom advancement of the tibial tuberosity may risk disturbing the growth in the anterior tibial apophysis and cause a recurvatum deformity. The technique is effective in correcting patella alta, extensor lag and improving stance phase knee extension. Also, there is no retained hardware in the knee extensor mechanism, which has to be removed or can cause secondary morbidity.

Guided growth

Children with spastic diplegia may present with severe crouch gait and progressive knee flexion contractures well before skeletal maturity. In this context, guided growth may be an attractive option because it is much less invasive than SEO-PTS. Klatt and Stevens[41] suggested guided growth for fixed knee flexion deformity of more than 10° with at least 12 months of predicted growth remaining.

The use of staples to the anterior part of the distal femoral growth plate for knee flexion contractures was first described by Kramer and Stevens.[42] Placed anteriorly, the staples cause differential growth of the distal femoral physis, with the anterior portion growing more slowly than the posterior portion. Over time, this may correct the flexion deformity. More recently, staples were replaced with eight-Plates (Orthofix Corporation, Lewisville, TX, USA). Klatt and Stevens reported preliminary results of eight-Plates applied to 13 knees in 8 patients with CP.[41] In this study, knee flexion deformity decreased by 0.9° per month, correcting knee flexion by an average of 12.7°.

The authors' preferred method In skeletally immature patients with knee flexion contractures greater than 10° to 20°, the authors consider applying the principles of guided growth, in combination with medial hamstring lengthening and semitendinosus transfers. In children with more than 2 years of growth remaining, the authors typically use eight-Plates. Once the correction is achieved, they often remove the proximal screw of the eight-Plate if the patient has growth remaining after complete correction, so that the plate may be reapplied if necessary in the future. The eight-Plates are applied outside the periosteum, and the effects are reversible once removed. One disadvantage of eight-Plates is that they are prominent and at times have been noted to cause a local bursitis, although the exact incidence is not well documented. It seems that patients with significant dystonia can be particularly affected. Staples are less prominent; however, as with the use of staples in any site, reversibility is not guaranteed. Therefore, the authors use staples in children who are within 2 years of reaching skeletal maturity and in whom bone age is known accurately, and consider that there would otherwise be a significant and unacceptable risk of recurvatum deformity at the knee. Recurvatum gait in the adolescent can be particularly difficult to correct.

MEASURING OUTCOMES

To date, there is no single measurement that reflects improvement or deterioration of knee function after intervention. All elements of the diagnostic matrix may be used in outcome assessment, including the patient's symptoms and findings on physical examination and instrumented gait analysis. Functional outcome measurements include the Gillette Functional Assessment Questionnaire (FAQ)[43] and the FMS.[44] GMFCS is not an outcome measure and usually remains stable, although some patients may improve by a level.[45,46] Deterioration in GMFCS level is of great concern and may suggest an incorrect diagnosis, an inappropriate intervention, or ineffective rehabilitation.

CASE EXAMPLES

The authors have chosen several clinical cases to illustrate both favorable and unfavorable outcomes after various surgical techniques for knee dysfunction in children and adolescents with spastic diplegia. The authors carefully considered the diagnostic matrix in deciding their surgical management of children with knee dysfunction with the goal of achieving sagittal plane balance. To achieve sagittal plane balance after surgery, the entire sagittal plane must be considered, which includes the pelvis, hip, knee, and ankle. It is not enough to improve knee extension if this means unacceptable deterioration in pelvic position as in the first case. In fact, all the 3 planes need to be considered, but the emphasis in this article remains on sagittal plane knee dysfunction.

Sagittal Plane Imbalance: Recurvatum Knee After Multilevel Surgery for Apparent Equinus

At the time of index surgery, patient A was an 8-year-old girl with spastic diplegia; GMFCS level III; FMS 4,4,1; and FAQ 6+5. Her presenting symptoms were anterior knee pain, increasing fatigue, and decreasing walking endurance. Physical examination revealed knee flexion contractures of 15° bilaterally with a positive Duncan-Ely test. According to the Silfverskiöld test there were contractures of the gastrocnemii but not of the soleus. Gait analysis confirmed a severe, flexed, and stiff knee gait with apparent equinus at the ankles (**Fig. 5**A). The patient underwent multilevel surgery, which included bilateral medial and lateral hamstring lengthening, bilateral Strayer calf lengthening, and bilateral os calcis lengthening.

Twelve months postoperatively, knee kinematics showed significant bilateral knee recurvatum throughout stance and increased anterior pelvic tilt throughout the gait cycle (see **Fig. 5**B). The surgical prescription had failed to achieve sagittal plane balance. Excessive ankle plantar flexion/knee extension coupling resulted in

recurvatum of the knees. Excessive hamstring lengthening resulted in marked anterior pelvic tilt. Salvage of this very poor outcome included injections of BoNT-A to the soleus and the use of AFOs with a plantar flexion stop to reduce the excessive ankle plantar flexion/knee extension coupling. Sagittal plane balance improved, with decreased anterior pelvic tilt, improved hip extension, reduced recurvatum at the knees, improved swing phase knee kinematics, and more appropriate dynamic ankle function (see **Fig. 5**C). At a 3-year follow-up, the patient remained at GMFCS level III; with FMS 4,2,2; and with FAQ 7+5.

Practice learning point

Achieving the correct "balance" between the ankle and knee level is paramount in multilevel surgery. In this example, the "surgical dose" at the knee (combined medial and lateral hamstring lengthening) was too much and the dose at the ankle was too little (gastrocnemius recession). The conservative calf-lengthening surgery combined with the bony surgery resulted in an excessively effective foot and ankle lever. With the weakness of the medial and lateral hamstrings, the result of surgery was severe recurvatum of the knees combined with a marked increase in anterior pelvic tilt. The authors no longer lengthen the lateral hamstrings to avoid recurvatum, and they use the semitendinous transfer to avoid increased pelvic tilt.

Mild Jump Knee in a Child with High Functional Expectations

At the time of evaluation, patient B was a 10-year-old boy with spastic diplegia and at GMFCS level II, who reported increased in-toed gait, toe scuffing, tripping, and falling, especially when playing sport. Physical examination showed increased femoral neck anteversion (40° bilaterally), spastic hamstrings with popliteal angles of 55° bilaterally, no fixed flexion deformity at the knees, and a moderately positive Duncan-Ely (prone rectus) test. Kinematics showed a mild jump gait pattern, with increased knee flexion at initial contact but full knee extension in late stance (**Fig. 6**A). In swing phase, the knees showed delayed and reduced peak flexion. Anterior pelvic tilt was increased, and both ankles were in equinus but with asymmetric kinematics and asymmetric calf contractures. According to the Silfverskiöld test, the contracture involved the gastrocnemius alone on the right side and the gastrocnemius and soleus on the left.

In the context of multilevel surgery, the patients' knee dysfunction was managed by distal medial hamstring lengthening and transfer

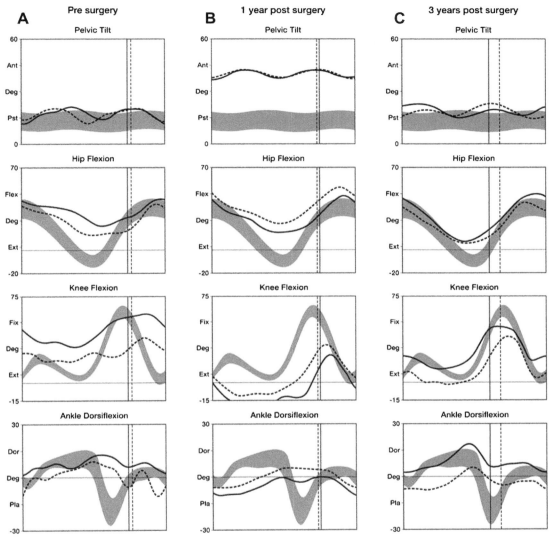

Fig. 5. Iatrogenic recurvatum knee caused by unbalanced multilevel surgery. In this and all subsequent kinematic traces, the solid line is the patient' right side and the dotted line is the patient's left side. The light grey band represents ± 1 standard deviation of the laboratory's normal database. (*A*) Preoperative kinematics shows apparent equinus gait, with increased knee flexion and a near-normal ankle ROM. (*B*) Sagittal plane imbalance from excessive hamstring lengthening (combined medial and lateral distal hamstring lengthening) and an overly effective foot-and-ankle lever arm (gastrocnemius lengthening combined with os calcis lengthening) resulted in increased anterior pelvic tilt and recurvatum at the knee. (*C*) Salvage included controlling the ankle plantar flexion/knee-extension coupling with BoNT-A injections to the soleus and AFO with a plantar flexion stop.

of the rectus femoris to the semitendinosus. The patient also had bilateral proximal femoral derotation osteotomies, with adductor longus tenotomy and bilateral Strayer calf lengthening with a left-sided soleal fascia lengthening. Five years after multilevel surgery, the patient achieved normal sagittal plane balance, including first rocker at the ankle and normal swing phase knee (see **Fig. 6**B). Such improvements in gait are difficult to achieve in spastic diplegia, but these improvements are possible when the patient has good underlying strength and selective motor control. The patient improved to GMFCS level I; FMS 6,6,6; and FAQ 10+21; and achieved his goals of increased participation in school sports.

Practice learning point

The strongest predictor of the outcome of multilevel surgery and knee dysfunction is the

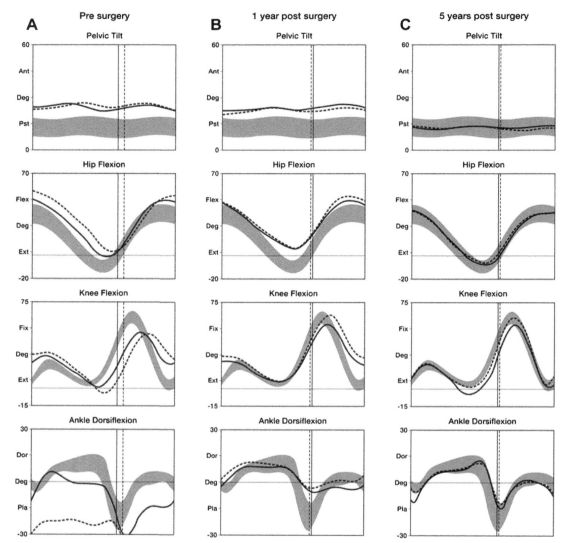

Fig. 6. Jump gait in a boy with high functional expectations. (*A*) Preoperative kinematics show jump knee gait, with increased knee flexion in early stance and increased ankle equinus. (*B*) Surgical intervention included distal medial hamstring lengthening and a rectus femoris transfer to the semitendinosus, combined with proximal femoral varus derotation osteotomies with adductor longus tenotomy and bilateral Strayer calf lengthenings plus a soleal fascial lengthening on the left leg. (*C*) Five years after multilevel surgery, there is near-normal sagittal plane kinematics, which is a reflection of the patient's high preoperative function, good strength, and good selective motor control.

patient's starting point. This patient had high preoperative function with mild jump knee gait, underlying good strength, and selective motor control. At 12 months after multilevel surgery, before plate removal, the main improvements were at the knee and ankle. However, at 5 years after surgery, with no interval intervention, the patient's sagittal plane kinematics was close to normal. He acquired first rocker at the ankle bilaterally and no longer needed AFOs.

Severe Crouch Gait (Iatrogenic), Close to Skeletal Maturity

Patient C was presented at 14 years of age, at GMFCS level III; with FMS C,3,1; and with FAQ 8.

Before evaluation in the authors' gait laboratory, the patient had been managed by bilateral percutaneous Achilles tendon lengthening combined with bilateral medial hamstring lengthening at 8 years of age. The patient and his parents were concerned about increasing fatigue and deteriorating function. Initially, the patient had walked independently but later required Canadian crutches for short distances and a wheelchair for longer distances. Ambulation was considered not sustainable into adult life. On physical examination, there were mild flexion deformities at both hips and severe flexion deformities of bilateral knees measuring 20°. Severe lever arm deformities were present distally with 30° of external tibial torsion bilaterally, combined with pes planovalgus. Soleal length was noted to be excessive bilaterally, although gastrocnemius length was closer to normal by the Silverskiöld test. Radiographs showed the patient to be close to skeletal maturity, with marked patella alta and fragmentation of the inferior pole of the patella. Kinematics revealed a severe crouch gait pattern with incomplete hip extension in late stance, severe flexion at the knees throughout stance, and swing varying from 60° to 75° (**Fig. 7**A). Both ankle traces were in the calcaneus range, although first rocker was noted to be present bilaterally and the ankle traces showed good modulation. The pelvis was tilted posteriorly during gait.

Because the patient was nearly skeletally mature, an SEO of the distal femur and a PTS procedure were performed to address the fixed flexion deformity of the knee. These procedures were combined with revision medial hamstring lengthening. In addition, bilateral psoas lengthening were performed to address the mild hip flexion deformity. The lever arm dysfunction of the lower leg was corrected by supramalleolar derotation osteotomies of the tibia and bilateral os calcis lengthening.

Outcomes at 18 months showed improvement of sagittal kinematics, with better hip and knee extension in midstance and pelvic and ankle kinematics within normal range, as seen in **Fig. 7**B. Eighteen months later, the patient functioned at GMFCS level II; with FMS 5,5,5; and with FAQ 8. The fatigue fractures of the patellae had healed, the patella alta remained corrected, and the patient no longer required crutches or a wheelchair.

Practice learning point

Percutaneous lengthening of the Achilles tendon causing weakness of the gastrocsoleus complex may contribute to crouch gait[47,48] and should be avoided in patients with spastic diplegia. When both the knee flexion deformity

and the quadriceps lag are severe, the most direct, but most invasive, technique is to correct the flexion deformity by SEO and the excessively long quadriceps by PTS. As observed in this case, these techniques are powerful and can result in dramatic improvements in gait and function. In severe crouch gait, the hip extensors, knee extensors, and ankle plantar flexors are usually excessively long, although only the knee extensor mechanism was shortened. The ankle kinematics suggests some retensioning of the gastrocsoleus complex, perhaps because of the correction of severe lever arm deformities.

Severe Flexed Knee Gait in a Skeletally Immature Patient

At presentation, patient D was a 9-year-old boy with a diagnosis of hereditary spastic paraplegia (HSP) and deteriorating gait. He could walk independently (GMFCS level II) but only for short distances, and had FMS 5,2,2 and FAQ 6. On physical examination, the patient was noted to have substantial weakness in his antigravity muscles with marked quadriceps lag bilaterally. The more involved knee, the right knee, had a popliteal angle of 65° and a fixed knee flexion deformity of 13°. The left knee had a popliteal angle of 54° and a fixed flexion deformity of 4°. Duncan-Ely test result was positive bilaterally. Gait analysis showed a jump gait pattern of the right leg and an apparent equinus gait pattern of the left leg (**Fig. 8**A).

Multilevel surgery included bilateral medial hamstring lengthening and bilateral semitendinosus transfers to the adductor tubercle. eight-Plates were applied anteriorly across the growth plate of the right distal femur to correct the more severe right knee flexion deformity. No form of calf lengthening was performed because of the patient's diagnosis of HSP and the apparent equinus pattern on the left leg. In consideration of the patient's underlying weakness and the probability of progression, it was decided not to perform a rectus femoris transfer but to consider it at a later stage if indicated.

On follow-up at 12 months, the patient maintains independent ambulation, with GMFCS level II; FMS 5,5,5; and FAQ 7. Sagittal kinematics is improved at all levels, especially at the knee (see **Fig. 8**B). There is residual reduced peak knee flexion in swing and a rectus femoris transfer will be considered. Removal of the eight-Plates are planned when the right knee extension equals 10° of recurvatum.

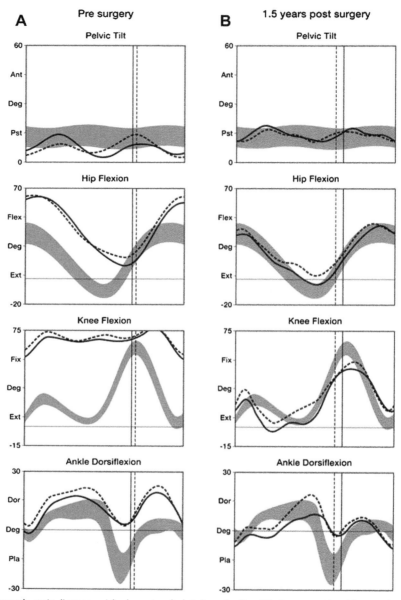

A Pre surgery

B 1.5 years post surgery

Pelvic Tilt

Hip Flexion

Knee Flexion

Ankle Dorsiflexion

Fig. 7. Severe crouch gait (iatrogenic) close to skeletal maturity. (*A*) Preoperative kinematics demonstrating crouch gait, with increased knee flexion and excessively long calf muscles from previous percutaneous lengthening of the Achilles tendon. (*B*) Surgical intervention included an SEO and a PTS. Follow-up gait analysis shows marked improvement in sagittal kinematics.

Practice learning point

In the child with severe flexed knee gait who presents at an earlier age, a wider range of surgical options may be considered. Combining soft tissue surgery for the spastic contracted hamstrings, in combination with distal femoral growth plate surgery, may offer marked improvements in gait and function through less invasive surgery and with less risk to the patient. In this example, the semitendinosus transfers to the adductor tubercle were instrumental in promoting knee extension while simultaneously preserving the strength of the hamstrings to extend the hip and place the pelvis in the appropriate amount of anterior tilt. eight-Plate application to the right knee for guided growth was intended to address the preoperative

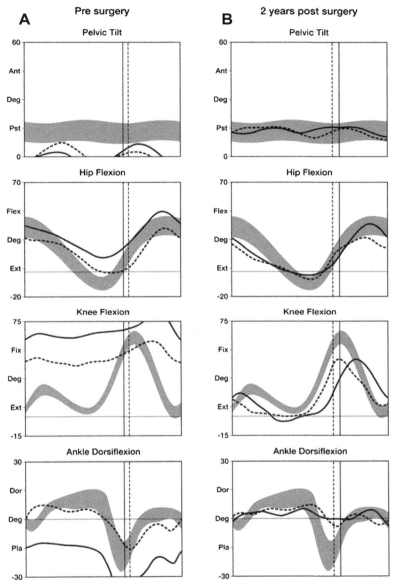

Fig. 8. Severe flexed knee gait in a skeletally immature patient. (*A*) Weakness of antigravity muscles contributes to the severe flexed knee gait demonstrated here. The right knee (*solid line*) demonstrates a jump gait pattern and the left knee (*dotted line*) demonstrates an apparent equinus gait pattern. (*B*) Treatment consisted of a combination of distal medial hamstring lengthening, semitendinosus transfers, and eight-Plate application to the right knee. At a younger age, a wider range of surgical options may be considered.

asymmetric knee flexion deformity. In this patient, the interventions chosen focused on improving stance phase knee function (semitendinosus transfer, medial hamstring lengthening, insertion of eight-Plate to the right knee). The problems with swing phase knee function were recognized, but management was deferred until the long-term gait and function of the patient with HSP were more clearly understood. Isolated transfer of the rectus

femoris to the fascia lata can be considered if symptoms dictate, closer to skeletal maturity.

SUMMARY

This article discusses the sagittal gait patterns in children with spastic diplegia, with an emphasis on the knee, as well as the concept of the "dose" of surgery required to correct different gait pathologies. Although clinical trials and comparative data are often lacking, the authors think that it is reasonable to list the interventions in the order of increasing dose and that the concept is useful in the consideration of the management of knee dysfunction. In the order of increasing dose,, the interventions for improving knee extension include:

- Injections of BoNT-A as a temporizing measure for hamstring spasticity
- Medial hamstring lengthening for mild knee dysfunction, usually in younger patients with mild jump gait and less than 5° knee flexion deformity
- Medial hamstring lengthening combined with semitendinosus transfer to the adductor tubercle for more severe flexed knee gait and mild to moderate knee flexion deformities, ranging from 5° to 15°
- Transfer of the semitendinosus combined with growth plate surgery for severe flexed knee gait, combined with knee flexion deformities of 10° to 25°, in the patients with at least 2 years of growth remaining
- SEO combined with PTS for severe flexed knee gait, combined with knee flexion deformities of 10° to 30°, in patients with severe quadriceps lag who are either close to or already at skeletal maturity.

REFERENCES

1. Chin TYP, Graham HK, Selber P, et al. Muscle-tendon surgery in cerebral palsy: what's the dose? American Academy of Cerebral Palsy and Developmental Medicine 58th Annual Meeting. Los Angeles (CA), September 30, 2004:10.
2. Davids JR, Ounpuu S, DeLuca PA, et al. Optimization of walking ability of children with cerebral palsy. J Bone Joint Surg Am 2003;85(11):2224–34.
3. Keenan WN, Rodda J, Wolfe R, et al. The static examination of children and young adults with cerebral palsy in the gait analysis laboratory: technique and observer agreement. J Pediatr Orthop B 2004; 13(1):1–8.
4. Marks MC, Alexander J, Sutherland DH, et al. Clinical utility of the Duncan-Ely test for rectus femoris dysfunction during the swing phase of gait. Dev Med Child Neurol 2003;45(11):763–8.
5. Sutherland DH, Davids JR. Common gait abnormalities of the knee in cerebral palsy. Clin Orthop Relat Res 1993;288:139–47.
6. Rodda JM, Graham HK, Carson L, et al. Sagittal gait patterns in spastic diplegia. J Bone Joint Surg Br 2004;86(2):251–8.
7. Desloovere K, Molenaers G, Feys H, et al. Do dynamic and static clinical measurements correlate with gait analysis parameters in children with cerebral palsy? Gait Posture 2006;24(3):302–13.
8. Thompson NS, Baker RJ, Cosgrove AP, et al. Relevance of the popliteal angle to hamstring length in cerebral palsy crouch gait. J Pediatr Orthop 2001; 21(3):383–7.
9. Rodda JM, Graham HK, Nattrass GR, et al. Correction of severe crouch gait in patients with spastic diplegia with use of multilevel orthopaedic surgery. J Bone Joint Surg Am 2006;88(12): 2653–64.
10. Damiano DL, Abel MF. Functional outcomes of strength training in spastic cerebral palsy. Arch Phys Med Rehabil 1998;79(2):119–25.
11. Scholtes VA, Becher JG, Comuth A, et al. Effectiveness of functional progressive resistance exercise strength training on muscle strength and mobility in children with cerebral palsy: a randomized controlled trial. Dev Med Child Neurol 2010;52: e107–13.
12. Damiano DL, Arnold AS, Steele KM, et al. Can strength training predictably improve gait kinematics? A pilot study on the effects of hip and knee extensor strengthening on lower-extremity alignment in cerebral palsy. Phys Ther 2010;90(2):269–79.
13. Leonard J, Graham HK. Treatment of motor disorders in cerebral palsy with botulinum neurotoxin. In: Jankovic E, editor. Botulinum toxin: therapeutic clinical practice and science. Philadelphia: Saunders Elsevier, Inc; 2009. p. 172–91.
14. Hutchinson R, Graham HK. Management of spasticity in children. In: Barnes M, Johnson G, editors. Upper motor neurone syndrome and spasticity. 2nd edition. Cambridge (UK): Cambridge University Press; 2008. p. 214–39.
15. Corry IS, Cosgrove AP, Duffy CM, et al. Botulinum toxin A in hamstring spasticity. Gait Posture 1999; 10(3):206–10.
16. Molenaers G, Desloovere K, Fabry G, et al. The effects of quantitative gait assessment and botulinum toxin A on musculoskeletal surgery in children with cerebral palsy. J Bone Joint Surg Am 2006;88(1):161–70.
17. Delp SL, Arnold AS, Speers RA, et al. Hamstrings and psoas lengths during normal and crouch gait: implications for muscle-tendon surgery. J Orthop Res 1996;14(1):144–51.
18. Drummond DS, Rogala E, Templeton J, et al. Proximal hamstring release for knee flexion and crouched posture in cerebral palsy. J Bone Joint Surg Am 1974;56(8):1598–602.
19. Elmer EB, Wenger DR, Mubarak SJ, et al. Proximal hamstring lengthening in the sitting cerebral palsy patient. J Pediatr Orthop 1992;12(3):329–36.
20. Kay RM, Rethlefsen SA, Skaggs D, et al. Outcome of medial versus combined medial and lateral

hamstring lengthening surgery in cerebral palsy. J Pediatr Orthop 2002;22(2):169−72.

21. DeLuca PA, Ounpuu S, Davis RB, et al. Effect of hamstring and psoas lengthening on pelvic tilt in patients with spastic diplegic cerebral palsy. J Pediatr Orthop 1998;18(6):712−8.

22. Majestro TC, Ruda R, Frost HM. Intramuscular lengthening of the posterior tibialis muscle. Clin Orthop Relat Res 1971;79:59−60.

23. Gage JR. Surgical treatment of knee dysfunction in cerebral palsy. Clin Orthop Relat Res 1990;253:45−54.

24. Gage JR, Perry J, Hicks RR, et al. Rectus femoris transfer to improve knee function of children with cerebral palsy. Dev Med Child Neurol 1987;29(2):159−66.

25. Kay RM, Rethlefsen SA, Kelly JP, et al. Predictive value of the Duncan-Ely test in distal rectus femoris transfer. J Pediatr Orthop 2004;24(1):59−62.

26. Sutherland DH, Santi M, Abel MF. Treatment of stiff-knee gait in cerebral palsy: a comparison by gait analysis of distal rectus femoris transfer versus proximal rectus release. J Pediatr Orthop 1990;10(4):433−41.

27. Perry J. Distal rectus femoris transfer. Dev Med Child Neurol 1987;29(2):153−8.

28. Ounpuu S, Muik E, Davis RB 3rd, et al. Rectus femoris surgery in children with cerebral palsy. Part II: a comparison between the effect of transfer and release of the distal rectus femoris on knee motion. J Pediatr Orthop 1993;13(3):331−5.

29. Muthusamy K, Seidl AJ, Friesen RM, et al. Rectus femoris transfer in children with cerebral palsy: evaluation of transfer site and preoperative indicators. J Pediatr Orthop 2008;28(6):674−8.

30. Ounpuu S, Muik E, Davis RB 3rd, et al. Rectus femoris surgery in children with cerebral palsy. Part I: the effect of rectus femoris transfer location on knee motion. J Pediatr Orthop 1993;13(3):325−30.

31. Miller F, Cardoso Dias R, Lipton GE, et al. The effect of rectus EMG patterns on the outcome of rectus femoris transfers. J Pediatr Orthop 1997;17(5):603−7.

32. Saw A, Smith PA, Sirirungruangsarn Y, et al. Rectus femoris transfer for children with cerebral palsy: long-term outcome. J Pediatr Orthop 2003;23(5):672−8.

33. Rethlefsen S, Tolo VT, Reynolds RA, et al. Outcome of hamstring lengthening and distal rectus femoris transfer surgery. J Pediatr Orthop B 1999;8(2):75−9.

34. Rethlefsen SA, Kam G, Wren TA, et al. Predictors of outcome of distal rectus femoris transfer surgery in ambulatory children with cerebral palsy. J Pediatr Orthop B 2009;18(2):58−62.

35. Moreau N, Tinsley S, Li L. Progression of knee joint kinematics in children with cerebral palsy with and without rectus femoris transfers: a long-term follow up. Gait Posture 2005;22(2):132−7.

36. Eggers GW. Transplantation of hamstring tendons to femoral condyles in order to improve hip extension and to decrease knee flexion in cerebral spastic paralysis. J Bone Joint Surg Am 1952;34(4):827−30.

37. Evans EB. The status of surgery of the lower extremities in cerebral palsy. Clin Orthop Relat Res 1966;47:127−39.

38. Ma FY, Selber P, Nattrass GR, et al. Lengthening and transfer of hamstrings for a flexion deformity of the knee in children with bilateral cerebral palsy: technique and preliminary results. J Bone Joint Surg Br 2006;88(2):248−54.

39. Stout JL, Gage JR, Schwartz MH, et al. Distal femoral extension osteotomy and patellar tendon advancement to treat persistent crouch gait in cerebral palsy. J Bone Joint Surg Am 2008;90(11):2470−84.

40. Ferraretto I, Machado PO, Rolim Filho EL, et al. Preliminary results of patellar tendon shortening, as a salvage procedure for crouch gait in cerebral palsy. Pediatric Orthopaedic Society of North America Annual Meeting. Vancouver, British Columbia, Canada, May 1−4, 2000.

41. Klatt J, Stevens PM. Guided growth for fixed knee flexion deformity. J Pediatr Orthop 2008;28(6):626−31.

42. Kramer A, Stevens PM. Anterior femoral stapling. J Pediatr Orthop 2001;21(6):804−7.

43. Novacheck TF, Stout JL, Tervo R. Reliability and validity of the Gillette Functional Assessment Questionnaire as an outcome measure in children with walking disabilities. J Pediatr Orthop 2000;20(1):75−81.

44. Harvey A, Graham HK, Morris ME, et al. The Functional Mobility Scale: ability to detect change following single event multilevel surgery. Dev Med Child Neurol 2007;49(8):603−7.

45. Palisano R, Rosenbaum P, Walter S, et al. Development and reliability of a system to classify gross motor function in children with cerebral palsy. Dev Med Child Neurol 1997;39(4):214−23.

46. McCormick A, Brien M, Plourde J, et al. Stability of the gross motor function classification system in adults with cerebral palsy. Dev Med Child Neurol 2007;49(4):265−9.

47. Segal LS, Thomas SE, Mazur JM, et al. Calcaneal gait in spastic diplegia after heel cord lengthening: a study with gait analysis. J Pediatr Orthop 1989;9(6):697−701.

48. Dietz FR, Albright JC, Dolan L. Medium-term follow-up of Achilles tendon lengthening in the treatment of ankle equinus in cerebral palsy. Iowa Orthop J 2006;26:27−32.

The Foot and Ankle in Cerebral Palsy

Jon R. Davids, MD

KEYWORDS

• Foot • Ankle • Cerebral palsy • Management

Foot and ankle problems are common in children with cerebral palsy (CP). In ambulatory children, the efficiency of gait may be compromised. Nonambulatory children may have problems with orthotic and shoe wear. Surgical interventions are frequently performed to address these issues. This article presents the current paradigm for clinical decision making for surgery about the foot and ankle in children with CP. This approach is built on a standardized assessment and classification of disruption of foot alignment and function in these children. Surgical treatment principles and options are considered, and preferred surgical techniques for the most common foot and ankle problems in children with CP are described.

CLINICAL DECISION MAKING

Clinical decision making for the management of foot deformities in children with CP can be standardized by the use of a diagnostic matrix (**Table 1**). This paradigm is based on the collection and integration of data from 5 sources: the clinical history, physical examination, plain radiographs, observational gait analysis, and quantitative gait analysis (which includes kinematic/kinetic analyses, dynamic electromyography [EMG], and dynamic pedobarography).[1]

Clinical History

The most common complaints related to foot deformity in children with CP are pain with ambulation, shoe wear, or use of orthoses; tripping because of poor clearance in swing phase; and in-toeing or out-toeing.

Physical Examination

Foot segmental alignment is assessed in both weight-bearing and non—weight-bearing conditions. Manual examination is performed to determine intra- and intersegmental flexibility, active and passive range of motion, and individual muscle strength and selective control. The static standing alignment of the foot is best assessed from the front, behind, and both sides. The plantar and medial margins of the foot should be examined for the presence of inadequate or excessive skin callous formation, which indicates disrupted loading patterns or problems with shoe or orthotic wear.

Plain Radiographs

Standardized radiographic analysis of foot deformity in children with CP should include 3 weight-bearing views: standing anteroposterior (AP) and lateral views of the foot, and AP view of the ankle. Foot deformities are best identified and classified by dividing the foot into 3 segments and 2 columns, then determining the relative alignment of each segment and the relative length of each column (**Fig. 1**). A comprehensive technique of quantitative segmental analysis of the ankle and foot, with normative values, has been developed, based on qualitative techniques derived from the foot model originally developed by Inman and colleagues.[2,3] This approach uses 10 radiographic measurements to determine the alignment of the 3 segments and the lengths of the 2 columns of the ankle and foot. Individual measures of segmental alignment that are beyond 1 standard deviation from the normal mean value are considered to be abnormal and can be used to describe malalignment patterns.

The author received no funding support related to this manuscript.

Motion Analysis Laboratory, Shriners Hospital for Children, 950 West Faris Road, Greenville, SC 29605, USA

E-mail address: jdavids@shrinenet.org

Orthop Clin N Am 41 (2010) 579–593

doi:10.1016/j.ocl.2010.06.002

Table 1
The diagnostic matrix

Source	Information
Clinical history	• Pain • Tripping • In-/out-toeing
Physical examination	• Gross foot shape weight bearing/non−weight bearing • Flexible/rigid • Plantar callous pattern
Radiographic examination	• Segmental alignment weight-bearing, anteroposterior, and lateral views
Observational gait analysis	• Foot contact with floor (3 rockers) • Foot progression angle • Foot clearance in swing phase
Quantitative gait analysis	• Kinematics • Kinetics • Dynamic electromyography • Pedobarography

Observational Gait Analysis

Ambulation is best observed from multiple viewpoints in the coronal and sagittal planes. This observation is most effectively achieved by having the child walk toward, away from, and past the examiner. The subject should be barefoot and wearing short pants, which allows for adequate visualization of the thigh, knee, lower leg, ankle, and foot. The key events of the gait cycle related to dynamic foot function that may be appreciated on observational gait analysis include foot position at initial contact (heel strike, flat foot, or toe strike), foot alignment in midstance (varus or valgus in the coronal plane; internal or external in the transverse plane, described as the foot progression angle), foot alignment at toe-off (varus or valgus in the coronal plane, dorsiflexed or plantarflexed in the sagittal plane), and foot clearance in swing phase.[4,5]

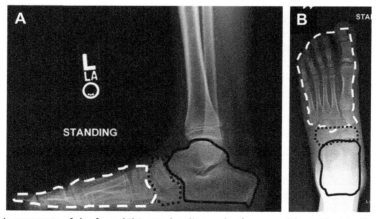

Fig. 1. Radiographic segments of the foot. (*A*) Lateral radiograph of a normal foot. The hindfoot (talus and calcaneus) is outlined by the solid black circle. The midfoot (navicular and cuboid) is outlined by the dotted black circle. The forefoot (cuneiforms, metatarsals, and phalanges) is outlined by the dashed white circle. (*B*) AP radiograph of the foot. The hindfoot (talus and calcaneus) is outlined by the solid black circle. The midfoot (navicular and cuboid) is outlined by the dotted black circle. The forefoot (cuneiforms, metatarsals, and phalanges) is outlined by the dashed white circle. The medial column (not outlined) consists of the talus, navicular, cuneiforms, and great toe metatarsal and phalanges. The lateral column (not outlined) consists of the calcaneus, cuboid, and lesser toe metatarsals and phalanges.

Quantitative Gait Analysis

The calculation of foot and ankle kinematics and kinetics involves modeling assumptions and approximations concerning the relationship between the skin markers and the underlying skeletal anatomy. The standard ankle and foot model most commonly used in clinical gait analysis was developed in the early 1980s, uses markers at the malleoli and forefoot, and considers the foot as a single segment.[6] It is assumed that the foot segment is rigid from the hindfoot to the forefoot. Ankle motion in the sagittal plane is calculated from the location of the foot axis relative to the tibial axis. Any movement between the 3 segments of the foot (eg, hindfoot to midfoot, midfoot to forefoot) that occurs between the malleolar and forefoot markers is captured by this simple foot model and described as ankle motion. Significant measurement artifact occurs when the normal foot segmental alignment is disrupted (eg, equinoplanovalgus foot malalignment in children with CP). This artifact creates apparent discrepancies within the diagnostic matrix between the data derived from the physical examination, observational gait analysis, and quantitative gait analysis. Failure to appreciate the causes for these apparent discrepancies may result in confusion for clinicians and compromise clinical decision making.

Technological improvements have allowed for the development of more sophisticated, multisegment foot models that more accurately approximate the complex anatomy and biomechanics of the foot.[7] However, these models are difficult to apply to children with CP, because of small foot size (intermarker distances are reduced beyond the ranges of resolution) and deformity (segmental malalignment obscures anatomic landmarks and compromises accurate marker placement). A foot model that is useful for clinical decision making for children with CP, with respect to orthotic prescriptions, surgical planning, and post-intervention outcome assessment, is currently being developed.[8]

Dynamic EMG is most relevant in the evaluation of specific foot deformities such as equinocavovarus segmental malalignment.[9] The use of surface and fine-wire EMG provides information on the timing of muscle activity during the gait cycle. This is most helpful in sorting out the relative activity of the tibialis anterior and posterior muscles in both stance and swing phases. This information facilitates clinical decision with respect to the selection of a particular muscle tendon unit for lengthening or transfer.[10,11]

Dynamic pedobarography measures the spatial and temporal distribution of force over the plantar aspect of the foot during the stance phase of the gait cycle. Pedobarography provides quantitative information regarding dynamic foot function, consisting of foot contact patterns, pressure distribution and magnitude, and progression of the center of pressure. In children with CP, foot function during gait is disrupted by several common patterns of skeletal segmental malalignment. All 3 rockers in stance phase may be affected. This biomechanical disruption has been termed lever arm deficiency, and is best characterized by the center of pressure progression (COPP) relative to the foot. Normative values for the COPP in children have been established.[12] Deviation in the location and duration of the COPP relative to the segments of the foot can be used to describe common abnormal loading patterns (**Fig. 2**). Displacement of the COPP medially in a particular segment of the foot describes a valgus loading pattern, which is usually the consequence of an everted, abducted, or pronated segmental malalignment of the foot segment. Displacement of the COPP laterally in a particular segment of the foot describes a varus loading pattern, which is usually the consequence of an inverted, adducted, or supinated segmental malalignment of the foot segment. Prolonged duration of the COPP in the forefoot segment describes an equinus foot loading pattern. Prolonged duration of the COPP in the hindfoot segment describes a calcaneus loading pattern. This standardized approach to the determination of foot loading patterns can be used to characterize abnormal foot loading patterns, assist in clinical decision making, and contribute to the assessment of outcome following a variety of interventions.[13]

DISRUPTION OF FOOT FUNCTION IN CHILDREN WITH CP

Foot deformities in children with CP are usually the result of a dynamic imbalance between the extrinsic muscles of the lower leg that control segmental foot and ankle alignment. This imbalance may be a consequence of spasticity, disrupted motor control, and/or impaired balance function. Typically, the ankle plantar flexor muscles are overactive, and the ankle dorsiflexor muscles are ineffective. Variable imbalance patterns may be seen between the foot and ankle supination and pronation muscle groups. These motor imbalances result in 3 common coupled foot and ankle segmental malalignment patterns in children with spastic type CP. Equinus is characterized by excessive plantar flexion of the

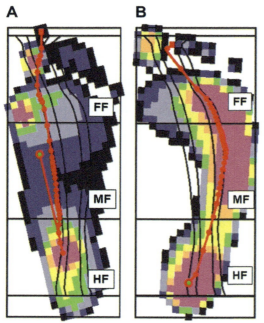

Fig. 2. Qualitative display of pedobarographic data. (*A*) The foot contact pattern is divided into 3 segments by the horizontal solid black lines; the hindfoot (HF), midfoot (MF), and forefoot (FF). The mean value for the normal COPP is shown by the solid red line. The ±1 and 2 standard deviations for the mean value of the COPP are shown by the vertical solid black lines. (*A*) Pedobarograph of an 11-year-old girl with diplegic type CP and equinoplanovalgus segmental malalignment on plain radiographs. The COPP is deviated medially, indicating a valgus loading pattern. (*B*) Twelve-year-old boy with CP and equinocavovarus segmental malalignment on plain radiographs. The COPP is deviated laterally, indicating a varus loading pattern.

hindfoot relative to the ankle, with normal midfoot and forefoot alignment. Equinoplanovalgus is characterized by equinus deformity of the hindfoot, coupled with pronation deformities of the midfoot and forefoot. The lateral column of the foot is functionally and/or structurally shorter than the medial column. Ankle valgus and hallux valgus deformities are frequently seen in association with equinoplanovalgus foot segmental malalignment. Equinocavovarus is characterized by equinus deformity of the hindfoot, coupled with supination deformity of the midfoot and variable malalignment of the forefoot. The lateral column is functionally and/or structurally longer than the medial column. Compensatory ankle valgus deformity may be seen in association with equinocavovarus foot segmental malalignment. Other, more complex, or uncoupled segmental alignments may occur, but are less common. These common

segmental malalignments of the foot and ankle are usually supple and correctible on manipulation in younger children with less severe CP. However, with increasing age and growth, the muscles develop fixed shortening or myostatic deformity, the bones develop permanent structural accommodations to the malalignment pattern, and the foot and ankle deformities become rigid and uncorrectable on manipulation.

Foot and ankle segmental malalignment may disrupt function during both the stance and swing phases of the gait cycle. In all 3 segmental malalignment patterns, heel strike at initial contact does not occur, disrupting the first or hindfoot rocker and shock absorption function in loading response. Equinus and equinocavovarus malalignment patterns disrupt the second or ankle rocker by blocking ankle dorsiflexion, compromising stability function in midstance. Equinoplanovalgus malalignment maintains the mid- and forefoot segments in an unlocked alignment, compromising stability function in midstance, which may result in excessive loading of the plantar, medial portion of the midfoot. All 3 segmental malalignments may compromise the ability of the ankle plantar flexor muscles to generate an adequate internal plantar flexion moment during third or forefoot rocker. The hindfoot malalignment associated with equinus and equinocavovarus malalignment patterns shortens the length of the plantar flexor muscles, compromising their ability to generate tension, as described by the length-tension curve for skeletal muscle. With equinoplanovalgus, the moment-generating capacity of the ankle plantarflexor muscles is further compromised by the malalignment of mid- and forefoot segments, which effectively shortens the lever arm available to this muscle group during the third or forefoot rocker. In addition, increased external tibial torsion, which may be associated with equinoplanovalgus segmental malalignment, may contribute to an external foot progression angle, further compromising the lever arm available to the ankle plantar flexor muscles in terminal stance. All 3 segmental malalignment patterns of the foot and ankle may inhibit ankle dorsiflexion in swing phase, compromising clearance in midswing and proper positioning of the foot and ankle in terminal swing.

SURGICAL TREATMENT: PRINCIPLES AND OPTIONS
Treatment Goals

Interventions to correct foot deformities in children with CP may be selected to improve function and cosmesis. These goals may be achieved by surgeries that are designed to improve foot shape. It is presumed that improved foot shape following soft tissue and skeletal surgery can restore both the stability function of the foot during the second or ankle rocker in midstance and the skeletal lever arm function of the foot during the third or forefoot rocker in terminal stance. However, increased foot stiffness associated with many skeletal surgical procedures (eg, arthrodesis) used to improve foot shape may compromise the shock absorption function of the foot during the first or ankle rocker in loading response. Cosmetic improvements following foot surgery are related to improved visual assessment of static standing foot alignment (particularly restoration of the medial longitudinal arch and toe alignment) and improved foot progression angle during stance phase.

Pain may be associated with foot deformities in children with CP and is usually the consequence of poor alignment and instability during stance phase. Equinoplanovalgus segmental malalignment of the foot may cause excessive loading of the medial midfoot during the second or ankle rocker in midstance, leading to the development of painful callosities that may compromise orthotic and shoe wear.[14–16] Equinocavovarus segmental malalignment of the foot may cause excessive loading of the lateral mid- and forefoot segments, resulting in instability during the second or ankle rocker in midstance and during the third or forefoot rocker in terminal stance, which may lead to frequent inversion injuries of the ankle and hindfoot.[9,17] It is presumed that surgically improved foot shape can correct pain by improving foot loading and stability in stance phase. Younger children with CP may tolerate mild or moderate foot deformities, with little complaint of pain or sense of impairment. However, such deformities may be poorly tolerated in teenage and adult life, where the magnitude of the abnormal loading is much greater (because of increased body mass), and the cumulative effect over time results in premature degenerative changes of the joints of the foot and ankle. It is presumed that surgery to improve foot shape in childhood will improve the loading of the foot and decrease the possibility of early degenerative arthritis in adulthood.

Levels of Deformity

Foot deformities in children with CP are sequential and progressive with growth and development. These deformities may be classified into 3 levels (**Table 2**). Level I deformities are the characterized by dynamic soft tissue imbalance. Skeletal anatomy is normal. Level II deformities are characterized by fixed or myostatic soft tissue imbalance. Skeletal segmental malalignments are flexible and correctable on manipulation. Level III deformities are characterized by structural skeletal deformities that are usually associated with fixed or myostatic soft tissue imbalance.

Treatment Principles

Level I foot deformities are best treated with pharmacologic (eg, botulinum toxin injection) or neurosurgical (eg, selective dorsal rhizotomy, intrathecal baclofen) interventions designed to manage muscle tone and spasticity. Early management of spasticity by pharmacologic, neurosurgical, and orthotic interventions is favored to avoid the development of fixed deformities of the muscle tendon

Table 2
Levels of deformity and treatment options

Level of Deformity	Treatment Options		
	Pharmacologic/ Neurosurgery	Muscle Tendon Surgeries	Skeletal Surgeries
Dynamic soft tissue imbalance, no skeletal deformities	• Botulinum toxin injection • Selective dorsal rhizotomy • Intrathecal baclofen	• Partial/complete tendon transfers	• Not appropriate
Fixed soft tissue imbalance, no skeletal deformities	• Not appropriate as isolated intervention	• Serial stretch casting • Lengthening (multiple possible techniques)	• Not appropriate
Fixed soft tissue imbalance, with skeletal deformities	• Not appropriate as isolated intervention	• Appropriate in conjunction with skeletal surgery	• Osteotomy (multiple possible techniques) • Arthrodesis

unit. Soft tissue (ie, muscle tendon unit) surgery, consisting of split or complete transfer of the muscle tendon unit, may also be appropriate for specific dynamic muscle imbalance problems. Level II foot deformities are best treated with soft tissue (ie, muscle tendon unit) surgery. Surgical options include release, lengthening, or transfer of the muscle tendon unit. Selective surgical lengthening techniques that minimize the subsequent weakness of the muscle tendon unit are favored. Level III foot deformities, in which the segmental malalignments are fixed and not correctable on manipulation, are best treated with a combination of soft tissue and skeletal surgeries. Skeletal surgical options include osteotomy and arthrodesis. These procedures may correct deformity by addition (ie, lengthening), subtraction (ie, shortening), angulation, or rotation. Whenever possible, osteotomy is preferred to arthrodesis to restore foot skeletal segmental alignment and maintain intra-and intersegmental motion, to optimize both shock absorption and lever functions of the foot.[15] Soft tissue and skeletal procedures are typically performed in a sequential fashion to restore or optimize foot segmental alignment.

SURGICAL TREATMENT: TECHNIQUES

As noted earlier, there are 3 common coupled foot and ankle segmental malalignment patterns in children with spastic type CP: equinus, equinoplanovalgus, and equinocavovarus. In addition there are 2 common secondary malalignments, ankle valgus and hallux valgus, which may be associated with any of the 3 principle malalignment patterns. The preferred techniques for the surgical management of these 5 common problems are discussed here.

Ankle Valgus

The alignments of the tibiotalar and talocalcaneal joints determine overall hindfoot alignment.[18,19] Valgus malalignment at both levels is usually the result of tightness of the ankle plantar flexor muscles group. Hindfoot valgus malalignment may disrupt alignment of the midfoot and forefoot, compromising loading and stability in stance phase.[4] Ankle valgus should be corrected when it contributes to overall hindfoot valgus deformity, as seen with equinoplanovalgus foot segmental malalignment. In some cases, ankle valgus deformity may be accepted when it occurs in compensation for talocalcaneal varus, as seen in mild cases of equinocavovarus foot segmental malalignment.

Tibiotalar joint alignment is best determined by AP radiograph of the ankle (**Fig. 3**). Long cassette

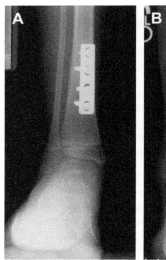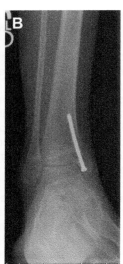

Fig. 3. Ankle valgus deformity. (*A*) AP radiograph of the ankle in an 11-year-old boy with hemiplegic type CP, showing ankle valgus deformity. The child has had a previous tibial rotation osteotomy. (*B*) AP radiograph 2 years and 3 months after placement (and immediately before removal) of a medial malleolar screw. Note the slight overcorrection of the ankle valgus deformity and the bending of the screw.

limb alignment views introduce parallax at the ankle and cannot be used to accurately assess tibiotalar joint alignment. Ankle valgus is best measured by the tibiotalar angle (defined by the anatomic axis of the tibia and the axis across the dome of the talus). Narrowing of the lateral distal tibial epiphysis, and shortening of the distal fibula (described as a high fibular station), are frequently associated with ankle valgus.[20]

By definition, ankle valgus is a level III deformity. Guided growth strategy is the treatment of choice for ankle valgus in children with open physes and sufficient (≥ 2 years) remaining growth.[20,21] Reversible hemiepiphyseodesis using a medial malleolar screw is preferred to the use of plates or staples (see **Fig. 3**). The medial malleolar screw may be placed and removed percutaneously and minimizes the chance of unintentional tibiotalar joint penetration associated with the plates and staples. A fully threaded screw should be placed across the medial quarter of the distal tibial physis on the AP radiograph view, and across the middle third of the distal tibial physis on the lateral radiograph view. The principle technical challenge is correct placement of the screw within the bone and across the physis. This is facilitated by the use of a cannulated screw system with intraoperative fluoroscopic guidance. In addition to assessing the position of the screw on orthogonal AP and lateral views, an approach withdrawal technique, achieved by rotating the ankle under real-time fluoroscopy to establish that the implant is within the bone, should be performed to confirm the final position. Slight bending of the screw as the valgus deformity corrects is common. Slight overcorrection (up to 5 degrees) is preferable before removal because rebound deformity can be anticipated in children with growth remaining. Percutaneous removal and resumption of longitudinal growth are predictable when the medial malleolar screw is removed within 2 years of placement. Placement of a medial malleolar screw may be safely repeated when treatment is initiated in younger children who have recurrent deformity following the initial procedure.

Equinus

Pure plantar flexion malalignment is usually the consequence of overactivity (level I) or tightness (level II) of the ankle plantar flexor muscle group. Assessment of foot segmental alignment with plain radiographs is essential to establishing that there are no associated deformities at the level of the mid- or forefoot. Apparent extreme equinus deformity may be a combination of both hind- and forefoot plantar flexion malalignments (**Fig. 4**). Failure to appreciate the forefoot component, and attempts to achieve a plantigrade foot through isolated plantar flexor muscle group lengthening, may result in hindfoot calcaneous malalignment. By definition, level III equinus deformity does not exist.

Level I deformity is best treated with intramuscular injection of the gastrocnemius muscle with botulinum toxin.[22–24] However, international dosing guidelines have not been established.[25,26]

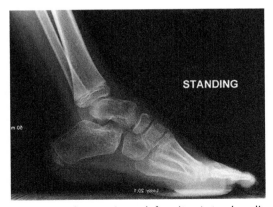

Fig. 4. Complex equinus deformity. Lateral radiograph of the foot in an 8-year-old boy with hemiplegic type CP. The overall equinus deformity is a combination of both hindfoot and midfoot plantar flexion.

Direct injection into each head of the muscle is possible in the clinic or outpatient setting, using topical anesthetic agents on the skin and, if necessary, conscious sedation for children with significant anxiety. A short course of casting, or use of ankle foot orthoses, initiated several weeks after the injection, may be used to potentiate and preserve the time-limited pharmacologic effect.

Treatment of level II deformity requires careful assessment to determine the relative contributions of the gastrocnemius and soleus muscles to the fixed shortening of the plantar flexor muscle group. This is best achieved by assessing ankle dorsiflexion range of motion with the knee both flexed and extended. Isolated limitation of dorsiflexion with the knee flexed suggests involvement of the soleus muscle; limitation only with the knee extended suggests gastrocnemius muscle involvement; limitation regardless of knee position suggests involvement of both muscles. The goal of surgical lengthening of the plantar flexor muscle group is to achieve 5 degrees of ankle dorsiflexion when the knee is extended. When only the gastrocnemius muscle is involved, a selective fractional lengthening is best performed proximally at the level of the muscle belly (zone I). When both muscles are involved, and 15 degrees or less of correction is required, selective fractional lengthening midcalf at the level of the myotendinous junction is preferred (zone II). When both muscles are involved, and greater than 15 degrees of correction is required, nonselective lengthening distally at the conjoined tendon (tendo Achilles) level is necessary (zone III). In most cases, zones I and II lengthening procedures are sufficient. However, with proper patient selection and careful surgical technique, all 3 techniques may be effective and excessive lengthening and weakness of the ankle plantar flexor muscle group can be avoided.[27,28]

Equinoplanovalgus

Equinoplanovalgus segmental malalignment (also known as pes planus or flat foot) is usually the consequence of overactivity (level I) or tightness (level II) of the ankle plantar flexor and evertor muscle groups. Physical examination is required to determine whether the muscle tendon unit deformities are dynamic or myostatic. Fixed skeletal segmental malalignment (level III) is assessed with plain radiographs, which is essential to preoperative planning. Radiographic findings may include hindfoot valgus, midfoot pronation, and forefoot eversion and valgus.

Level I deformity is best treated with intramuscular injection of the gastrocnemius muscle with botulinum toxin, as described earlier. Injection of the peroneus brevis muscle should also be considered.

Level II deformity (myostatic muscle shortening without fixed skeletal malalignment) is usually seen in children between 4 and 7 years of age (**Fig. 5**). The treatment of choice is lengthening of the ankle plantar flexor muscle group, as described earlier. In addition, transfer of the peroneus brevis muscle to the peroneus longus muscle (distal to the level of the lateral malleoleus) should be performed when fixed deformity of the former is present. At the time of surgery, it is essential to determine that normal foot segmental alignment has been restored following the soft tissue surgeries. This confirmation is best achieved by using intraoperative stress radiographs of the foot (**Fig. 6**). Failure to restore normal skeletal alignment should result in reclassification of the deformity to level III, which requires skeletal surgery as described later.

The primary procedure used to correct level III equinoplanovalgus malalignment is lateral column

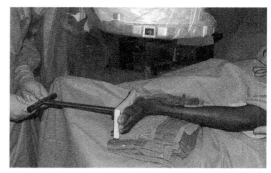

Fig. 6. The technique for the intraoperative stress assessment of foot segmental alignment. The assistant (*right*) stabilizes the knee while the surgeon loads the foot and ankle with the foot pusher (*left*). A fluoroscopic image is taken in the loaded position and is used to assess the segmental alignment.

lengthening.[13,14,16,29,30] This procedure may be performed at the neck of the calcaneus, through the calcaneocuboid joint, or in the body of the cuboid. This procedure allows for correction of all 3 segments of the foot, presumably as a result of ligamentotaxis (**Fig. 7**).[31] Sequential correction of equinoplanovalgus segmental malalignment includes initial correction of hindfoot soft tissue contractures. This correction is followed by addition osteotomy (lengthening) of the lateral column. In children who are 12 years of age or younger, lateral column lengthening is best performed through the neck of the calcaneus (**Fig. 8**). The lengthening is usually between 1 and 2 cm, and interposition grafting with tricortical iliac crest or patella allograft is preferred. The graft itself is usually stable, but longitudinal pin fixation may be used to control the calcaneocuboid joint subluxation that can occur during lateral column lengthening. In children who are more than 12 years of age, lateral column lengthening may also be performed through the calcaneocuboid joint (addition arthrodesis). The lengthening is usually between 1.5 and 2.5 cm, requiring a larger graft. The graft itself is usually stable, but internal fixation with a one-third tubular plate may be performed to minimize the possibility of graft collapse during the absorption and incorporation phases of healing.[30] The final step in the sequential correction of equinoplanovalgus malalignment involves assessment of the medial column. In some cases, lateral column lengthening alone results in adequate correction of all 3 segments of the foot. If there is residual forefoot varus deformity, or the medial column (ie, great toe metatarsal) is judged to be hypermobile in the sagittal plane, then a plantar based closing wedge (ie, plantar flexion) osteotomy is performed, through the medial

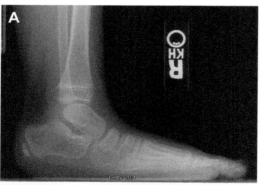

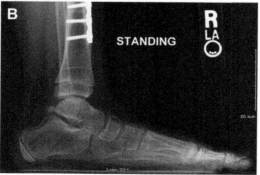

Fig. 5. Correction of level II equinus deformity. (*A*): Lateral radiograph of the foot in a 5-year-old boy with hemiplegic type CP. Note the mild hind- and midfoot segmental malalignments. (*B*): Lateral radiograph of the foot 13 months after single-event multilevel surgery, which includes a gastrocsoleus fractional lengthening (zone II). The foot segmental alignment has been normalized following the soft tissue surgery.

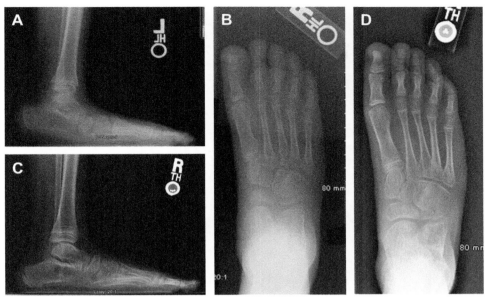

Fig. 7. Correction of moderate level III equinoplanovalgus deformity. (*A, B*): Lateral and AP (respectively) radiographs of the foot in a 7-year-old girl with diplegic type CP showing equinoplanovalgus segmental malalignment. (*C, D*): Lateral and AP (respectively) radiographs of the foot 13 months after gastrocsoleus fractional lengthening (zone II), and lateral column lengthening through the neck of the calcaneus. The foot segmental alignment has been normalized following the combined soft tissue and skeletal surgeries. Complete incorporation of the allograft and healing of the calcaneal osteotomy is best appreciated on the lateral view.

cuneiform or at the base of the great toe metatarsal (when the proximal physis has closed). If there is residual forefoot abduction deformity (ie, persistent talonavicular subluxation), as determined by palpation of the medial column or intraoperative radiographs of the foot, then a talonavicular arthrodesis is performed (**Fig. 9**). If lengthening of the lateral column fails to correct the hindfoot deformity, which is unusual, then subtalar, calcaneocuboid, and talonavicular arthrodeses (ie, triple arthrodesis) are required to achieve optimal realignment of the foot. Triple arthrodesis for equinoplanovalgus foot segmental malalignment is best performed through lateral and medial incisions (the latter are required to adequately visualize the talonavicular joint). Triple arthrodesis may be combined with lateral column lengthening through the calcaneocuboid joint to minimize the need for medial column shortening.[32]

Equinocavovarus

Equinocavovarus segmental malalignment (also known as varus foot) is usually the consequence of overactivity (level I) or tightness (level II) of the ankle plantar flexor and invertor muscle groups. Physical examination is required to determine whether the muscle tendon unit deformities are dynamic or myostatic. Fixed skeletal segmental

malalignment (level III) is assessed with plain radiographs, which are essential to preoperative planning. Radiographic findings may include hindfoot varus, midfoot supination, and forefoot inversion and varus.

Level I deformity in children 6 years of age and younger is best treated with intramuscular injection of the gastrocnemius muscle with botulinum toxin, as described earlier. Injection of the tibialis posterior muscle should also be considered. Because the tibialis posterior is a smaller muscle that is located in the deep posterior compartment, accurate injection of botulinum toxin requires either ultrasound or electrical stimulator guidance. In almost all cases, this needs to be performed with the child under general anesthesia. Children more than 6 years of age may be treated with muscle tendon transfer. Information from the physical examination, kinematics, kinetics, dynamic EMG, and pedobarography are used to determine the relative contributions of the tibialis anterior and tibialis posterior muscles to the dynamic varus deformity that occurs during stance and swing phases.[9–11,17] Split transfer of the tibialis anterior muscle should only occur when there is ankle dorsiflexion appreciated in midstance. Split transfer of the tibialis posterior should only occur when the dynamic EMG shows that the timing of the activation of this muscle corresponds with

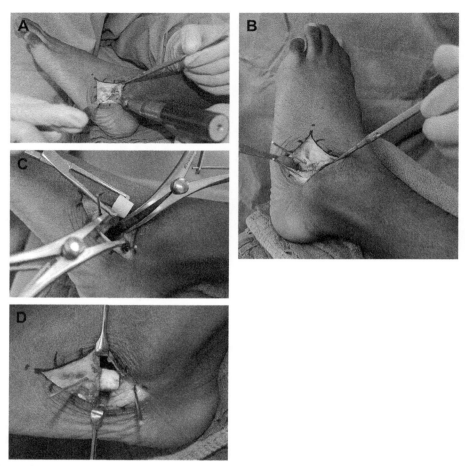

Fig. 8. The preferred technique for lateral column lengthening of the calcaneus. (*A*) The inferior portion of the sinus tarsi is exposed through a lateral approach. Care is taken to avoid disruption of the calcaneocuboid joint capsule and minimize the release of the extensor digitorum brevis muscle. The osteotomy is performed with an oscillating saw, from lateral and proximal to medial and distal. (*B*) Mobilization of the calcaneal fragments is facilitated by placing parallel wires (*solid black arrows*) proximal and distal to the osteotomy. (*C*) A modified, cannulated lamina spreader (*A*) is placed over the wires and used to distract the calcaneal osteotomy. Rotation of the distal fragment with lengthening is controlled by the distal wire. A modified, smooth lamina spreader (*B*) is also used to distract the calcaneal osteotomy. Care should be taken not to crush the calcaneus with the smooth lamina spreader. A tricortical iliac crest allograft (*solid back arrow*) is properly contoured to fit into the calcaneal osteotomy. (*D*) The allograft is pressed into the calcaneal osteotomy using a tamp and mallet. Control of rotation of the distal fragment is indicated by the wires remaining parallel.

the presence of varus malalignment during specific subphases of the gait cycle. When kinematics and dynamic EMG assessments are not available, dynamic varus deformity is best treated by concomitant split transfer of the tibialis anterior muscle and fractional lengthening of the tibialis posterior muscle.[33]

Level II deformity correction involves sequential correction of hindfoot and midfoot soft tissue contractures (**Fig. 10**). Fractional lengthening of the ankle plantar flexor muscle group and the tibialis posterior muscle are performed through a medial incision at the distal third of the calf.

Fractional lengthening of the flexor hallucis longus and flexor digitorum longus muscles are rarely necessary, but may be performed through the same incision. Fractional lengthening of the abductor hallucis muscle is performed on the medial border of the foot, at the distal third of the great toe metatarsal. Sequential release of the plantar fascia and the short intrinsic muscles of the foot may be performed through a plantar, medial, or lateral approach. At the time of surgery, it is essential to determine that normal foot segmental alignment has been restored following the soft tissue surgeries. This confirmation is best achieved with

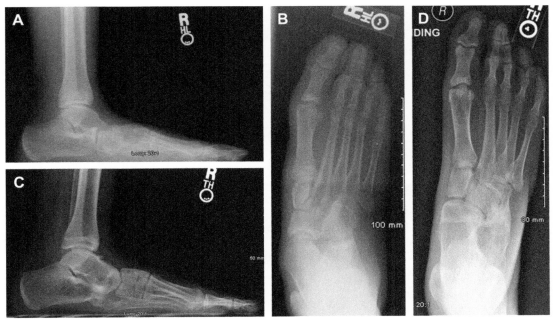

Fig. 9. Correction of severe level III equinoplanovalgus deformity. (*A, B*): Lateral and AP (respectively) radiographs of the foot in a 13-year-old boy with diplegic type CP showing severe equinoplanovalgus segmental malalignment. (*C, D*) Lateral and AP (respectively) radiographs of the foot 12 months after tendo Achilles lengthening (zone III), lateral column lengthening/arthrodesis through the calcaneocuboid joint, and talonavicular arthrodesis. Foot segmental alignment has been greatly improved following the combined soft tissue and skeletal surgeries. The hindfoot alignment is restored through the lateral column lengthening, obviating the need for subtalar arthrodesis.

intraoperative stress radiographs of the foot. Failure to restore normal skeletal alignment should result in reclassification of the deformity to level III, which requires skeletal surgery as described later.

Correction of level III equinocavovarus segmental malalignment is fundamentally different from correction of equinoplanovalgus malalignment, because there is no single skeletal procedure (ie, lateral column lengthening) that can achieve adequate correction of all 3 segments of the foot. Complete restoration of normal skeletal segmental alignment in the presence of level III equinocavovarus deformity by osteotomy is usually not possible. However, gross alignment and dynamic loading of the foot may be greatly improved by performing sequential osteotomies that create deformities to compensate for segmental malalignments (**Fig. 11**). Residual hindfoot varus malalignment may be corrected by calcaneal slide or laterally based closing wedge osteotomies (or a combination of both techniques).[34] Residual midfoot supination deformity may be corrected by lateral column shortening through the cuboid (ie, dorsolaterally based closing wedge osteotomy). Residual forefoot

inversion and varus deformities may be corrected by dorsiflexion osteotomy of the medial column (dorsally based closing wedge osteotomy of the medial cuneiform, or great toe metatarsal when the proximal physis has closed). Arthrodesis strategy is reserved for the most severe cases of level III equinocavovarus segmental malalignment. Triple arthrodesis of the subtalar, calcaneocuboid, and talonavicular joints may be required to achieve optimal foot alignment. Triple arthrodesis for equinocavovarus foot segmental malalignment is best performed through a lateral incision, which usually provides adequate exposure of all 3 joints. Segmental alignment is restored from proximal to distal. Hindfoot varus alignment is corrected by subtalar arthrodesis. Midfoot supination deformity is then corrected by calcaneocuboid arthrodesis. Forefoot inversion and valgus deformities are corrected by talonavicular arthrodesis.

Hallux Valgus

Hallux valgus deformity in children with CP may be the consequence of intrinsic and/or extrinsic

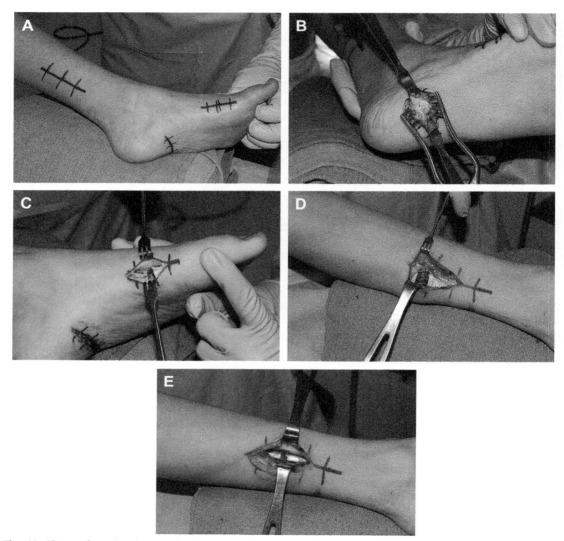

Fig. 10. The preferred technique for the correction of level II equinocavovarus deformity. (*A*) Three incisions (medial calf, plantar, and distal medial) are used to lengthen the appropriate soft tissue structures. (*B*) The plantar fascia and intrinsic muscles of the foot are released through the plantar incision, which is located distal to weight-bearing heel pad. (*C*) Fractional lengthening of the abductor hallucis muscle is performed through the distal medial incision. (*D*) Fractional lengthening of the gastrocsoleus muscle group (zone II) is performed through the medial calf incision. (*E*) Fractional lengthening of the tibialis posterior muscle is performed through the same medial calf incision.

factors. Examples of the former include spasticity and imbalance between the intrinsic muscles of the foot (eg, abductor and adductor hallucis muscles, and extensor hallucis longus muscle), which may result in both phalangeal valgus and metatarsal varus malalignments. Significant extrinsic factors include abnormal loading (eg, as a consequence of multilevel disruption of normal gait caused by spasticity and skeletal

malalignments) of the forefoot during the third or forefoot rocker in terminal stance. These deviations tend to medialize the forces across the great toe metatarsophalangeal (MTP) joint, resulting in an external abduction or valgus moment, which results in hallux valgus deformity. Radiographic assessment is essential for determining the elements and magnitude of deformity at the great toe MTP joint, and the presence of associated foot

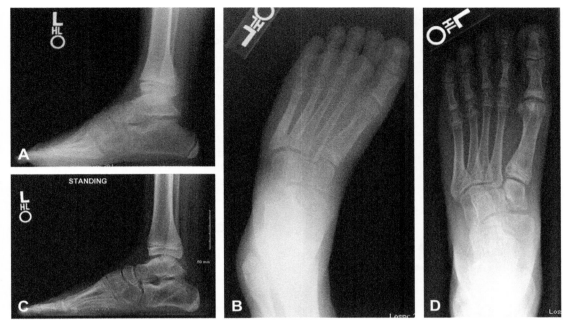

Fig. 11. Correction of level III equinocavovarus deformity. (*A, B*) Lateral and AP (respectively) radiographs of the foot in a 10-year-old boy with left hemiplegic type CP showing equinocavovarus segmental malalignment. (*C, D*) Lateral and AP (respectively) radiographs of the foot 13 months after gastrocsoleus fractional lengthening (zone II), posterior tibialis muscle fractional lengthening, radical plantar fascia release, calcaneal slide osteotomy, and medial cuneiform osteotomy. Overall foot shape is greatly improved, despite residual subtalar joint varus alignment and midfoot supination deformity.

segmental malalignments (**Fig. 12**). Correction of hallux valgus deformity is indicated to address pain at the great toe MTP joint, treat hygiene problems related to over- or underlapping of the great and second toes, and/or to facilitate shoe wearing and the use of orthotics. Correction of hallux valgus deformity is rarely performed in isolation. Associated etiologic factors (eg, foot segmental malalignment, multilevel causes of jump or crouch gait) should be addressed simultaneously to prevent recurrence of deformity.

Although theoretically appealing, there is little evidence to support early soft tissue botulinum injection, lengthening, or release to correct or improve foot intrinsic muscle overactivity (level I) or tightness (level II) that contributes to neuromuscular hallux valgus deformity.[35] Poor results of soft tissue balancing procedures are most likely a consequence of the failure to address significant extrinsic causes of hallux valgus deformity in children with CP.

The preferred treatment of level III hallux valgus deformity in children with CP is great toe MTP arthrodesis (see **Fig. 12**).[36,37] Because of the proximal location of the physis of the proximal phalanx,

MTP arthrodesis is performed in older children with no more than 2 years of growth remaining. Following a standard a dorsomedial approach, the articular cartilage and subchondral bone from both surfaces of the MTP joint are excised using a rongeur (see **Fig.10**). The cam contour of the joint is maintained, to preserve length and promote stability. As a result, cross-pin fixation is usually sufficient. Optimal alignment of the MTP arthrodesis is determined by the shape of the foot and the child's gait pattern. Correction in the coronal plane should, at a minimum, align the phalanges of the great toe with the lesser toes. Slight overcorrection at the level of the MTP joint, to compensate for associated hallux valgus interphalangeus deformity, is effective. Associated metatarsus varus deformity has been shown to correct in time following great toe MTP arthrodesis. Sagittal plane alignment of the arthrodesis should include between 15 and 20 degrees of dorsiflexion to facilitate the third or forefoot rocker. Dorsiflexion alignment should be determined relative to the plantar aspect of the foot, not relative to the alignment of the medial column, which may be compromised by foot segmental malalignment.

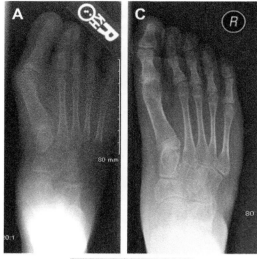

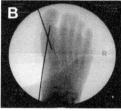

Fig. 12. Correction of hallux valgus deformity. (*A*) Standing AP radiograph of the foot in a 10-year-old girl with diplegic type CP. The great toe deformity consists of metatarsus varus, and MTP joint valgus. Overall foot alignment (not shown) is equinoplanovalgus, which is commonly associated with hallux valgus. (*B*) Intraoperative fluoroscopy AP view at the time of gastrocsoleus fractional lengthening (zone II), lateral column lengthening through the neck of the calcaneus, and great toe MTP joint arthrodesis. The cross-pin fixation is placed so that both the proximal and distal pins exit on the medial side of the foot. (*C*) Standing AP radiograph of the foot 1 year after great toe MTP arthrodesis. Metatarsus varus deformity has corrected spontaneously following MTP arthrodesis.

SUMMARY

Clinical decision making for the management of foot deformities in children with CP is based on the collection and integration of data from 5 sources: the clinical history, physical examination, plain radiographs, observational gait analysis, and quantitative gait analysis (which includes kinematic/kinetic analyses, dynamic EMG, and dynamic pedobarography). The 3 most common foot segmental malalignments in children with CP are equinus, equinoplanovalgus, and equinocavovarus. The 2 most common associated deformities are ankle valgus and hallux valgus. Level I foot and

ankle deformities (caused by dynamic overactivity and imbalance of muscles) are best treated with pharmacologic or neurosurgical interventions designed to manage muscle tone and spasticity, or muscle tendon unit transfers. Level II deformities (caused by fixed or myostatic soft tissue imbalance without fixed skeletal malalignment) are best treated with muscle tendon unit lengthening surgery. Level III deformities (consisting of structural skeletal malalignment associated with fixed or myostatic soft tissue imbalance) are best treated with a combination of soft tissue and skeletal surgeries.

REFERENCES

1. Davids JR, Ounpuu S, DeLuca PA, et al. Optimization of walking ability of children with cerebral palsy. Instr Course Lect 2004;53:511–22.
2. Davids JR, Gibson TW, Pugh LI. Quantitative segmental analysis of weight-bearing radiographs of the foot and ankle for children: normal alignment. J Pediatr Orthop 2005;25(6):769–76.
3. Inman VT, Ralston HJ, Todd F. Human walking. Baltimore (MD): Williams & Wilkins; 1981.
4. Davids JR. Normal function of the ankle and foot: biomechanics and quantitative analysis. In: Drennan J, McCarthy J, editors. Drennan's the child's foot and ankle. 2nd edition. Philadelphia: Lippincott Williams and Wilkins; 2009. p. 54–63.
5. Perry J. Gait analysis: normal and pathological function. Thorofare (NJ): Slack Inc; 1992.
6. Davis RB, Tyburski D, Gage JR. A gait analysis data collection and reduction technique. Hum Mov Sci 1991;10:575–87.
7. MacWilliams BA, Cowley M, Nicholson DE. Foot kinematics and kinetics during adolescent gait. Gait Posture 2003;17(3):214–24.
8. Davis RB, Jameson EG, Davids JR, et al. The design, development, and initial evaluation of a multisegment foot model for routine clinical gait analysis. In: Harris GF, Smith P, Marks R, editors. Foot and ankle motion analysis: clinical treatment and technology. Boca Raton (FL): CRC Press; 2007. p. 425–44.
9. Sutherland DH. Varus foot in cerebral palsy: an overview. Instr Course Lect 1993;42:539–43.
10. Scott AC, Scarborough N. The use of dynamic EMG in predicting the outcome of split posterior tibial tendon transfers in spastic hemiplegia. J Pediatr Orthop 2006;26(6):777–80.
11. Hoffer MM, Barakat G, Koffman M. 10-year follow-up of split anterior tibial tendon transfer in cerebral palsied patients with spastic equinovarus deformity. J Pediatr Orthop 1985;5(4):432–4.
12. Jameson EG, Davids JR, Anderson JP, et al. Dynamic pedobarography for children: use of the

center of pressure progression. J Pediatr Orthop 2008;28(2):254–8.

13. Davids JR. Orthopaedic treatment of foot deformities. In: Gage J, Schwartz M, Koop S, et al, editors. The identification and treatment of gait problems in cerebral palsy. 2nd edition. London: MacKeith Press; 2009. p. 514–33.

14. Mosca VS. Calcaneal lengthening for valgus deformity of the hindfoot. Results in children who had severe, symptomatic flatfoot and skewfoot. J Bone Joint Surg Am 1995;77(4):500–12.

15. Mosca VS. The child's foot: principles of management. J Pediatr Orthop 1998;18(3):281–2.

16. Yoo WJ, Chung CY, Choi IH, et al. Calcaneal lengthening for the planovalgus foot deformity in children with cerebral palsy. J Pediatr Orthop 2005;25(6): 781–5.

17. Mosca VS. The cavus foot. J Pediatr Orthop 2001; 21(4):423–4.

18. Stevens PM. Effect of ankle valgus on radiographic appearance of the hindfoot. J Pediatr Orthop 1988; 8(2):184–6.

19. Beals RK, Skyhar M. Growth and development of the tibia, fibula, and ankle joint. Clin Orthop 1984;182: 289–92.

20. Davids JR, Valadie AL, Ferguson RL, et al. Surgical management of ankle valgus in children: use of a transphyseal medial malleolar screw. J Pediatr Orthop 1997;17(1):3–8.

21. Stevens PM, Belle RM. Screw epiphysiodesis for ankle valgus. J Pediatr Orthop 1997;17(1):9–12.

22. Preiss RA, Condie DN, Rowley DI, et al. The effects of botulinum toxin (BTX-A) on spasticity of the lower limb and on gait in cerebral palsy. J Bone Joint Surg Br 2003;85(7):943–8.

23. Boyd RN, Pliatsios V, Starr R, et al. Biomechanical transformation of the gastroc-soleus muscle with botulinum toxin A in children with cerebral palsy. Dev Med Child Neurol 2000;42(1):32–41.

24. Bjornson K, Hays R, Graubert C, et al. Botulinum toxin for spasticity in children with cerebral palsy: a comprehensive evaluation. Pediatrics 2007;120(1):49–58.

25. Ade-Hall RA, Moore AP. Botulinum toxin type A in the treatment of lower limb spasticity in cerebral palsy. Cochrane Database Syst Rev 2000;2:CD001408.

26. Bakheit AM. Botulinum toxin in the management of childhood muscle spasticity: comparison of clinical practice of 17 treatment centres. Eur J Neurol 2003;10(4):415–9.

27. Etnyre B, Chambers CS, Scarborough NH, et al. Preoperative and postoperative assessment of surgical intervention for equinus gait in children with cerebral palsy. J Pediatr Orthop 1993;13(1):24–31.

28. Tylkowski C, Horan M, Oeffinger D. Outcomes of gastrocnemius-soleus complex lengthening for isolated equinus contracture in children with cerebral palsy. J Pediatr Orthop 2009;29(7):771–8.

29. Mosca VS. Flexible flatfoot and skewfoot. Instr Course Lect 1996;45:347–54.

30. Danko AM, Allen B Jr, Pugh L, et al. Early graft failure in lateral column lengthening. J Pediatr Orthop 2004;24(6):716–20.

31. Sangeorzan BJ, Mosca V, Hansen ST Jr. Effect of calcaneal lengthening on relationships among the hindfoot, midfoot, and forefoot. Foot Ankle 1993; 14(3):136–41.

32. Horton GA, Olney BW. Triple arthrodesis with lateral column lengthening for treatment of severe planovalgus deformity. Foot Ankle Int 1995;16(7): 395–400.

33. Barnes MJ, Herring JA. Combined split anterior tibial-tendon transfer and intramuscular lengthening of the posterior tibial tendon. Results in patients who have a varus deformity of the foot due to spastic cerebral palsy. J Bone Joint Surg Am 1991;73(5): 734–8.

34. Koman LA, Mooney JF 3rd, Goodman A. Management of valgus hindfoot deformity in pediatric cerebral palsy patients by medial displacement osteotomy. J Pediatr Orthop 1993;13(2):180–3.

35. Jenter M, Lipton GE, Miller F. Operative treatment for hallux valgus in children with cerebral palsy. Foot Ankle Int 1998;19(12):830–5.

36. Davids JR, Mason TA, Danko A, et al. Surgical management of hallux valgus deformity in children with cerebral palsy. J Pediatr Orthop 2001;21(1): 89–94.

37. Bishay SN, El-Sherbini MH, Lotfy AA, et al. Great toe metatarsophalangeal arthrodesis for hallux valgus deformity in ambulatory adolescents with spastic cerebral palsy. J Child Orthop 2009;3(1):47–52.

The Adult with Cerebral Palsy

Kevin P. Murphy, MD[a,b]

KEYWORDS

• Cerebral palsy • Adult • Lifetime care • Transition

Advances in medical and surgical care over the past 20 years have resulted in children who formerly would have died at birth or infancy now surviving well into adulthood, many with permanent physical disabilities,[1] including those caused by cerebral palsy (CP). Increased awareness of these problems is needed by adult health care providers of these individuals and also by pediatric providers who may be able to intervene and prevent some of the long-term problems. Orthopedic issues prevalent in the child with CP have long-term lifetime sequela being further defined at this time. Before any specific musculoskeletal intervention, the primary, secondary, and associated conditions of CP need to be considered in addition to comorbidities. The primary condition of CP, by definition, is nonprogressive over time in the neurologic sense.[2–4] Secondary conditions are those that develop as a result of the primary conditions and include causes such as soft tissue contractures, degenerative arthritis, hip dysplasia, and equinovalgus foot deformities. These conditions can often be prevented with early diagnosis and appropriate intervention before problematic sequelae develop.[5,6] Associated conditions are those that occur with increased prevalence in individuals with CP, such as visual or auditory impairment, seizure disorder, learning disability, and gastroesophageal reflux. These conditions are not necessarily preventable, but their impact may be lessened by early diagnosis and intervention during the developmental years. Comorbidities are those conditions unrelated to the primary disability and appearing with similar frequency whether one has CP or not (eg, diabetes, appendicitis, hypertension). In the author's experience medical care providers often blame the primary condition for just about all the symptoms and problems that can develop in the adult with CP. Symptoms such as leg pain, discomfort in the neck or lower back, and headaches are too often misattributed to the underlying condition of CP, giving no further pursuit to more specific and definitive diagnosis. For example, a person with CP presenting with a headache may be erroneously told that all people with CP develop headaches eventually, with no additional diagnostics being pursued. Strauss and colleagues[7] reviewed the public health record for the state of California and reported up to 9 times higher risk of brain cancer in people with CP, both young and old. As with any evaluation of an individual presenting with medical or surgical symptoms, the main initial goal should be to establish a correct diagnosis. This goal is less frequently achieved if medical symptoms and loss of function in individuals with CP are attributed to the primary condition.

Adults with CP are living longer, with an estimated population in the United States of between 400,000 and 500,000, depending on the defined age of an adult.[8–15] In addition to a possible higher risk of brain cancer in people with CP, Strauss and colleagues[7] also reported a 3 times higher risk of breast cancer and up to 4 times increased risk of cardiovascular death. A busy clinician might easily blame persistent back pain in an adult with CP on the primary condition without detecting breast cancer and a spinal metastasis in this higher-risk population. Most of the higher risk is believed to be secondary to inadequate medical screening in the adult with CP. Inadequate screening in part relates to a lack of education of the medical

[a] Gillette Specialty Healthcare Northern Clinics, 1420 East London Road, Suite 210, Duluth, MN 55805, USA
[b] Department of Physical Medicine and Rehabilitation, University of Minnesota Medical School, Duluth, MN 55803, USA
E-mail address: KMurphy@gillettechildrens.com

Orthop Clin N Am 41 (2010) 595–605
doi:10.1016/j.ocl.2010.06.007

provider, undersized and inaccessible medical examination rooms and equipment, and not enough time being allotted to the provider for adequate history taking and physical evaluation. This is especially so for those of increased physical involvement and with more challenging communication needs. Communication barriers are especially significant for those adults who are nonverbal, require augmentative communication devices, or have expressions of pain that are not recognized by the busy clinician. Adults with CP surviving well past 60 years of age and maintaining a functional lifestyle with or without caregiver assistance are not uncommon.[16–19] Higher survival rates have been found in those adults with increased functional levels, both ambulatory and mat mobility, and in individuals with gastrostomy tube feedings. Rimmer[20] was one of the first investigators to report that regular exercise improves functional status, decreases the level of required assistance, and reduces the incidence of secondary conditions in people with disability. Obesity is a secondary condition of concern in the adult with decreased metabolic rate and lack of exercise. Heller and colleagues[21] subsequently reported that participation in and frequency of exercise depend mostly on the care provider's attitude; if the care provider believed that exercise was important to the individual with physical disability, then exercise occurred.

A major functional premise in the care for the adult with CP is that functional deterioration is almost always secondary to something other than the primary condition. Multiple diagnoses always need to be considered. Adults with CP, not uncommonly, develop multiple sclerosis, Alzheimer disease, Parkinson disease, depression, cerebral vascular accident, and other associated or comorbid conditions.

The natural history of CP and musculoskeletal function is of utmost importance and needs further definition and lifetime perspective. Primitive reflexes, as well as a gradual trend toward more dystonia,[22] may be more noticeable with aging in this population. About 50% to 80% of individuals with cerebral palsy are able to walk in some manner during their lifetime.[23] The gross motor functional measure (GMFM) may be the most reliable method for predicting ultimate walking ability and gross motor function classification system (GMFCS) level.[24] The GMFM and GMFCS levels have been discussed previously in this text and therefore not repeated here for the sake of brevity. The loss of ambulatory skills in the adult with CP seems to occur at 2 peaks of age.[10,23] The first peak is around the age of 20 to 25 years, commonly associated with progressive crouch gait and inability of the young adult to keep up with peers efficiently in the community, workplace, and academic settings. The second peak is around the age of 40 to 45 years, with progressive fatigue, pain, and possibly accelerated joint degeneration, making further functional ambulation not possible. To date there are no studies of accelerated arthritis or joint degeneration in adults with CP, although anecdotal evidence is supportive.[23,25] Individuals with minimal to no ambulatory limitations (GMFCS level I) or those requiring just an ankle-foot orthosis (AFO) or simple gait aid for longer distances (GMFCS level II) are at less risk for gait deterioration and not uncommonly are ambulatory in the seventh decade of life.[23] Individuals who require more extensive gait aids for exercise or in-home walking and those just able to stand or take a few steps with transfers (GMFCS levels III and IV, respectively) are at greatest risk for loss of ambulatory function or weight-bearing skills over the lifetime.[23,25]

Too often, specialists who deal with children having CP focus inordinately on ambulatory function at the neglect of other more lifetime functional skills. Such skills include those dealing with social engagement, academics, and home and workplace participation. More emphasis should be placed on the concept of functional weight bearing over the lifetime, of which functional ambulation is just one component. In this manner, functional weight bearing becomes particularly more concerning for adults with CP having more physical involvement (GMFCS levels III and IV), whereby a loss of weight-bearing posture in any form can take away functional in-home or community participation. These individuals often crawl throughout their home or alternative living environment. Not uncommonly they ambulate 3 or 4 steps at a time into and out of a bathroom or pull to stand from a wheelchair allowing overhead reach into cupboards or preparation of meals on countertops. Taking a step or two often eliminates the need for a Hoyer lift, ceiling track, or similar hydraulic device while also sparing the care provider's spinal column from chronic stress, strain, and debility. These are all vital functions, not to exclude others, precluded without effective weight-bearing postures of the extremities. Any intervention by the treating orthopedist to preserve functional weight bearing over the lifetime is precious in keeping the adult as independent as possible in the community, home, and other chosen environments. Functional extension through the hips and knees and positioning of the feet are important for functional weight bearing over the lifetime and, when threatened, should be addressed aggressively at any age. The natural history of ambulation in CP (untreated outcomes) over the lifetime seems to be on a downward spiral, beginning around the time of early adolescence.[23,26,27] It is therefore important for parents, therapists, surgeons, and young adults with CP to realize that ambulation may already be on a slow downward trajectory when multilevel surgery (hips, knees, and ankles) is being considered. Surgical intervention to maintain gait at the present level of function might well be an improvement over the natural history. In this regard, further improvements in gait parameters compared with presurgical baseline could represent an even greater gain of function.[23] Comprehensive computerized functional gait laboratory assessment is still the best way to define, measure, and record gait function over time, pre- and postsurgically, and is the norm for all functional gait surgery in both young and older people with CP.[23,25] With this in mind, a brief discussion regarding spasticity management along with specific review of certain conditions identified as more common in the adult with CP is in order.

SPASTICITY

Botulinum toxin A (BTX-A) continues to have a positive role in adults for relaxing hypertonic muscles for functional gain in the absence of fixed contractures. The toxin can be particularly helpful for individuals with dystonia in relieving painful spasms, improving vertical posture, and controlling unwanted upper extremity motions or tremors that interfere with functional tasks. BTX-A inhibits the release of acetylcholine from the nerve terminal, causing partial paralysis of the muscle lasting up to 3 to 4 months at a time. Repeat BTX-A injections may not be needed every 3 months if appropriate stretching and splinting with home exercise is in place after the procedure. In individuals with dystonia, the botulinum toxin injections often need to be repeated every 3 months for inhibition of the recurrent movement patterns.

Adults may benefit from intrathecal baclofen, more commonly but not exclusively, those of nonambulatory status. It is not uncommon to see catheter tip placements as high as the midcervical spine in individuals with more dystonia or upper extremity involvement.[22] Baclofen acts at the level of the spinal cord; it binds to $GABA_B$ receptor sites, agonizes the site, and suppresses the release of excitatory neurotransmitters. Augmenting $GABA_B$ activity reduces spasticity. Medical management can include levodopa and/or trihexyphenidyl (a centrally acting anticholinergic) in those individuals with dystonia.[28,29] Diazepam,

oral baclofen, and α_2-adrenergic agonists such as tizanidine or clonidine can be helpful at the brain and spinal level (clonidine is often used in those with spinal cord injury). Dantrolene sodium works at the level of the muscle, inhibiting the release of calcium ions from the sarcoplasmic reticulum. It acts on nonspastic muscles as well and may cause some unwanted weakness in the ambulatory patient. The medication carries a "black box" warning for hepatotoxicity, which is seen in about 1.8% of patients treated. Monitoring the levels of liver enzymes is recommended (as for tizanidine) at least every 6 months, and the medication is weaned if drug-related abnormalities are identified. Phenol (a 5% or 7% solution) injected into motor nerves can still be helpful, particularly around the hip, to decrease unwanted adduction posture in the absence of contracture. With good positioning and exercise postprocedure, the partial phenol obturator neurectomy should not result in unwanted abduction and external rotation hip contracture. Phenol can also be useful at the level of the shoulder. Injections into the pectoralis major, latissimus dorsi, and biceps (musculocutaneous neurectomy) can improve upper extremity function and overhead reach, facilitating upper torso dressing and outer garment donning and doffing.

SPINE

Scoliosis can be present in up to 60% of adults with CP and is particularly likely in those with nonambulatory status having spastic quadriparesis.[25] Progression with aging can occur to approximately 1° per year and should be monitored carefully over time. Decompensation can be accompanied by loss of function, improved somewhat with custom molded seating or postural thoracolumbar orthosis, depending on the individual. Pain, when it occurs, is often associated with thoracolumbar soft tissue strain on the convex side and degenerative changes in the facet joints on the concave side. Scoliotic pain can be a new experience for the adult, as scoliosis in children is generally pain free. Episodic bolus physical therapy and nonsteroidal antiinflammatory drugs can be helpful. Despite conservative care, decompensating curvatures beyond 50° often require posterior fusion to prevent future compromise to the cardiopulmonary and gastrointestinal systems.

Spondylolysis has a prevalence of approximately 4.4% at 6 years of age, increasing to 6% in able-bodied adults.[30] Reports in the literature have identified spondylolysis in weight-bearing adults with CP, having an estimated prevalence of between 21% and 30%, with or without dystonia.[31–33] The prevalence may be higher in individuals who had a selective posterior rhizotomy and associated increased anterior pelvic tilt.[34–36] In a series of 143 patients who had never walked, in whom the condition of CP was predominant, no case of spondylolysis or spondylolisthesis was detected radiographically.[37] Dystonic movements in the lumbosacral spine, particularly into extension and axial rotation, seem to be contributing to the higher incidence of spondylolysis in patients with CP.[32,38] It is not uncommon to see adults with CP having chronic back pain, followed by their primary care providers for years. The back pain has usually been attributed to their primary condition of CP; it is believed to be expected and usual and elicits no further diagnostic evaluation. Simple radiographs of the lumbar spine, including an oblique view, often reveal spondylolysis with low-grade spondylolisthesis, commonly improving with basic conservative care. Efforts to minimize significant anterior pelvic tilt in weight-bearing children may be helpful in preventing these potential stress fractures later in life. These efforts would seem particularly important in those undergoing selective posterior rhizotomy or aggressive hamstring lengthening, especially in the presence of tight hip flexors.[39] Surgical options including segmental fusion in the presence of failed conservative intervention and any neurologic compromise should be used when necessary. Toe walking should be minimized with the use of appropriate orthosis when indicated. Medical history should also include a review of any falls or injuries to the lumbar and pelvic region because more distant traumatic causes may not be considered relevant by the individual at the time of medical evaluation.

Cervical stenosis has been found to occur with a higher incidence in adults with CP and dystonia than in normal controls.[40] In a study of 180 patients with CP and dystonia compared with 417 control subjects, Harada and colleagues[40] found an 8-fold increase of the frequency of cervical disk degeneration and a 6- to 8-times increased frequency of listhetic instability in the midcervical spine in the CP group. The combination of disk degeneration and listhetic instability with a narrowed spinal canal was believed to be predisposing individuals to rapid progressive loss of function and devastating neurologic deficit. In approximately 35% of adults with CP, Ando and Ueda[41] identified functional deterioration with higher frequency in those having involuntary movements of the head and neck. Symptoms often occur over a 6- to 18-month period and include neck pain, loss of ambulation, and progressive hypertonicity, as well as loss of bladder control and upper extremity function. Additional studies focused on adults with CP have associated the higher incidence of cervical spondylosis and myelopathy with dystonic neck and head postures.[42–50] **Fig. 1** is a magnetic resonance imaging (MRI) scan of a 38-year-old man with CP, spastic quadriparesis, and cervical dystonia. Encroachment of the spinal canal can be noted particularly at the C4-C5 level. This individual was independent with his self-care, toileting, and mobility including limited community ambulatory ability with a gait aid (GMFCS level III), 1 year before the discovery of his cervical stenosis. Over a 6- to 12-month period, he gradually lost his ambulatory skills, displayed increased hypertonicity in the trunk and lower extremities, and progressed toward inability to assist with his dressing and upper extremity hygienes. Bladder control was lost with spontaneous incontinence about 10 months after onset of symptoms. Anterior surgical decompression with posterior fusion was provided, and the patient regained his former ability to walk and participate in self-care activities within 8 months. Thirteen years after surgery, he continues to maintain independent living skills and ambulation at GMFCS level III and requires just minimal supervision within his community group home residence.

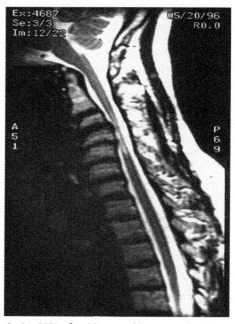

Fig. 1. An MRI of a 38-year-old man with CP, spastic quadraparesis, and cervical dystonia. Segmental encroachment is noted, particularly at the C4 and C5 levels with canal compromise.

In individuals with higher risk beginning in young adulthood, serial MRI scans every 2 years may facilitate early identification of cervical spondylosis and stenosis, allowing for more proactive intervention and prevention of sequelae. Botulinum toxin injections can be helpful in minimizing cervical dystonia, particularly excessive movements into extension and axial rotation.[51] Medications for control of dystonia, including intrathecal baclofen therapy, should be considered in carefully selected individuals. Calmer environments, use of sensory biofeedback techniques, and stress-reduction strategies can be helpful in reducing some regional dystonia. The author recalls a patient who, when flying alone in her glider plane, was completely relieved of all her dystonic movements until touchdown, when the ground support staff would come to her assistance. Cervical discomfort of any sort should be taken seriously in this population, as it may be the only prodrome recognizable before more devastating neurologic compromise. Serial neurologic examinations adapted for individuals with CP are encouraged. Reproducible voluntary motor functions measured over time along with a clinically reproducible spasticity measure are suggested. Close monitoring of bowel and bladder functions is not to be neglected. If conservative care fails, surgical decompression of the stenotic cervical canal may be required. A trend toward more anterior approach with interbody fusion and posterior wiring has been noted in the literature.[46,49,52–54] Regional dystonia postoperatively in the surgical zone, with potential for aspiration and bleeding, is a higher risk of such surgical procedures. Cervical immobilization devices are of limited use in this population. Cervical stenosis with major functional loss over time seems to be rapidly progressive in this population of patients with dystonic CP. For this reason, surgical intervention, despite the higher risk, seems warranted when conservative care has failed to maintain function and comfort.

SURGICAL PROCEDURES AND INDICATIONS
Hip

Hip displacement occurs in approximately 1% of patients with spastic hemiplegia, up to 15% of those with diplegia, and more than 50% of those with quadriplegia.[23,55,56] It has been shown that children who function at GMFCS level I have almost no chance of hip subluxation[57,58] and those who function at GMFCS levels IV and V have up to a 70% to 90% chance of hip dysplasia. As the GMFCS level increases, the degree of hip abnormality increases and the ability to walk decreases.[23] Pain with degenerative arthritis and joint space incongruity can occur in at least 50% of individuals with CP who have dislocated hips or pseudoacetabulum formation over time.[59–62] This problem is of particular concern in individuals having functional weight bearing in the lower extremities. Weight bearing can be limited but is important in standing pivot transfers, standing table usage, household or community ambulation, or crawling. Mild hip displacement, which is asymptomatic in the teenager, may develop into painful premature degenerative arthritis, leading to a loss of functional weight bearing and the need for additional reconstructive surgery later in life.[23,25] Early identification of hip dysplasia and appropriate intervention in the younger child should hopefully prevent most of this hip abnormality in subsequent years. Intra-articular injections with long-acting steroid and anesthetic can provide relief in the dysplastic, dislocated, or osteoarthritic hip for up to 6 months or longer in certain individuals. These injections combined with periarticular BTX-A injections and phenol obturator neurectomies in individuals having more dynamic adduction preference can alter joint articulating surfaces, reduce spasms, and provide further relief. Intrathecal baclofen, oral medications to reduce tone, and therapy interventions including seating adjustments are still valuable and always need to be considered in the adult with a painful hip.

Total hip arthroplasties have been reported as safe and effective in selected individuals with CP having severe degenerative arthritis and pseudoacetabular formation.[31,63–65] Long-term follow-up studies have shown more than 90% pain relief and improved function with time, even when operated on at a young age of 30 years.[66,67] Wear and tear to the arthroplastic joint seems to be minimal, which may relate to fewer steps per day and over time in the adult with CP. **Fig. 2** shows severe

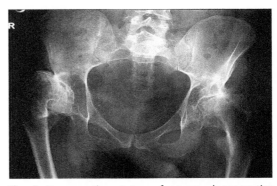

Fig. 2. Preoperative status of severe degenerative arthritis with pseudoacetabular formation in a 42-year-old adult with CP and spastic diplegia.

degenerative arthritis with pseudoacetabular formation in a 42-year-old man with spastic diplegia. Ambulatory function had markedly decreased 5 years before surgery, from more than a mile (GMFCS level II) to less than 10 steps (GMFCS level IV). Severe loss of hip motion was present, which limited hip abduction to less than 15° with near arthrodesis bilateral. **Fig. 3** shows the same individual 1 year after bilateral total hip arthroplasties.

The right hip was operated on first, and the left hip approximately 4 months later. The operation was performed by an adult and pediatric surgeon simultaneously, as neither felt comfortable doing the operation alone. Within a year of the first surgery, the patient regained his ability to walk almost a mile using a single-tip cane and returned to his independent home and limited community functions. Mixed results are still noted with hip arthroplasty in adults with CP,[23] especially in those having dystonia. When conservative management fails, proximal femoral head resection (Castle procedure) with or without interposition arthroplasty may be helpful in individuals having no functional weight bearing in the lower extremities.[68,69] The question of whether crawling is used for functional household mobility should be answered before surgical intervention because most individuals do not offer this information on their own. Once the proximal femur has been removed, crawling ceases and the adult may go from a household independent to community group home dependent status. Self-injurious behavior must also be assessed pre- and postoperatively because individuals can scratch their surgical incisions and disrupt traction units and immobilization devices if this problem is not carefully managed. Pain control needs to be carefully assessed, especially in those individuals with limited communication skills and variations of expression.

Nonetheless, end-stage hip disease in functional weight-bearing adults with CP is virtually certain to result in a loss of gait and mobility. For this reason, it is wise to prevent dysplasia as much as possible starting at an early age. Despite technical challenges, complications, and mixed results, aggressive surgery for the adult with symptomatic chronic hip dysplasia seems appropriate for certain individuals as a last resort in efforts to alter natural history, pain, and functional loss.

Knee

Patella alta is a common condition in ambulatory adults with CP, especially with spastic diplegia.[70,71] Residual knee flexion deformity and patella alta are associated with a constant overloading of the knee during gait, resulting from the continuous use of the quadriceps throughout the stance phase of gait. Recurrent anterior knee pain, patella femoral arthritis, and arthritis of the knee joint itself may occur in the younger adult, especially if crouch gait has not been fully corrected.[23] Patella alta is seen on lateral radiographs with an Insall ratio[72] greater than 1 (**Fig. 4**). The ratio is determined by dividing the length of the patellar tendon by the greatest diagonal length of the patella in 30° of knee flexion.[72] The ratio should be approximately 1, with less than 20% variation. The condition, common to the individual with

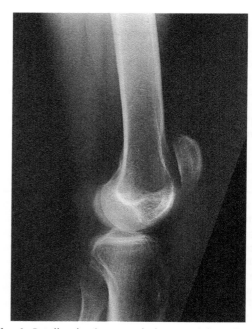

Fig. 4. Patella alta in an ambulatory adult with CP. Lateral view.

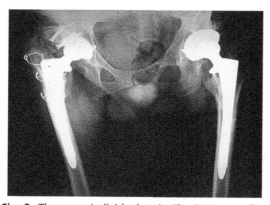

Fig. 3. The same individual as in **Fig. 2**, 1 year after bilateral total hip arthroplasty.

crouch gait, can limit ambulatory distance and contribute further to biomechanical and lever arm dysfunction on gait analysis.[39,73,74] Stress fractures through the patella are common, particularly at the inferior pole, with palpable tenderness and at times requiring excision, on failure of conservative care.[31] Patellar subluxations and dislocations are additional complications.[55,75] Medical and surgical efforts to minimize crouch gait during the developmental years can be helpful in preventing problems in the adult with CP. Interventions to maximize the knee-ankle-foot extension couple, with hamstring, quadriceps, and hip flexor stretching, in addition to strengthening the extensor muscles are of paramount importance.[34,76–78] Excessive tightness of the rectus femoris muscle can be contributory.[31] Quadriceps stretching in children with CP is often neglected but may be helpful in minimizing patella alta in adulthood. Efforts to minimize anterior pelvic tilt may also help, including increased prone lying along with abdominal wall and hip extensor strengthening. Efforts to improve patella tracking within the trochlear groove can be beneficial in the case of milder symptoms, including patellar taping techniques and neoprene patellar tracking orthoses. Intraarticular injections of long-acting steroid and anesthetic can provide more immediate relief, sometimes lasting 6 months or longer. A distal quadriceps elastic tension band placed about 2 to 3 cm above the superior patellar border can also provide significant relief in certain individuals with more mild to moderate discomfort. Physical therapy and nonsteroidal antiinflammatory drugs can be of additional help as part of an overall conservative care program. With the failure of conservative care in the more skeletally mature individual with CP and progressive crouch gait, more aggressive surgical options should be considered. Such options may include multilevel operative interventions to correct tibial and femoral torsion, equinovalgus foot deformities along with distal femoral extension wedge osteotomies, patellar and tibial tubercle advancements, hamstring lengthening, and rectus femoris transfers.[39,74] A focus on preventative strategy to minimize patella alta during the developmental years may well prevent symptomatic abnormality later in life and the need for more aggressive orthopedic surgical care.

Ankle and Foot

Foot pain in the adult with CP is a common scenario. Often asymptomatic in the teenager, aging degenerative changes in the hindfoot, midfoot, and forefoot region can result in limited mobility and dysfunctional weight bearing. Residual deformities in the foot include external tibial torsion and pes planoabductovalgus deformities.[23] Progressive equinovalgus and equinovarus of the foot and ankle are associated with rocker bottom deformity, subluxation of the talonavicular joint, and symptomatic hallux valgus.[31] A distal tibial valgus deformity always needs to be considered with significant valgus deformity of the hindfoot. The talocalcaneal angle reflects alignment of the hindfoot, whereas the talus-first metatarsal angle reflects alignment of the forefoot and the forefoot to the hindfoot. Equinus deformity (plantar flexed calcaneous) is still common in adults, seen best on measurement of the tibialcalcaneal angle.[23] As in childhood, it remains associated with excessive knee and hip flexion along with jump gait.[23] It needs to be carefully distinguished from true forefoot equinus best seen through the lateral talus-first metatarsal angle. Equinovalgus deformities are commonly associated with a vertical talus and eventual rocker bottom deformity.[31] Transient deformities gradually become fixed deformities with time as soft tissues contract and bones develop structural accommodations. Equinovalgus foot deformities are associated with an increased talocalcaneal angle, whereas equinovarus deformities are associated with a decreased talocalcaneal angle.[23] Valgus and varus deformities of the hindfoot carry similar influence into the midfoot and forefoot, including talonavicular subluxation and severe chondromalacia at the talocalcaneal, talonavicular, calcaneal cuboid, tarsal-metatarsal and phalangeal joints.[31] It is important to maintain as normal a medial and lateral column to the foot as possible.[79] If neglected, the lateral and medial columns shorten over time, respectively, with equinovalgus and equinovarus deformities, interfering with effective knee-ankle-foot extension coupling. Maintaining an effective knee-ankle-foot extension couple over the lifetime is crucial for functional weight bearing. Triple arthrodesis along with hindfoot and midfoot soft tissue releases and/or osteotomies can be helpful in achieving a functional weight-bearing position of the foot throughout the adult years. In the author's opinion, persistent pain over time after triple arthrodesis is not uncommon in community or household ambulators (GMFCS level II or III) requiring relief via floor-reaction AFOs, gait aids, or intermittent usage of powered mobility equipment. **Fig. 5** shows a 45-year-old adult with spastic diplegia after triple arthrodesis of the left foot and ankle. Severe mid- and forefoot pain continues despite solid fusion of the subtalar joint. Zigzag deformity is noted along with severe

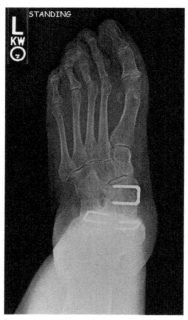

Fig. 5. A 45-year-old man with CP and limiting mid-foot pain after triple arthrodesis 1 decade prior. Severe degenerative arthritic changes, particularly talo lateral cuneiform and talo cuboid articulations.

degenerative changes in the mid- and forefoot regions. At present, the patient uses Lofstrand crutches and shoe inserts for limited and short distance ambulation (GMFCS level III) in the home and community and intermittent power mobility for longer distances. Functional foot positioning is of great importance no matter what the GMFCS level as long as weight bearing on the foot and ankle is a goal. Performing safe standing pivot transfers, short steps into and out of a bathroom, or standing at a countertop reaching overhead cannot be completed without a safe and tolerant position of the foot. The more independent the adult can be the higher the self-esteem and personal dignity usually achieved. In addition, the elimination of medical costs that can be associated with troublesome foot and ankle decubiti, unnecessary ceiling tracks, or hydraulic transfer equipment is essential in the present health care environment. Certainly the goal continues to be early identification and corrective intervention for the younger patient with limiting foot position, facilitating optimal functional weight bearing throughout the adulthood years.

SUMMARY

The conditions that have been discussed in this article are not uncommon to the adult with CP

and should be anticipated by the specialty medical provider. Other yet-to-be-identified secondary and associated conditions are most certainly present in the adult and require further clinical definition and research. Interventions to the child with CP need to be weighed carefully over the lifetime, with functional outcome variables presenting themselves into the adulthood years. The need to look beyond the primary condition of CP for correct diagnosis of secondary and associated conditions in addition to comorbidities cannot be overemphasized. An adult with CP may have a surgical rotator cuff tear or internal derangement of the knee not uncommon particularly in those with dystonia.[10] Surgical evaluation may sometimes be slow to recognize the surgical need because of focusing more on the primary condition of CP and the recommendation for observation. Further discussion and review can lead to corrective surgical intervention that facilitates lifetime functional upper and lower extremity self-care, mobility, and recreation. Decreased physical activity and participation in physical therapy and fitness programs are prevalent in the adult population, which, along with loss of strength, contractures, and pain, are common factors in the loss of functional weight bearing, self-care, and daily performance over time.[23] It is the responsibility of all to advocate augmentation of surgical and nonsurgical interventions in addition to home exercise for the adult with CP. Early identification and intervention in the child and younger adult remain the ideal in the pursuit of optimal musculoskeletal function and lifestyle throughout the adult years.

REFERENCES

1. Hallum A. Disability and the transition to adulthood: issues for the disabled child, the family and the pediatrician. Curr Probl Pediatr 1995;25:12–50.
2. Ropper AH, Brown RH. Adam's and Victor's principle of neurology. 8th edition. Columbus (OH): McGraw-Hill Companies Inc; 2005.
3. McCormick A, Brien M, Plourde J, et al. Stability of Gross Motor Function Classification System in adults with cerebral palsy. Dev Med Child Neurol 2007;49: 265–9.
4. Rosenbaum P, Paneth N, Leviton A, et al. A report: the definition and classification of cerebral palsy April 2006. Dev Med Child Neurol Suppl 2007;109: 8–14.
5. Turk MA, Scandale MS, Rosenbaum PF, et al. The health of women with cerebral palsy. Phys Med Rehabil Clin N Am 2001;12(1):153–68.
6. Turk MA, Geremski CA, Rosenbaum PF, et al. The health status of women with cerebral palsy. Arch Phys Med Rehabil 1997;78:10–7.

7. Strauss D, Cable W, Shavelle R. Causes of excess mortality in cerebral palsy. Dev Med Child Neurol 1999;41:580–5.

8. Murphy KP. Medical problems in adults with cerebral palsy: case examples. Assist Technol 1999;11: 97–104.

9. Granet KM, Balaghi M, Jaeger J, et al. Adults with cerebral palsy. N J Med 1997;94:51–4.

10. Murphy KP, Molnar GE, Lankasky K. Medical and functional status of adults with cerebral palsy. Dev Med Child Neurol 1995;37:1075–84.

11. Murphy KP, Molnar GE, Lankasky K. Employment and social issues in adults with cerebral palsy. Arch Phys Med Rehabil 2000;81:807–11.

12. Young NL, Steele C, Fehlings D, et al. Use of health-care among adults with chronic and complex disabilities of childhood. Disabil Rehabil 2005;27 (23):1455–60.

13. Rimmer JH. Physical fitness levels of persons with cerebral palsy. Dev Med Child Neurol 2001;43: 208–12.

14. Hemming K, Hutton JL, Pharoah PO, et al. Long-term survival for a cohort of adults with cerebral palsy. Dev Med Child Neurol 2006;48:90–5.

15. Rapp CE, Torres MM. The adult with cerebral palsy. Arch Fam Med 2000;9:466–72.

16. Strauss D, Shavelle R. Life expectancy of adults with cerebral palsy. Dev Med Child Neurol 1998;40: 369–75.

17. Strauss D, Ojdana K, Shavelle R, et al. Decline in function and life expectancy of older persons with cerebral palsy. NeuroRehabilitation 2004;19:69–78.

18. Strauss D, Shavelle R, Reynolds R, et al. Survival in cerebral palsy in the last 20 years: signs of improvement? Dev Med Child Neurol 2007;49:86–92.

19. Strauss D, Brooks J, Rosenbloom L, et al. Life expectancy in cerebral palsy: an update. Dev Med Child Neurol 2008;50:487–93.

20. Rimmer JH. Health promotion for people with disabilities. Phys Ther 1999;79(5):495–502.

21. Heller T, Ying G, Rimmer JH, et al. Determinants of exercise in adults with cerebral palsy. Public Health Nurs 2002;19(3):223–31.

22. Albright AL. Principles & practice of pediatric neuro-surgery. 2nd edition. New York: Thieme Medical Publishers, Inc; 2008.

23. Gage JR, Schwartz MH, Koop SE, et al. The identification and treatment of gait problems in cerebral palsy. Clinics in Developmental Medicine Nos 180-181. 2nd edition. London: Mac Keith Press; 2009.

24. Rosenbaum P, Walter S, Hanna SE, et al. Prognosis for gross motor function in cerebral palsy: creation of motor development curves. J Am Med Assoc 2002; 288:1357–63.

25. Michaud LJ, Kraft GH. Cerebral palsy. Physical Medicine and Rehabilitation Clinics of North America, vol. 20, 3. Philadelphia: WB Saunders; 2009.

26. Bell KJ, Ounpuu S, DeLuca PA, et al. Natural progression of gait in children with cerebral palsy. J Pediatr Orthop 2002;22:677–82.

27. Hanna SE, Rosenbaum PL, Bartlett DJ, et al. Stability and decline in gross motor function among children and youth with cerebral palsy aged 2 to 21 years. Dev Med Child Neurol 2009;51:295–302.

28. Hoon AH Jr, Freese PO, Reinhardt EM, et al. Age-dependent effects of trihexyphenidyl in extrapyramidal cerebral palsy. Pediatr Neurol 2001;25:55–8.

29. Sanger TD, Bastian A, Brunstrom J, et al. Prospective open-label clinical trial of trihexyphenidyl in children with secondary dystonia due to cerebral palsy. J Child Neurol 2007;22:530–7.

30. Fredrickson BE, Baker D, McHolick WJ, et al. The natural history of spondylolysis and spondylolisthesis. J Bone Joint Surg Am 1984;66:699–707.

31. Morrell DS, Pearson FM, Sauser DD, et al. Progressive bone and joint abnormalities of the spine and lower extremities in cerebral palsy. Radiographics 2002;22:257–68.

32. Sakai T, Yamada H, Nakamura T, et al. Lumbar spinal disorders in patients with athetoid cerebral palsy: a clinical and biomechanical study. Spine 2006;31(3):E66–70.

33. Harada T, Ebara S, Anwar MM, et al. Lumbar spine and patients with spastic diplegia. J Bone Joint Surg Br 1993;75:534–7.

34. Peter JC, Hoffman EB, Arens LJ, et al. Incidence of spinal deformity in children after multiple level laminectomy for selective posterior rhizotomy. Childs Nerv Syst 1990;6:30–2.

35. Li Z, Zhu J, Liu X. Deformity of lumbar spine after selective dorsal rhizotomy for spastic cerebral palsy. Microsurgery 2008;28:10–2.

36. Peter JC, Hoffman EB, Arens LJ, et al. Spondylolysis and spondylolisthesis after five level lumbosacral laminectomy for selective posterior rhizotomy in cerebral palsy. Childs Nerv Syst 1993;9:285–8.

37. Rosenberg NJ, Bargar WL, Friedman B, et al. The incidence of spondylolysis and spondylolistheses in non-ambulatory patients. Spine 1981;6(1):35–8.

38. Wang JP, Shou-Yu C, Yates P. Finite element analysis of the spondylolysis in lumbar spine. Biomed Mater Eng 2006;16:301–8.

39. Gage JR. The treatment of gait problems in cerebral palsy. Clinics in developmental medicine #165-165. London: Mac Keith Press; 2004.

40. Harada T, Ebara S, Anwar MM, et al. The cervical spine in athetoid cerebral palsy, a radiologic study of 180 patients. J Bone Joint Surg Br 1996;78(4): 613–9.

41. Ando N, Ueda S. Functional deterioration of adults with cerebral palsy. Clin Rehabil 2000;14:300–6.

42. Reese ME, Msall ME, Owen S, et al. Acquired cervical spine impairment in young adults with cerebral palsy. Dev Med Child Neurol 1991;33:153–66.

43. Anderson WW, Wise BL, Itabashi HH, et al. Cervical spondylosis in patients with athetosis. Neurology 1962;72:410–2.

44. Levine RA, Rosenbaum AE, Waltz JM, et al. Cervical spondylosis and dyskinesias. Neurology 1970;20:1194–9.

45. Angelinie L, Broggi G, Nardocci M, et al. Subacute cervical myelopathy in a child with cerebral palsy. Secondary to torsion dystonia. Childs Brain 1982;9:354–7.

46. Fuji T, Yonenobu K, Fujiwara K, et al. Cervical radiculopathy or myelopathy secondary to athetoid cerebral palsy. J Bone Joint Surg Am 1987;69:815–21.

47. Nokura K, Hashizume Y, Inagaki T, et al. Clinical and pathological study of myelopathy accompanied with cervical spinal canal stenosis with special reference to complication of mental retardation or cerebral palsy. Rinsho Shinkeigaku 1993;33:121–9.

48. Hrose G, Kadoya S. Cervical spondylitic radiculo-myelopathy in patients with athetoid-dystonic cerebral palsy: clinical evaluation and surgical treatment. J Neurol Neurosurg Psychiatry 1984;47:775–80.

49. Pollak L, Schiffer J, Klein C, et al. Neurosurgical intervention for cervical disc disease in dystonic cerebral palsy. Mov Disord 1998;13(4):713–7.

50. Ebara S, Harada T, Yamamoto Y, et al. Unstable cervical spine in athetoid cerebral palsy. Spine 1989;14:1154–9.

51. Gallien P, Nicolas B, Petrilli S, et al. Role for Botulinum toxin in back pain treatment in adults with cerebral palsy: report of a case. Joint Bone Spine 2004;71:76–8.

52. Nishihara N, Tanabe G, Nakahara S, et al. Surgical treatment of cervical spondylitic myelopathy complicating athetoid cerebral palsy. J Bone Joint Surg Br 1984;66:504–8.

53. Bishop RS, Moore KA, Hadley MN, et al. Anterior cervical interbody fusion using autogenic and allogenic bone graft sub straight. J Neurosurg 1996;85:206–10.

54. Connolly PJ, Esses SI, Kostuik JP. Anterior cervical fusion outcome analysis of patients fused with and without anterior cervical plates. J Spinal Disord 1996;9:202–6.

55. Morrissy RT, Weinstein SL. Lovell and Winter's pediatric orthopedics. 6th edition. Philadelphia: Lippencott, Williams and Wilkins; 2006.

56. Laplaza FJ, Root L, Tassanawipas A, et al. Femoral torsion and neck shaft angles in cerebral palsy. J Pediatr Orthop 1993;13:192–9.

57. Soo B, Howard JJ, Boyd RN, et al. Hip displacement in cerebral palsy. J Bone Joint Surg Am 2006;88:121–9.

58. Hagglund G, Lauge-Pedersen H, Wagner P. Characteristics of children with hip displacement in cerebral palsy. BMC Musculoskelet Disord 2007;8:101.

59. Cooperman DR, Bartucci E, Dietrick E, et al. Hip dislocations in spastic cerebral palsy: long-term consequences. J Pediatr Orthop 1987;7:268–76.

60. Moreau M, Drummond DS, Rogala E, et al. Natural history of the dislocated hip in spastic cerebral palsy. Dev Med Child Neurol 1979;21:749–53.

61. Pritchett JW. Treated and untreated unstable hips in severe cerebral palsy. Dev Med Child Neurol 1999;32:3–6.

62. Hodgkinson I, Jindrich ML, Duhaut P, et al. Hip pain in adults with cerebral palsy. Dev Med Child Neurol 2001;43:806–8.

63. Koffman M. Proximal femoral resection or total hip replacement in severely disabled cerebral spastic patients. Orthop Clin North Am 1981;12:91–100.

64. Root L, Spero CR. Hip adductor transfer compared with adductor tenotomy in cerebral palsy. J Bone Joint Surg Am 1981;63:767–72.

65. Root L, Goss JR, Mendes J. The treatment of the painful hip in cerebral palsy by total hip replacement or hip arthrodesis. J Bone Joint Surg Am 1986;68:590–8.

66. Buly RL, Huo M, Root L, et al. Total hip arthroplasty in cerebral palsy. Long-term follow-up results. Clin Orthop Relat Res 1993;296:148–53.

67. Bradley S, Raphael MD, Dines JS, et al. Long term follow-up of total hip arthroplasty in patients with cerebral palsy. Clin Orthop Relat Res 2010;468:1845–54. DOI:10.1007/sl 1999-009-1167-1.

68. McCarthy RE, Douglas B, Zawacli RP, et al. Proximal femoral resection to allow adults who have severe cerebral palsy to sit. J Bone Joint Surg Am 1988;70:1011–6.

69. Widmann RF, Do TT, Doyle SM, et al. Resection arthroplasty of the hip for patients with cerebral palsy: an outcome study. J Pediatr Orthop 1999;19:805–10.

70. Able MF. Orthopedic knowledge update. Rosemont (IL): American Academy of Orthopedic Surgeons; 2006.

71. Insall JN, Aglietti P, Tria AJ Jr. Patellar pain and incongruence, clinical application. Clin Orthop Relat Res 1983;176:225–32.

72. Aglietti P, Insall JN, Cerulli G. Patellar pain and incongruence, measurements of incongruence. Clin Orthop Relat Res 1983;176:217–24.

73. Hoffinger SA, Rad GT, Abou-Ghaida H. Hamstrings in cerebral palsy crouched gait. J Pediatr Orthop 1993;13:722–6.

74. Rodda JM, Graham HK, Carson L, et al. Correction of severe crouched gait in patients with spastic diplegia with use of multilevel orthopedic surgery. J Bone Joint Surg Am 2006;88(12):2653–64.

75. Simmons E, Cameron JC. Patella alta and recurrent dislocation of the patella. Clin Orthop Relat Res 1992;274:265–9.

76. Andersson C, Grooten W, Hellsten M, et al. Adults with cerebral palsy: walking ability after progressive strength training. Dev Med Child Neurol 2003;45:220–8.

77. Taylor NF, Dodd KJ, Larkin H. Adults with cerebral palsy benefit from participating in a strength training program and a community gymnasium. Disabil Rehabil 2004;26(19):1128–34.

78. Allen J, Dodd K, Taylor NF, et al. Strength training can be enjoyable and beneficial for adults with cerebral palsy. Disabil Rehabil 2004;26(19):1121–7.

79. Davids JR, Gibson TW, Pugh LI. Quantitative segmental analysis of weight-bearing radiographs of the foot and ankle for children: normal alignment. J Pediatr Orthop 2005;25:769–76.

Index

Note: Page numbers of article titles are in **boldface** type.

A

Activity limitation, in cerebral palsy, classification of, 460–466

Adductor tenotomy, in hip deformity management, 552–553

Adolescent idiopathic scoliosis, spinal deformity in cerebral palsy vs., 532

Adult(s), cerebral palsy in, **595–605.** See also *Cerebral palsy, in adults.*

Ankle, in cerebral palsy, **579–593**
  clinical decision related to, 579–581
  in adults, surgical procedures for, 601–602
  observational gait analysis in, 580
  physical examination in, 579
  plain radiographs in, 579
  quantitative gait analysis in, 581

Ankle dorsiflexion, described, 475

Ankle eversion, described, 476

Ankle inversion, described, 475–476

Ankle plantarflexion, described, 475

Ankle valgus deformity, in cerebral palsy, surgical treatment of, 584–585

Antifibrinolytic agents, in spinal deformity in cerebral palsy management, 540

B

Balance, in cerebral palsy examination, 485

Benzodiazepine(s), in spasticity management, 511

Bone deformity, assessment of, in cerebral palsy examination, 478–485. See also specific types, e.g., *Tibial torsion.*

C

Cerebral palsy
  classification systems in, **457–467**
    activity limitation—related, 460–466
    dystonia, 458–459
    FMS, 461, 464–465
    functional classification, 490–491
    GMFCS, 460–461
    hyperkinetic movements, 459–460
    hypertonia, 458–459
    ICF, 458
    impairments-related, 458–460
    MACS, 465–466
    motor abnormalities, 458
    negative signs, 460
    spasticity, 458
    topography or limb distribution, 460
  clinical descriptions of, 444–445
  defined, 457–458
  described, 441–442
  diagnosis of, 444–445
  epidemiology of, **441–455**
  examination of child with, **469–488**
    balance in, 485
    bone deformity assessment in, 478–485
    clinical evaluation in, 469
    foot-related, 480–485
    functional outcome measures in, 469–470
    gait by observation in, 485–486
    leg-related, 485
    medical history in, 469
    muscle strength evaluation in, 470–472
    muscle tone assessment in, 472
    physical examination in, 470
    posture in, 485
    ROM in, 473, 476–478
    selective motor control assessment in, 472, 474–476
  foot and ankle in, **579–593.** See also *Ankle, in cerebral palsy; Foot (feet), in cerebral palsy.*
  functional gait patterns in, 492–493
  gait abnormalities in, treatment of, gait analysis in, **489–506.** See also *Gait analysis, in treating gait abnormalities in cerebral palsy.*
  hip deformities in, management of, **549–559.** See also *Hip deformities, in cerebral palsy.*
  impairments related to, classification of, 458–460
  in adults, **595–605**
    described, 595–597
    life expectancy, 595–596
    prevalence of, 595
    scoliosis in, 597
    spasticity in, 597
    spondylolysis in, 597–598
    surgical procedures for, 599–602
      ankle- and foot-related, 601–602
      hip-related, 599–600
      knee-related, 600–601
  levels of, 446
  malnutrition in, 448–449
  management of, 449
  movement disorders in children with, **507–517.** See also *Movement disorders, in children with cerebral palsy.*

doi:10.1016/S0030-5898(10)00083-0

Cerebral (*continued*)
   neuromusculoskeletal pathology in, 507, 508
   pathophysiology of, 447–448
      cerebral, 447–448
      musculoskeletal, 448
   pneumonia in, 448–449
   prevalence of, 442–443
   prevention of, 449–450
   risk factors for, 443–444
   spinal deformity in, management of, **531–547.**
      See also *Spinal deformity, in cerebral palsy,
      management of.*
   upper extremity in patients with, surgery of,
      519–529. See also *Upper extremity(ies), in
      cerebral palsy, surgery of.*
Cervical stenosis, in adults with cerebral palsy,
   598-599
Children, with cerebral palsy. See *Cerebral palsy.*
Classification systems, in cerebral palsy, **457–467.**
      See also *Cerebral palsy, classification systems in.*
Contracture, in cerebral palsy examination, 473,
   476-478

D

Dantrolene, in spasticity management, 511–512
Diazepam, in spasticity management, 511–512
Diplegia, spastic. See *Spastic diplegia.*
Dislocation(s), hip, painful, treatment of, 556–557
Distal hamstring lengthening, in spastic diplegia, 566
Duncan-Ely test, 473, 477
Dystonia
   defined, 509
   in cerebral palsy, classification of, 458–459
   management of, 514–515
   measurement of, 510

E

Elbow deformity, surgery for, 521–522
Equinocavovarus deformity, in cerebral palsy,
   surgical treatment of, 587–589
Equinoplanovalgus deformity, in cerebral palsy,
   surgical treatment of, 585–587
Equinus
   deformity of, in cerebral palsy, surgical treatment
      of, 585
   true vs. apparent, 494–497

F

Femoral anteversion, in cerebral palsy examination,
   478
Femoral rotation, 502
Finger(s), deformity of, in cerebral palsy, surgery for,
   524–525
Finger flexion deformity, in cerebral palsy, surgery of,
   524–525

Flexed knee gait, severe, in skeletally immature
   patient, case example, 573–575
FMS. See *Functional Mobility Scale (FMS).*
Foot (feet), in cerebral palsy, 480–485, **579–593**
   clinical decision related to, 579–581
   compensations, 482
   developmental trends, 485
   forefoot equinus, 485
   forefoot position in, 481–482
   forefoot valgus, 483–485
   forefoot varus, 482–483
   functional disruption of, 581–582
      surgical treatment of, 582–584
         ankle valgus deformity, 584–585
         equinocavovarus deformity, 587–589
         equinoplanovalgus deformity, 585–587
         equinus deformity, 585
         hallus valgus deformity, 589–591
         techniques, 584–592
   in adults, surgical procedures for, 601–602
   observational gait analysis in, 580
   physical examination in, 579
   plain radiographs in, 579
   quantitative gait analysis in, 581
   rearfoot position in, 481
Foot rotation, 503
Forearm deformity, in cerebral palsy, surgery for, 523
Forefoot equinus, in cerebral palsy examination, 485
Forefoot valgus, in cerebral palsy examination,
   483-485
Forefoot varus, in cerebral palsy examination,
   482-483
Functional classification, in cerebral palsy, 490–491
Functional gait patterns, 492–493
Functional Mobility Scale (FMS), 461, 464–465
Functional outcome measures, in cerebral palsy
   examination, 469–470

G

Gait
   abnormalities of, in cerebral palsy, treatment of,
      gait analysis in, **489–506.** See also *Gait
      analysis, in treating gait abnormalities in
      cerebral palsy.*
   by observation, in cerebral palsy examination,
      485–486
   grouch, 497
      severe, case example, 572–574
   jump knee, 493–494
   knee, severe flexed, in skeletally immature patient,
      case example, 573–575
   stiff knee, 497–499
Gait analysis. See also *Jump knee gait; specific types
   of gait, e.g., Grouch gait.*
   fundamentals of, 491–492
   in spastic diplegia, 563

in treating gait abnormalities in cerebral palsy, **489–506**
  described, 489–490
  equinus, true vs. apparent, 494–497
  functional gait patterns, 492–493
  fundamentals of, 491–492
  grouch gait, 497
  IGA in, 503–504
  jump knee gait, 493–494
  normal gait cycle, 491–492
  normal gait patterns, 492
  rotational abnormalities, 499–503
    femoral rotation, 502
    foot rotation, 503
    lever arm disease, 499–500
    pelvic rotation, 500–502
    tibial torsion, 502–503
  stiff knee gait, 497–499
  observational, in foot and ankle evaluation in cerebral palsy, 580
  quantitative, in foot and ankle evaluation in cerebral palsy, 581
Gait cycle, normal, 491–492
Gait patterns, normal, 492
Gillette Children's Specialty Healthcare Physical Assessment, form used in, 471
GMFCS. See *Gross Motor Function Classification Score (GMFCS).*
GMFCS-ER. See *Gross Motor Function Classification System—Expanded and Revised (GMFCS-ER).*
Great toe extension, described, 476
Great toe flexion, described, 476
Gross Motor Function Classification System (GMFCS), 460–461, 549
Gross Motor Function Classification System—Expanded and Revised (GMFCS-ER), 461–463
Grouch gait, 497
  severe, case example, 572–574

H

Hallus valgus deformity, in cerebral palsy, surgical treatment of, 589–591
HAT. See *Hypertonia Assessment Tool (HAT).*
Hip(s)
  dislocated, painful, treatment of, 556–557
  ROM and contracture of, in cerebral palsy examination, 473
  surgical procedures for, in adults with cerebral palsy, 599–600
Hip abduction, described, 474
Hip adduction, described, 474
Hip deformities, in cerebral palsy
  clinical evaluation of, 550–552
  hip flexion deformities, 553
  incidence of, 549

management of, **549–559**
  comprehensive, 555–556
  GMFCS in, 549
  nonsurgical, 552
  postoperative, 554–555
  reconstructive procedures, 553–554
  surgical, 552–553
  natural history of, 549–550
  rotational deformities, reconstructive procedures for, 553–554
  spectrum of, 549
Hip extension, described, 474
Hip flexion
  deformities of, in cerebral palsy, 553
  described, 474
Hyperkinetic movements
  hypertonia vs., 510
  in cerebral palsy, classification of, 459–460
Hypertonia
  hyperkinetic disorders vs., 510
  in cerebral palsy, classification of, 458–459
  symptoms of, 507, 508
Hypertonia Assessment Tool (HAT), 472, 477
Hypertonic syndromes, in children with cerebral palsy, discriminating between, 507–510

I

ICF. See *International Classification of Functioning, Disability, and Health (ICF).*
Idiopathic scoliosis, adolescent, vs. spinal deformity in cerebral palsy, 532
Infection(s), wound, after spinal deformity in cerebral palsy management, 541–542
International Classification of Functioning, Disability, and Health (ICF), 458
International Workshop on Definition and Classification of Cerebral Palsy, 457

J

Jump knee, in child with high functional expectations, case example, 570–572
Jump knee gait, 493–494

K

Knee(s)
  in spastic diplegia, management of, **561–577.** See also *Spastic diplegia, knee management in.*
  jump
    gait of, 493–494
    in child with high functional expectations, case example, 570–572
  ROM and contracture of, in cerebral palsy examination, 473, 476–478
  surgical procedures for, in adults with cerebral palsy, 600–601

Knee extension, described, 474–475
Knee flexion, described, 475

L

Leg(s), in cerebral palsy examination, 485
Lever arm disease, 499–500
Limb distribution, in cerebral palsy, classification
    of, 460

M

MACS. See *Manual Ability Classification System
    (MACS)*.
Malnutrition, in cerebral palsy, 448–449
Manual Ability Classification System (MACS),
    465-466
Medial hamstring lengthening, with semitendinosus
    transfer to adductor tubercle, in spastic diplegia,
    567–568
Motor control
    assessment of, in cerebral palsy examination, 472
    definitions associated with, 476–478
Movement disorders, in children with cerebral palsy,
    507–517. See also Spasticity; *specific disorders,
    e.g.,* Dystonia.
    described, 507
    hypertonic syndromes in, discriminating between,
        507–510
    oral medications for, 511–512
Muscle strength, in cerebral palsy examination,
    470-472
Muscle tone, in cerebral palsy examination, 472

N

Negative signs, in cerebral palsy, classification of,
    460

P

Patella alta, in cerebral palsy examination, 479–480
Patellar tendon shortening, supracondylar extension
    osteotomy and, in spastic diplegia, 568–569
Pelvic rotation, 500–502
Pneumonia(s), in cerebral palsy, 448–449
Posture, in cerebral palsy examination, 485
Pseudoarthrosis, after spinal deformity in cerebral
    palsy management, 541–542

R

Radiography, in foot and ankle evaluation in cerebral
    palsy, 579
Range of motion (ROM), in cerebral palsy
    examination, 473, 476–478

Rectus femoris transfer, in spastic diplegia, 566–567
Rigidity, defined, 509–510
ROM. See *Range of motion (ROM)*.
Rotational abnormalities, gait-related, 499–503. See
    also *Gait analysis, in treating gait abnormalities in
    cerebral palsy, rotational abnormalities*.

S

Sagittal plane imbalance, case example, 570, 571
Scoliosis
    idiopathic adolescent, vs. spinal deformity in
        cerebral palsy, 532
    in adults with cerebral palsy, 597
Shoulder deformity, in cerebral palsy, surgery for,
    520–521
Silverskiöld test, 473, 477
Spastic diplegia
    described, 561–562
    evaluation of, 562–563
    gait analysis in, 563
    knee management in, **561–577**
        case examples, 570–575
        distal hamstring lengthening in, 566
        guided growth in, 569
        medial hamstring lengthening in, with
            semitendinous transfer to adductor tubercle,
            567–568
        musculoskeletal strengthening in, 563–564
        nonoperative methods, 563–565
        outcomes of, measurement of, 569–570
        rectus femoris transfer in, 566–567
        spasticity management in, 564–565
        supracondylar extension osteotomy and
            patellar tendon shortening in, 568–569
        surgical correction of knee gait dysfunction in,
            565–569
    physical examination in, 562–563
    sagittal gait patterns in, 563, 598
    sagittal knee patterns in, 563
Spasticity
    defined, 509
    in cerebral palsy
        classification of, 458
        in adults, 597
    management of, 510–514
        intramuscular medications in, 512–513
        neurosurgical, 513–514
        physical treatment methods in, 511
    measurement of, 510
Spinal deformity, in cerebral palsy
    causes of, 531–532
    incidence of, 531
    management of, **531–547**
        nonsurgical, 533
        patient outcomes after, 542–543
        surgical, 533–541

anterior approach in, 538–539
antifibrinolytic agents in, 540
author's preferred method, 540–541
bone graft choices in, 540
complications of, 541–542
fusion in, 536
instrumentation in, 536–538
neuromonitoring in, 539–540
perioperative traction in, 539
planning and perioperative considerations
  in, 536–540
preoperative evaluation in, 533–536
natural history of, 532–533
vs. adolescent idiopathic scoliosis, 532
Spondylolysis, in adults with cerebral palsy, 597–598
Stenosis(es), cervical, in adults with cerebral palsy,
  598–599
Stiff knee gait, 497–499
Supracondylar extension osteotomy, patellar tendon
  shortening and, in spastic diplegia, 568–569
Swan-neck deformity, in cerebral palsy, surgery
  of, 525

T

Tenotomy, adductor, in hip deformity management,
  552–553
Thumb deformity, in cerebral palsy, surgery for,
  525–527

Thumb-in-palm deformity, in cerebral palsy, surgery
  of, 525–527
Tibial torsion, 502–503
  in cerebral palsy examination, 478–479
Tizanidine, in spasticity management, 512
Topography, in cerebral palsy, classification of, 460

U

Upper extremity(ies), in cerebral palsy, surgery of,
  519–529
  elbow deformity, 521–522
  evaluation before, 519–520
  forearm deformity, 523
  general principles of, 520
  postoperative care, 527–528
  procedures, 520–527
  shoulder deformity, 520–521
  wrist deformity, 523–524

W

World Health Organization, on classification of
  cerebral palsy, 458
Wound infections, after spinal deformity in cerebral
  palsy management, 541–542
Wrist deformity, in cerebral palsy, surgery for,
  523–524

United States Postal Service

Statement of Ownership, Management, and Circulation
(All Periodicals Publications Except Requestor Publications)

1. Publication Title
Orthopedic Clinics of North America

2. Publication Number
9 5 0 - 9 2 0

3. Filing Date
9/15/10

4. Issue Frequency
Jan, Apr, Jul, Oct

5. Number of Issues Published Annually
4

6. Annual Subscription Price
$251.00

7. Complete Mailing Address of Known Office of Publication (Not printer) (Street, city, county, state, and ZIP+4®)
Elsevier Inc.
360 Park Avenue South
New York, NY 10010-1710

Contact Person
Stephen Bushing

Telephone (Include area code)
215-239-3688

8. Complete Mailing Address of Headquarters or General Business Office of Publisher (Not printer)
Elsevier Inc., 360 Park Avenue South, New York, NY 10010-1710

9. Full Names and Complete Mailing Addresses of Publisher, Editor, and Managing Editor (Do not leave blank)

Publisher (Name and complete mailing address)
Kim Murphy, Elsevier, Inc., 1600 John F. Kennedy Blvd. Suite 1800, Philadelphia, PA 19103-2899

Editor (Name and complete mailing address)
Deb Dellapena, Elsevier, Inc., 1600 John F. Kennedy Blvd. Suite 1800, Philadelphia, PA 19103-2899

Managing Editor (Name and complete mailing address)
Barbara Cohen-Kligerman, Elsevier, Inc., 1600 John F. Kennedy Blvd. Suite 1800, Philadelphia, PA 19103-2899

10. Owner (Do not leave blank. If the publication is owned by a corporation, give the name and address of the corporation immediately followed by the names and addresses of all stockholders owning or holding 1 percent or more of the total amount of stock. If not owned by a corporation, give the names and addresses of the individual owners. If owned by a partnership or other unincorporated firm, give its name and address as well as those of each individual owner. If the publication is published by a nonprofit organization, give its name and address.)

Full Name	Complete Mailing Address
Wholly owned subsidiary of	4520 East-West Highway
Reed/Elsevier, US holdings	Bethesda, MD 20814

11. Known Bondholders, Mortgagees, and Other Security Holders Owning or Holding 1 Percent or More of Total Amount of Bonds, Mortgages, or Other Securities. If none, check box. ☑ None

Full Name	Complete Mailing Address
N/A	

12. Tax Status (For completion by nonprofit organizations authorized to mail at nonprofit rates) (Check one)
The purpose, function, and nonprofit status of this organization and the exempt status for federal income tax purposes:
☐ Has Not Changed During Preceding 12 Months
☐ Has Changed During Preceding 12 Months (Publisher must submit explanation of change with this statement)

PS Form 3526, September 2007 (Page 1 of 3 (Instructions Page 3)) PSN 7530-01-000-9931 PRIVACY NOTICE: See our Privacy policy in www.usps.com

---

13. Publication Title
Orthopedic Clinics of North America

14. Issue Date for Circulation Data Below
July 2010

15. Extent and Nature of Circulation

		Average No. Copies Each Issue During Preceding 12 Months	No. Copies of Single Issue Published Nearest to Filing Date
a. Total Number of Copies (Net press run)		2300	2000
b. Paid Circulation (By Mail and Outside the Mail)	(1) Mailed Outside-County Paid Subscriptions Stated on PS Form 3541. (Include paid distribution above nominal rate, advertiser's proof copies, and exchange copies)	728	642
	(2) Mailed In-County Paid Subscriptions Stated on PS Form 3541 (Include paid distribution above nominal rate, advertiser's proof copies, and exchange copies)		
	(3) Paid Distribution Outside the Mails Including Sales Through Dealers and Carriers, Street Vendors, Counter Sales, and Other Paid Distribution Outside USPS®	717	704
	(4) Paid Distribution by Other Classes Mailed Through the USPS (e.g. First-Class Mail®)		
c. Total Paid Distribution (Sum of 15b (1), (2), (3), and (4))	▲	1445	1346
d. Free or Nominal Rate Distribution (By Mail and Outside the Mail)	(1) Free or Nominal Rate Outside-County Copies Included on PS Form 3541	93	90
	(2) Free or Nominal Rate In-County Copies Included on PS Form 3541		
	(3) Free or Nominal Rate Copies Mailed at Other Classes Through the USPS (e.g. First-Class Mail)		
	(4) Free or Nominal Rate Distribution Outside the Mail (Carriers or other means)		
e. Total Free or Nominal Rate Distribution (Sum of 15d (1), (2), (3) and (4))	▲	93	90
f. Total Distribution (Sum of 15c and 15e)	▲	1538	1436
g. Copies not Distributed (See instructions to publishers #4 (page #3))	▲	762	564
h. Total (Sum of 15f and g)	▲	2300	2000
i. Percent Paid (15c divided by 15f times 100)		93.95%	93.73%

16. Publication of Statement of Ownership

If the publication is a general publication, publication of this statement is required. Will be printed in the **October 2010** issue of this publication. ☐ Publication not required

17. Signature and Title of Editor, Publisher, Business Manager, or Owner

Stephen R. Bushing

Stephen R. Bushing – Fulfillment/Inventory Specialist

Date September 15, 2010

I certify that all information furnished on this form is true and complete. I understand that anyone who furnishes false or misleading information on this form or who omits material or information requested on the form may be subject to criminal sanctions (including fines and imprisonment) and/or civil sanctions (including civil penalties).

PS Form 3526, September 2007 (Page 2 of 3)

Printed and bound by CPI Group (UK) Ltd, Croydon, CR0 4YY

08/06/2025

01896875-0015